Trusting in Psychotherapy

Trusting in Psychotherapy

Jon G. Allen, Ph.D.

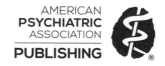

AMERICAN
PSYCHIATRIC
ASSOCIATION
PUBLISHING

To Susan, with gratitude for a half-century of trust

Contents

About the Author

Jon G. Allen, Ph.D., holds the position of Clinical Professor as a member of the voluntary faculty in the Menninger Department of Psychiatry and Behavioral Sciences at the Baylor College of Medicine in Houston, Texas. He is a member of the faculty emeriti at the Center for Psychoanalytic Studies in Houston and an adjunct faculty member of the Institute for Spirituality and Health at the Texas Medical Center. Dr. Allen received his B.A. degree in psychology at the University of Connecticut and his Ph.D. degree in clinical psychology at the University of Rochester. He completed postdoctoral training in clinical psychology at the Menninger Clinic. While remaining engaged in education and research, he retired from clinical practice after 40 years at the Menninger Clinic, where he taught and supervised fellows and residents along with conducting psychotherapy, diagnostic consultations, psychoeducational programs, and research on clinical outcomes. He is past editor of the *Bulletin of the Menninger Clinic* and a member of the editorial board of *Psychiatry: Interpersonal and Biological Processes.* His books include *Coping With Trauma: From Self-Understanding to Hope; Coping With Depression: From Catch-22 to Hope; Restoring Mentalizing in Attachment Relationships: Treating Trauma With Plain Old Therapy;* and, with coauthors Peter Fonagy and Anthony Bateman, *Mentalizing in Clinical Practice*, all published by American Psychiatric Publishing. He is also author of *Traumatic Relationships and Serious Mental Disorders* and coeditor, with Peter Fonagy, of *Handbook of Mentalization-Based Treatment*, both published by John Wiley and Sons, as well as author of *Mentalizing in the Development and Treatment of Attachment Trauma*, published by Karnac. He has authored and coauthored numerous professional articles and book chapters on trauma-related problems, psychotherapy, the therapeutic alliance, hospital treatment, and psychological assessment. He is also a jazz pianist and composer.

Foreword

To fall in love with a book is a new experience for me. I have been a deep admirer of Jon Allen for decades and have always appreciated his exceptional scholarship and almost unrivaled capacity to put things simply, no matter how intricate, controversial, complex, or multifaceted they might be. Perhaps it is because I manifestly lack this capacity (and have built my own career on making simple concepts unhelpfully complicated) that I have been in awe of Allen's ability to tackle such issues as depression (Allen 2006), attachment (Allen 2013a), trauma (Allen 2005), and psychotherapy (Allen 2013b) with a lightness of touch that reminds one of the most skillful of musicians recreating the sounds of the most intricate score with a facility that disguises the hours of painstaking practice behind it. (As an aside, besides being a brilliant scholar, Allen is exactly such a jazz pianist.) Allen advocates deliberate practice in psychotherapy, operationalized as systematic learning from experience, which for him consists of personal, jargon-free case formulations. But somehow I doubt that I will ever reach his virtuosity of scholarship and writing, despite years of practice. It takes something else—something less easily systematized— to write like Allen does. I guess it is called talent. I would never think of describing meta-analyses as "homogenizing fruit salads into smoothies" (p. 41).

I always knew that reading Allen's manuscript over the Christmas holiday was going to be a treat, which is why I left this seasonal present under the tree to be opened last, after a number of dissertations, papers to review, and commentaries to write. What I was not ready for (at my age) was being swept off my feet, admiration turning into something closer to passion (I stopped short of writing adoration because it seemed unseemly, although it would by no means be totally inaccurate). Scholarly books are not easy to fall in love with, yet, just like with the most intense of relationships I recall, I felt compelled to revisit again and again moments where I experienced an intense sense of identification with Allen's subtle narrative of a scientifically guided personal journey along the sometimes joyous but also quotidian route that psychological therapists carve through their professional careers. It is a wonderful book because it stands as proof of the case it intends to construct: that trust is the key to the privilege of changing lives, whether the lives of patients or readers of a scholarly volume. To testify in brief, this is the most theoretically clarifying and practically helpful book on psychotherapy I have read in decades, as will be evidenced by the numerous times colleagues and I will be able to refer to it in our writings.

Allen speaks to me—the book continuously addresses the audience—on what feels like first-name terms. Allen adopts a conversational style that disguises the weight of the issues he brings, presents, and solves. He establishes himself as a trustworthy source by this quality of communication, bringing his experience to the task and again and again evidencing that he knows the challenges faced by the practitioner from inside. As a result, we read the recommendations at the end of each chapter with a feeling of "Oh yes, of course, I always thought that. Well put, Dr Allen!" What he has communicated now forms part of my personal knowledge because as a writer, he has established the epistemic trust he describes. Without fanfare, he has opened our minds not just to learning (as the continuing professional development seminars he is skeptical about) but as a new part of our tacit knowledge about the world.

The book starts with a magisterial review of the psychotherapy process within its philosophical context, with Allen pointing to the irony of the theoretical fragmentation of even psychotherapy integration. As he poignantly notes, we should move "from developing therapies to developing therapists" (p. xxvii). He shows how personal experience (tacit or implicit) grounded in relational understanding manifesting in action, not insight, has a moral presence in the life of the therapist. At the heart of the book is a view of psychotherapy as a technique that is intertwined with the person of the therapist and his or her ethics, values, and personal knowledge along with his or her professional knowledge—all these domains are called on in the task of addressing mental distress through psychological means. Although research findings are relevant and helpful, the craft of therapy is essentially an interpersonal endeavor that requires a holistic perspective on human complexity and cannot be limited to understandings arising from quantifying interactions in the therapeutic setting alone. Thus, Allen acquaints the reader with half a century of psychotherapy research only to politely set it aside (as one might a cantankerous relative at a family celebration, settling him or her with a drink, reassurance, and a firm instruction to stop interfering) and proceed to create a novel and exciting dialogue between psychotherapy and more distant relations in philosophy, particularly ethics and epistemology.

Allen presents the complex ideas of others in a way that we can easily learn from and confidently integrate. How does he achieve that? Well, that is what the book is about; by the end you, too, will know. But here is a spoiler: he is able to attune to our reading of his book and captures (implicitly and unconsciously) our struggles and supports our imperfect reading with generous elaboration and well-placed examples, illustrations, and, yes, simplifications of complex philosophical ideas. We join him on a journey, and he guides us and ultimately persuades us that the issue of trust is the key issue of psychological therapy. By ceasing to take this idea for granted unthinkingly, we will be more helpful to our patients.

At the heart of the book is an account of current thinking around the origins of human social cognition, most notably described by Michael Tomasello (2018, 2019). Humans possess an evolutionarily unparalleled capacity to transfer information between agents, which enables remarkable levels of cooperation between partners across infinitely variable environments and knowledge domains (in other words, what we know as our culture). Allen places psychotherapy in line with a conception of the human mind not just as a product of the social, but rather as an intrinsically social formation (Gallotti and Frith 2013), and therefore psychotherapy might be considered a paradigmatic human activity. An adequate psychological treatment of the concept of trust needs to take into account the development of social as well as individual aspects of cultural behavior, considering a range of capacities including, but not limited to, human cooperation (Tomasello et al. 2012), group conformity (Claidière et al. 2014), memory (Causey and Bjorklund 2014), and the social transmission of information (Csibra and Gergely 2011). This is partly informed by evolutionary thinking: in order to protect the survival of our DNA, we are motivated to promote our children's adaptive fitness by supporting their social learning. Such social teaching and learning are driven by trust, which reflects our capacity for "thinking together"—joint attention, intellectual collaboration, empathic entanglements in relation to understandings and misunderstandings—that involves interpersonal engagement and functioning at quite a sophisticated level (O'Madagain and Tomasello 2019; Tomasello 2020).

Allen points out that these capacities require robust and at times highly reflective mentalizing, which remains for him at the center of the psychotherapeutic effort. Reflecting the assertion from evolutionary sociobiology that working together toward a shared goal is our essential species-specific attribute, Allen puts collaboration at the heart of his account of what psychotherapy is (Tomasello 2018). He shows, following Tomasello, that trust assumes joint attention: the experience when the infant and the infant's partner understand themselves to be attending to the same thing at the same time but to be doing so from different perspectives (Tomasello 2018). Allen suggests that in psychotherapy, as in any human interchange, this joining of minds is the crucial element of interpersonal trust in humans. Joint attention involves identifying a common object while also recognizing that our collaborators' view of that object will be different from our own. An awareness of difference in perspective is the essential first stage in reaching an alignment of attention, which in turn makes cooperation possible.

Allen's study of trust pinpoints the significance of the joining of minds in a particular cognitive mode, designated the "we" mode. Developmentalists (e.g., Tronick 2008), primatologists (Tomasello 2019), philosophers (Tuomela 2005), psychoanalysts (e.g., Winnicott 1956), and, more recently, neuroscientists (e.g., Gallotti and Frith 2013) have identified this mode as irreducibly collective. The we mode may be organized around cognitive and neural structures that are intrinsic to our individual makeup and are the product of a distinct developmental and evolutionary history (Tomasello 2019). When we build on joint intentionality—the shared focus on reaching a particular outcome—a joint, "we" agent appears, in which cognition is aligned for the purpose of reaching that shared objective and within which each individual has an agentive role (Tomasello 2016).

There is an important subtlety to Allen's conceptualization. The we mode remains individualistic in the sense that separate individuals are the possessors of we mode intentional states. However, these individually held but collectively existent "we" mode mental states are distinct from "I" states. The we mode is manifest only at the level of joint action. The we mode does not obliterate the I mode; rather, it qualifies it to be an I mode engaged in social action—more accurately, it is an "I with you" mode (Higgins 2020). The implication is not that the individual, while operating in the we mode, feels like a different person; it does not even necessarily involve reflective consideration of oneself as somehow socially modified. It simply assumes that one's epistemic stance (one's position in terms of communicating with the world) demands alignment with others and therefore implicates an awareness of one's position as both separate and joined with other minds. Thus, there is no mysterious leap into a mystical interpersonal space of "we-ness" (Di Paolo et al. 2013): the we mode is an individual state characterized by voluntary subsuming of the I mode into one where the dominant goal is joint action and collaboration, and it necessarily implies some level of interpersonal trust. At moments in psychotherapy, the content of individual intention is transformed so that patient and therapist each see themselves and the other as intending to play a mutually collaborative role in working together. Allen proposes that in the case of the formation of trust, we may assume the shared goal to be the well-being of the trusting person, which then requires trustworthiness on the part of the trusted person.

Allen links his ethical perspective of a "good life" with trustworthiness and trust via the shared intentionality described by developmentalists (Tomasello), attachment theory, and the epistemology of culture. In pointing to it he also reframes attachment theory, giving it a goal beyond secure emotional ties: the establishment of a capacity for basic trust and basic trustworthiness. At this point, I should declare that Dr. Allen and I have collaborated over some years around these issues (Allen and Fonagy 2014, 2019). He weaves our joint work into his beautiful conceptual tapestry, and it is as if it was always designed to be there. Mentalizing joins Tomasello; issues around the cultural competence of psychotherapy are woven in with the struggles of attachment theory in relation to its recent anthropological challenge (Keller 2018). The issue in contrasting Western with non-Western societies is not about promoting more or less instruction that is consistent with the Western, Educated, Industrialized, Rich, and Democratic (WEIRD) world. Rather, the questions are as follows: 1) Is it possible to have a model of socialization that is (rightly or wrongly) the dominant mode of cultural transmission globally? and 2) Can study of aspects of non-WEIRD approaches to mentalizing and shared intentionality highlight different expressions of these social-cognitive processes and inform a more sophisticated understanding of these mechanisms? Examples of such different ways of thinking together might involve a greater emphasis on mentalizing the other in more collectivist cultures, as opposed to a focus on the mentalizing the self in more individualistic cultures (Aival-Naveh et al. 2019) or a view of the infant as apprentice rather than master.

What comes across in this book is a curious combination of hyperclarity of thinking alongside a deep humility about the level of understanding and competence Allen experiences himself as having achieved—perhaps not surprising in light of his voracious appetite for enhancing his personal knowledge of current philosophers and researchers. The book opens a new chapter in our understanding of the process of psychological therapies: moving from what we have already accepted from infant research, it takes us to a completely new level of understanding about the nature of the social process of therapy from an evolutionary standpoint. By the final chapter, we see that trust itself is curative in therapy. Aligning the views of therapist and patient in a joint vision of an aspect of reality can restore faith and enhance the capacity to cope, not least by reviving the capacity to collaborate in individuals whose trust has been profoundly undermined by attachment trauma. Achieving a trusting relationship in therapy and generalizing that trust to others is critical if our patient is going to fully join the socially collaborative pursuits of the human race. The technical advice that follows each chapter is written in a style true to the principles of pedagogy Allen espouses—that didactic teaching has impact when directly connected to practice—and he supplies exactly this essential link. For example, Allen describes how writing personal formulations to articulate the therapist's understanding of the patient and the therapy is a potential means of promoting trust, and this whole book can be understood as a personal formulation and establishes Allen as a trustworthy interpreter of the many domains he covers.

Among the many unique features of this book are the fluidity and fluency with which Allen moves between psychological (psychotherapeutic) and philosophical discourse. In these discourses, Allen is bilingual. He brings depth to his psychological advice by reaching into ethics, moral philosophy, and epistemology. When we read about counseling couples, we are not used to reaching into some of the key philosophic contributions to understanding such concepts as communication (Paul Faulkner), the morality of reliance (Karen Jones), moral integrity (Carolyn McLeod), the decision to trust (Olli Lagerspetz), vigilance (Hugo Mercier), trusting relationships (Annette Baier), and the nature of hope (Adrienne Martin). What is extraordinary and massively enjoyable in reading Allen is that he has preprocessed the work of these thinkers for us and is presenting not a list of alien ideas but a well thought-out elaboration of issues exquisitely selected from the perspective of a practicing psychotherapist and immediately illustrated with an elaboration of an important clinical problem: couples therapy and John Gottman's extensive contribution. As you read the book, you will find yourself thinking more deeply about issues that you had been aware of (e.g., distrust among married couples) and issues that you may not have considered (e.g., the dichotomy between presumption and despair, which has hope at its point of equilibrium). With this book Allen opens the door to the depth of his own thinking and enables the reader to reap the benefit of a range of great intellects, and in this I include Allen's own.

In the final chapter, Allen cites the case of a patient unable to trust him until the moment, several sessions in, when she insists on turning the tables on him and interviewing him about his past. Beginning with relatively factual and easy questions, she then asks Allen what he found hardest in graduate school, and he admits finding learning to do psychotherapy difficult because of a lack of structure. She recognizes that his insistence on structure for their therapy may be rooted in this unease. Allen's patient was astute in her line of questioning. This book is beautifully structured. It grows from a close study of trust in developmental theory to a scrutiny of trust in adult relationships, leading to an examination of its organizing role in psychotherapy. Trust is core to our social nature, and its absence deprives us of our human agency. Trust is key to communication, which is our sole means of preserving accumulated knowledge. Trusting someone does not simply involve relying on that person: it implies that we can anticipate an affective commitment that justifies our dependence. The issue of trust is rarely all or nothing: Allen shows how qualified (three-place) trust restricted to a specific set of conditions can be distinguished from two-place trust, which may describe general relationships without situational qualifications. Therapy may then be thought of as a widening of the contexts or domains in which a person is able to feel trusting in relation to another. Building on the evolutionary social cognitive model he has adopted, Allen advocates that creating and maintaining an experience of "we"— including the capacity to reinstate it when it is lost—paves the road to a trusting relationship. The technical implication is that increasing the amount of time the patient spends in the "we" mode with the therapist in the room and the opportunity the patient has for shared intentionality may provide a basis for an empirically robust and potentially rigorous evaluation of the process (and progress) of a treatment and could be a useful predictor of therapeutic outcome. It is a small matter of being able to work out how we quantify that pesky synchronicity.

On the basis of insights from Kantian philosophy, Allen locates where productive psychotherapeutic exploration is most likely to be fruitful. The guiding lights of love and respect, closeness and distance will, in combination, generate the stance of optimal collaboration, and the clarity of Allen's advice will empower practitioners, regardless of their level of experience. Allen positions us as therapists with a ready acceptance of our limitations in living up to a therapeutic ideal. Although that is helpful in itself, identifying how to reach the balance between reacting and being distant as we inevitably make judgments, using natural curiosity as the antidote, is the kind of practical technical support this book offers. Taking us beyond the shared vision of the world curiosity can deliver, Allen illustrates the essential role of compassion without which curiosity may be experienced as persecution. Allen is an educator; you will leave this book a better person in terms of your knowledge but also, potentially, ethically and morally. It will set you standards that not only have positive impacts on your well-being but also enable you to assist your patients in a more effective manner.

What can be new in psychotherapy? After all, surely it has all been rehearsed before. The situation is the same: two people talking to each other in comfortable armchairs. What can be said about that room that has not already been said? But taking that attitude ignores one of the great mysteries of modern medicine. The talking cure remains in many instances the strongest intervention we have in the psychiatric armamentarium. Its effectiveness is underpinned by more randomized controlled trials than for any other medical therapy. Why is there a need for so many studies? The answer is that it is not trusted. Why not? Most likely, as Allen outlines in his excellent review, because its processes remain mysterious. For example, sometimes the benefits come faster than the supposedly effective component of the treatment was delivered (e.g., in the first five sessions). We are still uncertain about why and how psychotherapy works. The variability of components claimed to be the effective ingredient is large; the cumulative page numbers devoted to speculations about theories, techniques, and processes are probably comparable to, if they do not already outstrip, the number of patients who have benefited from these treatment methods. New therapies are developed, but the prevalence of mental disorder remains unchanged, regardless of supposed new discoveries. And each effort to produce something new spawns more attempts to reach new conclusions: a sure sign that we have not arrived at definitive answers.

Take my word for it. Without promising definitive answers, Allen offers clear guidance on how to become a (better) trustworthy therapist. However, he has produced something even more valuable: a way of thinking about what happens in psychotherapy that is pragmatically and philosophically robust and inspiring. You are holding in your hand a book that might, just might, focus the thinking of scholars and scientists, clinical researchers, and practicing therapists on a specific mechanism which could generate the next generation of psychotherapy development and training.

Peter Fonagy, OBE, FMedSci, FBA, FAcSS
University College London

References

Aival-Naveh E, Rothschild-Yakar L, Kurman J: Keeping culture in mind: a systematic review and initial conceptualization of mentalizing from a cross-cultural perspective. Clin Psychol Sci Pract 26(4):ee12300 2019

Allen JG: Coping With Trauma: Hope Through Understanding. Washington, DC, American Psychiatric Publishing, 2005

Allen JG: Coping With Depression: From Catch-22 to Hope. Washington, DC, American Psychiatric Publishing, 2006

Allen JG: Mentalizing in the Development and Treatment of Attachment Trauma. London, Routledge, 2013a

Allen JG: Restoring Mentalizing in Attachment Relationships: Treating Trauma With Plain Old Therapy. Arlington, VA, American Psychiatric Publishing, 2013b

Allen JG, Fonagy P: Mentalizing in psychotherapy, in Textbook of Psychiatry, 6th Edition. Edited by Hales RE, Yudofsky S, Roberts L. Washington, DC, American Psychiatric Publishing, 2014, pp 1095–1118

Allen JG, Fonagy P: Mentalizing in psychotherapy, in The American Psychiatric Association Publishing Textbook of Psychiatry, 7th Edition. Edited by Roberts LW. Washington, DC, American Psychiatric Association Publishing, 2019, pp 1019–1040

Causey KB, Bjorklund DF: Prospective memory in preschool children: influences of agency, incentive, and underlying cognitive mechanisms. J Exp Child Psychol 127:36–51, 2014 24813540

Claidière N, Bowler M, Brookes S, et al: Frequency of behavior witnessed and conformity in an everyday social context. PLoS One 9(6):e99874, 2014 24950212

Csibra G, Gergely G: Natural pedagogy as evolutionary adaptation. Philos Trans R Soc Lond B Biol Sci 366(1567):1149–1157, 2011 21357237

Di Paolo EA, De Jaegher H, Gallagher S: One step forward, two steps back—not the tango: comment on Gallotti and Frith. Trends Cogn Sci 17(7):303–304, 2013 23769302

Gallotti M, Frith CD: Social cognition in the we-mode. Trends Cogn Sci 17(4):160–165, 2013 23499335

Higgins J: Cognising with others in the we-mode: a defence of 'first-person plural' social cognition. Rev Phil Psychol September 7, 2020 Epub ahead of print

Keller H: Universality claim of attachment theory: children's socioemotional development across cultures. Proc Natl Acad Sci USA 115(45):11,414–11,419, 2018 30397121

O'Madagain C, Tomasello M: Joint attention to mental content and the social origin of reasoning. Synthese August 1, 2019

Tomasello M: A Natural History of Human Morality. Cambridge, MA, Harvard University Press, 2016

Tomasello M: How children come to understand false beliefs: a shared intentionality account. Proc Natl Acad Sci USA 115(34):8491–8498, 2018 30104372

Tomasello M: Becoming Human: A Theory of Ontogeny. Cambridge, MA, Belknap Press, 2019

Tomasello, M: The role of roles in uniquely human cognition and sociality. J Theory Soc Behav 50(1)2–19, 2020

Tomasello M, Melis AP, Tennie C, et al: Two key steps in the evolution of human cooperation: the interdependence hypothesis. Curr Anthropol 53(6):673–692, 2012

Tronick EZ: Emotional connections and dyadic consciousness in infant-mother and patient-therapist interactions: commentary on paper by frank m. Lachmann. Psychoanal Dialogues 11(2):187–194, 2008

Tuomela R: We-intentions revisited. Philos Stud 125(3):327–369, 2005

Winnicott DW: Mirror role of mother and family in child development, in Playing and Reality. Edited by Winnicott DW. London, Tavistock, 1956, pp 111–118

Preface

I saw my first psychotherapy patient more than 50 years ago, and it took me a decade thereafter to develop a modicum of trust in myself as a therapist. I did not know what I did not know, and I am still learning after having retired from clinical practice. I continue to be engaged in teaching and research as well as educating patients, but—abetted by being sequestered during the novel coronavirus pandemic—retirement has afforded me time to pursue a long-standing interest in integrating science with philosophical work in ethics insofar as both inform the practice of psychotherapy. My appreciation for the cardinal role of trusting in psychotherapy grew out of that interdisciplinary orientation.

Consistent with my training and identification as a psychologist, I have been invested in science and research throughout my career, but I also have become increasingly impressed with how indelibly personal the practice of psychotherapy must be. Accordingly, I have devoted much of this book to the personal as well as professional development of the therapist as it pertains to trusting in psychotherapy and being trustworthy in conducting it. Broadly knowledgeable and open-minded as we might aspire to be, each one of us psychotherapists brings an individual perspective to bear on our practice. Each perspective will have its strengths and limitations. Therefore, readers should be aware of my perspective because it bears on their trust in what I have to say.

I gravitated toward the social sciences quickly in college, homed in on psychology, and thought that clinical psychology would be the most practical specialty. My undergraduate teachers were academically oriented and critical of clinical practice, but by virtue of personal connections I entered a graduate program with a heavy clinical focus. I conducted psychotherapy but never felt a special knack for it and planned on an academic career, which I pursued for 4 years beyond my doctorate degree. Yet I continued to teach and practice psychotherapy as well as seeking ongoing supervision; alas, I discovered I had a limited knack for academia. The challenges of working with a few severely disturbed patients (whose disturbance I understood fully only many years later) led me to pursue postdoctoral training before shifting into a more clinically oriented career. I never gave up my interest in teaching and research.

I developed an interest in psychoanalysis even before I went to college, reading about Freud while sailing aboard an aircraft carrier. I maintained my interest in psychoanalysis despite academic antipathy toward it throughout my early career, such that I applied for a 2-year postdoctoral fellowship at the Menninger Clinic in Topeka, Kansas, which embraced the psychoanalytic orientation of its psychiatrist founders in the 1920s. Given the breadth of my interests, I never undertook psychoanalytic training, but the broad developmental orientation focused on the thorough understanding of individuals shaped my career over the course of the 40 years I practiced there.

I conducted long-term psychotherapy (sometimes lasting several years) throughout the first part of my career and shifted to short-term therapy during the latter years, largely as a result of the social shift to managed care. I gained considerable experience in outpatient therapy, but my practice was predominantly in the context of hospital psychiatry, engaging in long-term and then short-term therapy with inpatients. By contemporary standards, this shorter inpatient treatment (lasting several weeks) was lengthy, allowing for a dozen therapy sessions (and sometimes many more). Working in the Menninger hospital throughout the bulk of my career was both broadening and narrowing. I worked intensively with patients struggling with the full range of severe psychiatric disorders, acute and chronic. In collaboration with a group of colleagues, I developed an interest in trauma in attachment relationships that can begin in early life and persist into adulthood. As a group, we came to appreciate the profound role of attachment trauma in a wide spectrum of severe psychiatric disorders. Pervasive distrust and social alienation were common concomitants of this form of trauma and posed great challenges to developing therapeutic relationships.

Although long-term hospital treatment was narrow in its specialized role in the mental health landscape, it provided a rare opportunity to come to know patients thoroughly, consistent with its psychoanalytic orientation. In addition, hospital treatment provided a unique opportunity to work closely with the full range of mental health professionals, including nurses, psychiatrists, social workers, activities therapists, chaplains, and other psychologists. I did not fully understand my professional identity as a psychologist until I worked in an interprofessional setting. I found it especially valuable to my role as a psychotherapist to collaborate with social workers who were working intensively with the patient's family. For many of the patients I saw, the success of the treatment hinged on the family work, without which the psychotherapy would have been of limited benefit. Furthermore, in the context of both long-term and shorter-term inpatient treatment, I came to appreciate the immense value of a therapeutic community, which exemplified the ethos of the Menninger hospital from its inception.

Although I had shifted from an academic to a clinical setting early in my career, education and research were fundamental to the mission of the institution, such that I could pursue my enduring academic interests. I continued to do some university teaching and ultimately came to develop and conduct a wide range of educational groups for patients in the hospital. I began by educating patients about trauma (eventually coming to appreciate that they were educating me) and then developed other groups on depression, relationships, attachment, and mentalizing that spread throughout the hospital.

In other respects, working at Menninger for the bulk of my career narrowed my perspective. I never developed expertise in the multiplicity of short-term, symptom-focused treatments, which continue to play a major role in the practice of psychotherapy. I came to appreciate the value of contemporary versions of cognitive-behavioral therapy—the predominant form of psychosocial treatment—only later in my career as the practice of the hospital became more eclectic and I had the opportunity to work more closely with some of my cognitive-behavioral psychologist colleagues. Perhaps most significantly, consistent with the social context in which I grew up, the patients I worked with were predominantly white and from the middle and upper socioeconomic classes, owing largely to the costs of long-term intensive treatment (including the insurance that covered some of it). To put it plainly, with all the professional resources at Menninger—clinical, academic, and medical resources as well as extended time to work with hospitalized patients—working there was a luxury, as was obtaining treatment there. Only belatedly in the course of writing this book did I fully appreciate the influence of my narrow cultural perspective on my way of thinking about psychosocial development, including trust. I address the import of limited cultural diversity in this book.

To reiterate, I am interested in the personal aspects of psychotherapy, which I am addressing in this preface. I have begun with a conversational style that continues throughout this book, as I do when speaking with a group of therapists or patients. But the conversational style does not obscure the demanding nature of the substance, which includes reviews of research on psychotherapy as well as challenging conceptual material. I am fond of saying that I like simple ideas, but I like a lot of them. In my aim to give trust the full consideration it merits, I have packed this book tight, and parts of it will be slow going. With less than complete success, I have aspired to minimize technical language, and I have confined acronyms to one paragraph. Apart from the short introduction, the chapters are long. When I read a challenging book, I dislike having to wait a long time for a place to put my bookmark. Therefore, I've included numerous headings and subheadings not only to provide conceptual signposts but also to give you abundant places to rest. To help pull the material together as we go, I have included summaries of key points followed by recommendations for clinical practice at the end of each chapter.

Although psychotherapists are my primary audience, the book is intended to be accessible to those who are not mental health professionals, including patients who might wish to listen in on the conversation and who are the primary subject of it. More broadly, the book is about trusting relationships; psychotherapy is an exemplar, and anyone with a serious interest in trust will have much to learn.

Acknowledgments

A long professional developmental history will include a large cadre of mentors too numerous to mention, and mine is no exception. Amerigo Farina launched my research career when I was an undergraduate. Len Horwitz, who supervised and then hired me at Menninger, nurtured my continuing interest in research in the context of clinical work and continued his mentorship as I wrote this book. A great boon to my writing was Paul Pruyser's invitation to join the editorial board of the *Bulletin of the Menninger Clinic*, where I ultimately came to succeed him as editor. Along with Paul, the staff, including Mary Ann Clifft and Phil Beard, cultivated my skill in writing. As illustrated in this book, Paul's thinking also has played a large role in my appreciation for the role of hope in treatment. I also was fortunate as editor to have Karl Menninger's mentorship in turning cumbersome manuscript titles for articles awaiting publication into crisply worded headlines; no author ever objected to our intrusion.

In the late 1980s, when the psychiatric impact of trauma was becoming more widely apparent, Alice Brand Bartlett and Bonnie Buchele formed a study group with a focus on sexual abuse that captured and informed the interest of a group of us clinicians who had worked together in the hospital, including David Console (psychiatrist), Mike Keller (social worker), and Sondra Murray (nurse). We all found dissociative disturbance (including what was then called multiple personality disorder) to be most bewildering, and I relied heavily on Bill Smith (director of psychology) for his long-standing expertise in dissociation and hypnosis. As I was developing an interest in attachment theory and research, I was extremely fortunate that Peter Fonagy started to commute regularly to Topeka from London to direct research and shape clinical practice. Fortuitously, he arrived in 1995, coincident with the publication of my first book, *Coping With Trauma*. My 25-year friendship and collaboration with Peter in research and writing has played a formative role in my thinking about trauma and psychotherapy as well as psychological and social development more generally. His thinking has infused all the books I have written since 1995, including this one. I am also indebted to two successive chiefs of staff at Menninger, Richard Munich and John Oldham, for providing steadfast administrative support for my writing after the clinic's transition from Topeka to Houston, where the partnership with the Baylor College of Medicine was formed.

I am grateful to many colleagues who have read various parts of this manuscript in sundry drafts and provided helpful commentary and suggestions, including Estella Beale, Mel Berg, Tom Ellis, Chris Grimes, Michael Groat, Len Horwitz, Barton Jones, Jim Lomax, Susana McCollom, Cynthia Mulder, Shweta Sharma, Helen Stein, and Amanda Yoder. Numerous discussions with Michelle Patriquin informed my writing about treatment outcomes. I am also grateful to philosopher Adrienne Martin for exchanging ideas about hope and expanding my understanding of it. I thank Michael Tomasello and Jessica Benjamin for their careful reading of my account of their writing and their helpful comments. I am particularly grateful to two colleagues outside the mental health professions for reading the entire manuscript carefully and providing extensive feedback: Andy Achenbaum and Roger Verdon. They have bolstered my confidence that the book is understandable to a wider audience and has personal relevance; it hits home, as writing about trust should do. In addition, I am indebted to Carrie Farnham, Senior Editor at American Psychiatric Association Publishing, for her masterful and meticulous editing of the manuscript.

Finally, in the company of legions of authors, I am most grateful to my wife, Susan, for her careful reading of multiple drafts and for her intermingling of discerning criticism with unalloyed enthusiasm. Helpfully, she is not a mental health professional, although she has decades of relevant experience as a school counselor. Over the course of writing several books, I have come to trust her judgment to the point of giving her veto power: if she cannot understand something, does not see its relevance, thinks it is unduly technical, or finds it uninteresting, it goes into cyberspace and I rewrite it—sometimes more than once. Innumerable conversations with Susan about topics in this book have enabled me to articulate my thinking, consistent with one of the main themes of the book: minds need other minds. After extensive exploration, Susan also discovered the perfect evocative image for the cover. Most important, over the course of more than five decades of life, I have learned more from Susan about relationships, attachment, and trust than from any other source.

Introduction:

The Scope of Trust in Psychotherapy

In the course of writing this book, I spoke with diverse groups—therapists, students, and patients—about trust. In each group, I started by asking, "How many of you think trust is crucial or highly important in psychotherapy?" All hands went up. You will find the word *trust* sprinkled throughout the psychotherapy literature. Yet, to my knowledge, only two prominent leaders in the field of psychotherapy have homed in on trust, making it a primary concern in their treatment approach: Peter Fonagy (Fonagy et al. 2017) and John Gottman (2011). Bruce Wampold (Wampold and Imel 2015) placed trust at the starting point of his comprehensive contextual model of psychotherapy, but he did not elaborate on trust per se.

For the latter part of my career, I have taken a major interest in attachment theory, wherein secure attachment takes pride of place. If we were to locate the heart of trust anywhere, it would be in secure attachment relationships. Yet "trust" appears in the index of only one volume of John Bowlby's (1982) classic trilogy, in a reference to Erik Erikson's concept of basic trust. "Trust" is indexed only nine times in Jude Cassidy and Philip Shaver's most recent edition of the thousand-page *Handbook of Attachment* (Cassidy and Shaver 2016) and invariably is employed in passing, without elaboration. Do we therapists understand trust so well that we need not think about it in any depth?

When trust comes transiently into our therapeutic purview, we focus on the patient's problems with it. But trusting makes no sense unless the trusted person is trustworthy, and trustworthiness is almost entirely neglected in the psychotherapy literature. Perhaps our starting point should be: What makes a therapist trustworthy? Moreover, I think psychotherapy goes best when trust is reciprocal, that is, when the patient and therapist are trusting of each other and trustworthy to each other—as it should be in any close relationship.

I chose a deliberately ambiguous title for this book, *Trusting in Psychotherapy,* with two senses in mind. We can trust in psychotherapy as a *professional practice,* as we might trust in medication, surgery, or acupuncture. Of course, we would be more discriminating than that, trusting (or not) in some *types of* therapy, medication, surgery, or acupuncture. We are trusting in methods or procedures, often on the basis of their reputation and research support. Alternatively, we can *trust in the person* providing the treatment: the person conducting the therapy, prescribing the medication, performing the surgery, or inserting the needles. Ideally, we trust in both the practice and the practitioner, often trusting the practice on the basis of trusting the practitioner. Moreover, a trustworthy practitioner must trust in the practice, in effect, regarding the method as trustworthy. We might say that the patient borrows trust in the practice from the practitioner's trust in it—if the patient trusts the practitioner.

Trust and trustworthiness are prototypical examples of what philosopher Bernard Williams (1985) called *thick* concepts, comprising fact and value, objective description and ethical-moral judgment. We can describe someone informatively as untrustworthy, but this description carries heavy moral freight. We generally approve of trusting, aspiring to promote it in therapy. My commitment to understanding trust in depth stemmed substantially from my broader conviction that the practice of psychotherapy has been unduly dominated by science to the neglect of scholarly ethical thought; trust takes us straight into interdisciplinary territory with philosophy that psychotherapists explore too infrequently (Burston and Frie 2006). In the past three decades, philosophers—many of them women and brilliant writers—have generated a rich literature on trust and trustworthiness that is highly pertinent to our thinking about psychotherapy.

Once we dig into it, we discover many senses of the word *trust*: you can trust your car, your dog, your best friend, or your doctor. You can trust what someone says or what he or she will do—or you can trust the person. Trust has degrees and limits. Then we have distrust in various forms and levels. Just as we must learn to trust well (in proper relation to trustworthiness), we also must learn to distrust well (in proportion to untrustworthiness). To make a broad point, many of our patients have learned from past relationships to distrust well, but they overgeneralize from the past to the present, failing to trust others who are trustworthy. Trustworthy therapists can provide significant help with this pernicious problem. Philosophers think carefully about such distinctions, and we therapists might do well to consider them. I blend science and philosophy throughout this book.

This book's title, *Trusting in Psychotherapy,* might be misleading in implying that I am concentrating exclusively on psychotherapy relationships. On the contrary, this book is about trusting and trustworthiness as they pertain to our entire range of relationships. Certainly, we therapists aspire to create trust in psychotherapy, but the major value of doing so is fostering discerning trust as well as trustworthiness in relationships beyond psychotherapy. This book is about trust, full stop. But I wrote it with psychotherapy and psychotherapists in mind as the primary audience I am addressing directly (i.e., as "you").

We have already gone a considerable way from using the word *trust* merely in passing. Yet we have a long way to go, starting with Chapter 1, "From Trusting Therapies to Trusting Therapists." In this chapter, we take up the problem of trusting in the *practice* of psychotherapy and its primary source: Hundreds of brands of therapy have been developed in the context of competing schools of thought. The broader culture clash between academics and clinicians compounds the problem of knowing where to place our trust—a problem for patients as well as therapists. As a clinical psychologist, caught between science and practice, I have been in the middle of this conflict for several decades. I think trust in the practice of psychotherapy should be based in part on a broad knowledge of the field, the acquisition of which is no small feat. I provide an overview here with the invaluable help of several recent compendia synthesizing decades of research.

The broad exploration of the psychotherapy research literature in the first part of Chapter 1, necessarily guided by my personal predilections, led me to a simple conclusion: we should shift the balance of our efforts from developing therapies to developing therapists. This conclusion derives from research indicating that individual differences among therapists influence the outcome of the therapy more than the therapists' particular methods do. With both science and ethics in mind, I advocate thinking not only about professional development but also about personal development, proposing that a broad base of personal knowledge informs the practice of psychotherapy—more or less consciously. Accordingly, in Chapter 1 I include an account of the relevance of ethical thought to psychotherapy along with an overview of professional literature on the development of expertise in conducting psychotherapy. In subsequent chapters, I apply the ethical thought to various aspects of trusting and trustworthiness.

Throughout most of my career, I have employed a developmental approach in psychotherapy, and Chapter 2, "Developing Trust and Trustworthiness," reflects this mindset. A number of philosophers are mindful about the developmental origins of trust, but science rules here. Developmental psychologist Michael Tomasello's (2019) work anchors my thinking; although he does not focus on trust, he provides a detailed analysis of social-cognitive and moral development over the first 6 years of life that I use to articulate the basic capacities for trusting and trustworthiness. My interest in Tomasello's contributions stemmed from the influence of my long-standing collaboration with Peter Fonagy, with whom I became fully immersed in the literature and research on attachment theory; concomitantly, I came to appreciate the central role of mentalizing (i.e., understanding behavior in relation to mental states) in secure attachment. In the context of secure attachment and mentalizing, in Chapter 2 I highlight Fonagy's emphasis on the centrality of trust in psychotherapy and the significance he accords to epistemic trust in particular. Here we consider the role of attachment trauma in the development of distrust; my long-standing professional interest in attachment trauma has motivated and informed my thinking about trusting in psychotherapy when it is hardest to achieve. The chapter concludes on a disconcerting note: the cultural specificity of the work on attachment and mentalizing that I have enthusiastically embraced. Trenchant critiques of the ostensible universality of attachment theory have pointed to its disproportionate reliance on populations that are—by global standards—WEIRD (Western, Educated, Industrialized, Rich, and Democratic). Disconcerting as it may be, this cultural critique is consistent with the pressing need for psychotherapists to respect cultural diversity, and it also points our attention to trust beyond dyadic relationships.

Having established the developmental foundations, in Chapter 3, "Trusting," I focus on adulthood. Early in life, we develop the capacities to trust, but we do not employ them consistently or optimally, especially when there is a history of adverse experience in relationships. Although my main concerns are clinical, I make ample use of philosophers' thinking in elucidating the various forms of trust to which I have alluded thus far. Accordingly, the chapter has a broad scope, with topics including the ethical-moral basis of trust, trusting in the community, the distinction between trust and reliance, and varying degrees of trust. With psychotherapy in mind, I also make a broad distinction between trusting in care and trusting in competence. Here I review John Gottman's (2011) clinical and research contributions to promoting trust in couples therapy. I also address the challenges in trusting oneself. The chapter concludes with a way of thinking about hope that I find essential to understanding trust.

These first three chapters establish a framework for broaching my main point: We psychotherapists should move beyond concern with our patients' problems with trust to considering our own trustworthiness in the psychotherapy relationship. I am not questioning psychotherapists' character but rather advocating a different way of thinking about trust. Chapter 4 is titled "Becoming Trustworthy" to counter a natural tendency to take our trustworthiness for granted and to put the onus for trust on our patients. To a great extent, trusting and trustworthiness are relationship-specific, and they must be *created* anew in each relationship: developed, maintained, and repaired when disrupted. The creation is interpersonal. Again, I begin the chapter with the ethical-moral basis of trustworthiness, with a focus on the complex balance of closeness and distance in the psychotherapy relationship. This balance has been a highly controversial matter under the rubric of therapeutic *neutrality*. With this backdrop, I make extensive use of psychoanalyst Jessica Benjamin's theoretical and clinical work, which exemplifies the enormous challenges of becoming trustworthy in the treatment of patients with a history of attachment trauma. From the vantage point of my long-standing interest in attachment and mentalizing, I find remarkable consilience in Benjamin's and Tomasello's thinking inasmuch as both writers—coming from highly divergent backgrounds—explicitly incorporate a moral context into their understanding of development. I also include my experience in writing personal formulations for patients as a way of promoting trust in psychotherapy by means of making my understanding fully known to them.

With a cue from psychoanalyst Jeremy Holmes (2010), I was converted from thinking of psychotherapy as an art to considering it a *craft*. There is ample room for art as well as science in craft. In my view, coming from a developmental perspective, mastery of a craft is the work of a lifetime. This book reflects my current understanding of the craft of psychotherapy as viewed from the perspective of trusting and becoming trustworthy.

From Trusting Therapies to Trusting Therapists

As broached in the "Introduction," we can think of trusting in psychotherapy as a professional practice, and we can think of trusting in the therapist. In this chapter, I begin with the practice with the aim of shifting the focus from the therapy to the therapist. Be forewarned that in psychotherapy, the practice can be virtually inextricable from the practitioner. Yet, if we are to succeed, we therapists as well as our patients must trust in the practice, and the field of psychotherapy is inordinately complex as well as rife with disputes about best practices. We therapists need to discover what in the seemingly open-ended field of psychotherapy will we trust. For me, this has been a decades-long quest. You will not find consensus. Ultimately, you need to trust yourself in choosing the methods you consider trustworthy.

Not so blissfully ignorant of my ignorance, I entered the practice of psychotherapy unknowingly more than 50 years ago, in a way I assume would never happen these days. I was a senior undergraduate destined for graduate school in clinical psychology when my adviser suggested that I get my feet wet by working with a client in the university Psychology Clinic. His idea was not entirely crazy, only moderately so. The fact that I had already taken some graduate classes mattered less than the form of the therapy. The client was hampered by

1

a public speaking phobia that threatened his new job, and I could use a procedure that was highly structured: systematic desensitization.

As therapies go, desensitization was simple to conduct: teach progressive muscle relaxation and then guide the client through imagined speaking scenarios that are increasingly challenging, while ensuring that he or she remains relaxed throughout the imagined events. It was easy for the two of us to do, and it worked. But something else was developing in the background: As his phobia diminished, my client wanted increasingly to talk to me about problems in his life. Perhaps, opening with his phobia, he had entered into the process with an important but not particularly fraught concern. In wanting to talk, maybe he was beginning to trust me with more personal matters. I will never know because I was in over my head. As I recall, we referred him on for psychotherapy—not a bad outcome. Only after having forgotten it for decades did I appreciate how formative this first experience of psychotherapy was. What is the scientific procedure for talking to people about their life problems? How would I know? Could I learn?

Unknowingly, I had started my psychotherapy career as a specialist. I gradually developed into a generalist with some more specific areas of expertise—a decades-long career path that posed never-ending challenges to becoming reasonably trustworthy. When I use the term *psychotherapy* throughout this book, I have the generalist version in mind: therapists who work with patients presenting with a wide range of psychiatric disorders and personal problems. As I make plain in this chapter, however, the specialist-generalist distinction applies in varying degrees to a nearly unlimited variety of blends. For me, learning to blend was not easy, and, unlike systematic desensitization, generalist psychotherapy never came easy. I needed to figure out how to talk with people plagued by psychiatric illness about their extremely challenging problems in living—mostly, problems in close relationships. More specifically, how could I do this work with confidence and competence?

As knowledge goes, science gets high marks for trustworthiness, and I will take as much as I can manage to acquire. In addition to conducting psychotherapy, I devoted a great deal of time to educating patients. I needed to feel confident in what I was telling them. And, in addition to teaching at all levels, I was writing books. In this work, too, I wanted to feel confident in the soundness of what I was teaching and writing. I needed to trust myself. Scientific knowledge played a significant role in all this work, but, to go back to my beginnings: When I had to talk with patients about problems in their life, science was not enough. Where did that leave me?

Today, all therapists have a multitude of theories and hundreds of brands to choose from. With my first patient five decades ago, however, what I needed to learn was out of sync with the method of treatment that was on offer. Psychotherapy integration, a broad movement in the psychotherapy field that has developed over the past three decades, offers the best general guidance for navigating the thicket of therapy approaches and methods on offer over the entire course of a professional career. But the most substantial research on psychotherapy shows that interpersonal skill—which can be viewed broadly as the capacity to cultivate trusting relationships—plays the predominant role in the effectiveness of the treatment. That interpersonal skill is largely a matter of personal development that begins in infancy, although it can be refined in the course of professional training and practice over the course of a lifetime. The professional development of the therapist is a career-long process of mastering the craft.

When we move past specialized therapies to more generalist practice, we continue to need scientific knowledge, but we also need much broader knowledge, including skill in developing trusting relationships with persons who are loath to trust—for good reasons. To embrace a nontechnical term, I will refer to this as personal knowledge. In this broad domain of knowledge, I include knowledge of ethics, most of which we acquire from culture, which includes religious traditions for many people. Apart from religion, however, we have a magnificent scholarly literature on ethics in more than two millennia of philosophy, including a burgeoning contemporary literature on trust and trustworthiness that I rely on throughout this book.

I have filled this book with quotations. If you have room in your memory for only one, hold on to the first two sentences of Huston Smith's (1992) book, *Forgotten Truths*: "In envisioning the way things are, there is no better place to begin than with modern science. Equally, there is no worse place to end" (p. 1). This insight was entirely absent from my academic training in psychology, and, as an undergraduate, I had no appreciation for its application to psychotherapy. Along with Smith, I am not opposed to science; I am all for it. My foe is *scientism*—the view that science is the sole pathway to knowledge or, as applied to psychotherapy, to competent practice. I argue that scientism, under the banner of evidence-based treatments, has led us down a path to putting too much emphasis on developing therapies and too little on developing therapists. With some irony, I make a science-based case for going beyond science to fully inform the practice of psychotherapy. Seeking balance, I advocate *science-informed humanism* (Allen 2016). Along with predominantly ordinary language, we need some technical language and poetic language to talk about psychotherapy—utterly personal as it must be.

For orientation to this complex chapter, I outline the steps of my argument in Table 1–1. In the rest of this chapter, I elucidate the argument, with some anchors in the scientific and ethical literature. We delve more deeply into trust in subsequent chapters; here I provide a bird's-eye view of the scholarly justification for putting trust and trustworthiness in the foreground

Evidence-Based Practice

We compose much of our human life in the form of stories. In my first effort as a psychotherapist, I could treat a symptom, but I was not prepared to contend with a life story. My friend and colleague Tom Ellis, a cognitive-behavioral therapist, told me a story about a young therapist he was supervising. Exceptionally

---

TABLE 1–1.   Steps in the argument for shifting the focus from therapies to therapists

---

1. Over the course of a century, psychotherapists have developed hundreds of competing brands of therapy, tailored largely to treating specific psychiatric symptoms and disorders.

2. Research demonstrating efficacy has played a large role in developing and legitimizing many of these brands.

3. Researchers have had difficulty demonstrating that any one of these myriad treatment approaches is generally more effective than any other.

4. Concomitantly, extensive research on common factors has shown that a good therapeutic relationship contributes more substantially to the effectiveness of the therapy than do the particular theory, methods, or techniques employed.

5. A good patient-therapist relationship does not abrogate the need to provide some specific treatment for the patient's problems, but the choice of treatment often will be disconcertingly wide open.

6. Research shows that treatment outcomes are improved by going beyond symptoms and disorders to adapt therapies to patients' personal characteristics (e.g., ethnic or religious background, sexual orientation).

7. We should shift the balance of our efforts from developing therapies to developing therapists, that is, promoting therapists' knowledge, skills, effectiveness, and—from the broadest perspective—their trustworthiness as practitioners.

8. Short of narrowly specializing, therapists need to find ways of integrating theories and methods throughout their career.

9. Without abandoning specialized therapies, we need to broaden our purview to helping patients with their problems in living, which constitute the broader social context in which their symptoms and disorders develop; to a large extent, these problems in living are embedded in problems in relationships.

10. Addressing problems in living requires extensive personal knowledge beyond professional education, including ethical knowledge. Science-informed humanism provides a model for the knowledge base of psychotherapy.

11. Thinking about becoming increasingly trustworthy as a therapist provides a useful overarching framework for mastering the craft of psychotherapy over the course of a career.

---

adept, she had mastered many evidence-based procedures, but she was flummoxed about which one to employ with a patient whose problems were complicated and severe—not so simple as treating a phobia with systematic desensitization. The therapist could not see the forest for the trees: too many symptoms to match with too many procedures for an uncooperative and distrusting patient. Tom's suggestion: "How about starting by getting to know your patient?"

As I was writing this chapter, I talked with my daughter, Yvonne, about her work as a speech and language pathologist who specializes in treating children with autism spectrum disorder. I marveled at the sheer delight she takes in these children's extraordinary quirkiness—they are masters of individuality. But they need a great deal of help in finding commonality with adults and their peers. There is science behind Yvonne's work, along with plenty of technique, but she is not training these children to speak; she is striving to engage them in *communication*, which requires personal contact and recognition—an appreciation of individuality. In establishing contact, she is working on the ground floor of trust. Her work is not so different from mine; it is psychotherapeutic, not dominated by science but informed by it. She teaches the children to communicate by getting to know them and helping them get to know her and, more importantly, their peers—the function of speech.

Too Many Choices

Consider the number of brands of therapy now on the market. Of course, it depends on how you count, but the consensus would be in the hundreds (Wampold and Ulvenes 2019). Improbably, my colleague, Peter Fonagy (2020), counted more than 1,400. How did we get ourselves into this absurd situation? It reminds me of my first experience in a Texas-size liquor store where I had gone in search of some wine. I encountered aisle after aisle of wine racks, the likes of which I had never seen. I was overwhelmed and rushed out of the store with one bottle. It was cheap, and it was terrible. I hope this sort of thing does not happen to a patient who is looking for a therapist.

The abundance of acronyms heralds the real trouble. Two or four letters can be accepted (PE for prolonged exposure, EMDR for eye movement desensitization and reprocessing) but three letters are preferred: CBT (cognitive-behavioral therapy), DBT (dialectical behavior therapy), MBT (mentalization-based treatment), ACT (acceptance and commitment therapy), and so forth. But we can do better than that, combining types of therapy with the disorders for which they were developed, for example: PE for PTSD (prolonged exposure for post-traumatic stress disorder), ERP for OCD (exposure and response prevention for obsessive-compulsive disorder), and DBT for BPD (dialectical behavior therapy for borderline personality disorder).

I was pleased to discover a diagnosis for my malaise in the face of all these brands and acronyms: theoretical exhaustion (Norcross and Alexander 2019) exacerbated by antipathy toward empirical imperialism (Castonguay et al. 2019). Worn out with the spate of brands and protesting the narrow demands for experimental evidence, I declared myself a practitioner of *plain old therapy* (Allen 2013c). At least I was in step with my three-letter acronym.

What Constitutes Evidence?

Prominent in the quest for evidence were studies based on the gold standard medical model for drug (and vaccine) development: randomized controlled trials comparing the improvement of patients randomly assigned to a treatment group with those assigned to a control group (or horse race comparisons between different types of treatment). This gold standard research method was instrumental in establishing the effectiveness of specific therapies and the effectiveness of psychotherapy as a whole. But the gold standard also has become oppressive in its scientistic extension into the practice of therapy more generally. Drugs and vaccines, along with placebos, can be manufactured such that any one variant is identical to another.

To approximate this medical model (very roughly), therapies need to be highly structured such that they can be replicated from one patient to the next (and, ideally, from one treatment setting to another). For this purpose, researchers develop treatment manuals to structure the therapy, and they monitor therapists' adherence to the manuals. Moreover, the manuals typically are tailored for the treatment of specific psychiatric disorders and symptoms (akin to my treating the patient with a public-speaking phobia with systematic desensitization). Although essential for research, requiring therapists to practice by the controlled trial standards can put them in straitjackets. Most patients do not come with neatly packaged disorders or symptoms, and therapists must be flexible in many ways. At the price of a scolding conscience, therapists could simply ignore researchers' standards. The advent of managed care, however, has put economic pressure on therapists to practice treatments supported by research. It is utterly reasonable to restrict payment to demonstrably effective treatments. We will not get a large population to take a vaccine without convincing them that it is safe and will prevent infection and disease. But effective psychotherapy is a far more complex intervention that is jointly created in a trusting patient-therapist relationship.

One point bears emphasizing in conjunction with potentially confusing terminology: controlled trials have concentrated heavily on treatments developed for particular psychiatric disorders. I am not exaggerating the dominant role played by this approach to psychotherapy research: "we estimate that approximately 90% of federal research grants for psychotherapy goes to comparing and disseminating manualized treatments for specific mental disorders" (Norcross and Wampold 2019b, p. 336). Borrowing from the medical language, these experimentally validated treatments are regarded as having *efficacy*. The term *empirically supported treatments* was employed to identify treatments supported by controlled trials, which would (understandably) appeal to insurance companies.

The alternative term to efficacy, *effectiveness*, is far broader, applied to treatments supported by more naturalistic studies that demonstrate clinical improvement associated with a treatment. Helpfully removing the straitjackets of manualized treatments, the American Psychological Association (APA Presidential Task Force on Evidence-Based Practice 2006, p. 273) defined *evi-*

dence-based practice as "the integration of the best available research with clinical expertise in the context of patient characteristics, culture, and preferences." The task force noted this definition's similarity to one proposed by the Institute of Medicine: "the integration of the best research evidence with clinical experience and patient values" (p. 273). These definitions not only go beyond research evidence to take into account the broader context of treatment but also respect the value of research methods beyond controlled trials: "A sizable body of scientific evidence drawn from a variety of research designs and methodologies attests to the effectiveness of psychological practices" (pp. 273–274)—psychotherapy not least.

For starters, if we can accept the need for evidence-based practice, we are freed from linking therapies to specific theories and diagnoses, consistent with transtheoretical and transdiagnostic approaches to treatment that I discuss in this chapter. We can incorporate clinical experience and judgment into the process. We can shift our attention from treating the illness to treating the person who is ill, welcoming the individuality of the patient—and the therapist—into the process. In so doing, we have not simplified the problem of conducting trustworthy therapy; we have complicated it. And the complexity poses enormous challenges for conscientious therapists who aspire to be trustworthy.

Happily, decades of controlled research on efficacy along with more naturalistic studies on effectiveness have shown that diverse methods of psychotherapy result in substantial improvement. Yet this reassuring evidence comes with a disconcerting qualification: with the abundant competition in the horse races, researchers have not found a winner of the triple crown but rather have found a far-reaching, broad equivalence in effectiveness of diverse approaches. This finding has drawn much-needed attention to the limitations of the unbridled development of competing brands developed to treat psychiatric symptoms and disorders.

I must head off misunderstanding at this juncture. I am not arguing that we should ignore psychiatric disorders; on the contrary, spending a career working with serious mental illness, I could not have understood my patients' experience and struggles without a great deal of knowledge about psychiatric disorders, and no one should dispute the value of the wealth of knowledge that researchers and clinicians have accrued over more than a century (Roberts 2019). I am convinced that learning about psychiatric disorders—trauma-related disorders in particular—contributed substantially to my trustworthiness. As demanding as it is to acquire, knowledge of psychiatric disorders is not enough. We might begin there, but we should not end there. For an overview of factors beyond diagnosis to which psychotherapy is best adapted, see Table 1–2.

Common Factors and the Therapeutic Relationship

The idea that commonalities play a more important role in psychotherapy than specific methods long antedated the proliferation of psychotherapies. Barry

---

TABLE 1–2.   Adaptations of psychotherapy beyond psychiatric symptoms and disorders

Common factors	Individualizing therapy
Empathy	Ethnicity and race
Positive regard	Religion and spirituality
Genuineness	Treatment preferences
Emotional engagement	Sexual orientation and gender identity
Therapeutic alliance	Readiness for change
Repair of ruptures in the alliance	Reactance
	Internalizing-externalizing

Duncan (2010) reviewed this early history, featuring the prescient work of Saul Rosenzweig, who published the paper "Some Implicit Common Factors in Diverse Forms of Psychotherapy" in 1936. When he was a graduate student at Harvard, Rosenzweig created an elaborate panorama of psychotherapy depicting diverse forms of healing, from ancient to modern. His array of healers included a Hindu god, Jesus, priests in confessionals, medicine men, and Anton Mesmer (a progenitor of hypnosis) as well as Freud. Writing that "no form of psychotherapy is without cures to its credit" and that the "therapeutic result is not a reliable guide to the validity of the theory" (Duncan 2010, p. 9), Rosenzweig referred to the dodo bird's pronouncement from Lewis Carroll's *Alice in Wonderland*: "*Everybody* has won, and all must have prizes." As Duncan put it, Rosenzweig's provocative pronouncement became "a symbol of the raging controversy" (p. 8) between the advocates of common factors and the developers of specific treatments.

By and large, subsequent decades of psychotherapy research have reaffirmed Rosenzweig's conclusions, with ever-increasing methodological sophistication encompassing hundreds of studies with many thousands of patients. But we must be aware of qualifications to the dodo bird verdict, the most important being the following: *The research does not show that any type of therapy is as effective as any other.* The verdict pertains to well-established treatments that are supported by research—a multitude, but a fraction of all the therapies that have been promoted.

As psychotherapy research progressed, Rosenzweig acquired plenty of company. As Duncan put it, "If Rosenzweig wrote the first notes of the call to the common factors, Johns Hopkins University's Jerome Frank composed an entire symphony" (p. 6). As Frank (1961) put it in the first edition of *Persuasion and Healing:* "Much, if not all, of the effectiveness of different forms of psychotherapy may be due to those features that all have in common rather than to those that distinguish them from one another" (p. 104). Albeit 25 years later than Rosenzweig, Frank was writing before the extensive research supporting his view had been conducted. In a later edition coauthored with his daughter, Julia (Frank and Frank 1991), Frank identified one broad domain of specificity, namely, cognitive and behavioral approaches directed at "relieving anxieties that are linked to particular stimuli, situations, or persons" (p. 216) by means of repeated exposure to the feared situation (even in imagination, as occurs in systematic desensitization).

With common factors in mind, Frank articulated a common state of mind shared by psychotherapy patients: *demoralization* (Frank 1961; Frank and Frank 1991). Accordingly, restoring morale would be a common process by which diverse therapies achieve their effect. Frank's broad view of psychotherapy is consistent with the central emphasis I give to hope as it relates to trust (see Chapter 3, "Trusting"). Frank proposed four features common to effective therapy (Frank and Frank 1991): an emotionally charged confiding relationship, a healing setting, a conceptual framework that plausibly explains the patient's problems and procedures for resolving them, and a healing ritual or procedure in which both patient and therapist actively participate and which both believe will be a means of restoring the patient's health. Keep a caveat in mind, however: common factors exert their influence across brands of therapy, but we have no reason to believe that all therapies depend on all the common factors and certainly not all at the same levels (Weinberger 1995). *Common does not imply universal.* Empathy might be more important for some patients; a convincing rationale or credible technique might matter more to others.

What Are the Common Factors?

The research literature on common factors is voluminous, and I take as canonical those reviewed in Norcross and Lambert's (2019b) recent volume, *Psychotherapy Relationships That Work*. This volume, to which multiple research groups contributed, synthesized the work of the third Interdivisional American Psychological Association Task Force on Evidence-Based Relationships. Here is the editors' summary of the spirit of their work: "Most practice guidelines…depict interchangeable providers performing treatment procedures. This stands in marked contrast to the clinician's and client's experience of psychotherapy as an intensely interpersonal and deeply emotional experience" (Norcross and Lambert 2019a, p. 7).

Here I will confine myself to enumerating a set of common factors documented in a wealth of research based on *meta-analyses* designed to reveal broad patterns based on large data sets. You might liken these meta-analyses to fruit salads. For example, *empathy*, a familiar common factor, has been researched in dozens of studies with thousands of patients, rated from different perspectives (e.g., observers or patients), using different measures of empathy along with different measures of treatment outcome, in diverse types of therapy conducted by a multitude of therapists in an array of practice settings. After scouring the literature and carefully screening the studies for quality, researchers aggregate all the data and arrive at a statistic that quantifies the strength of the relationship between empathy and treatment outcomes. In so doing, they transform the fruit salad into a smoothie.

Readers will not be surprised that the *quality of the patient-therapist relationship* contributes substantially to the effectiveness of the therapy, regardless of the specific method employed. Three therapist characteristics that Carl Rogers (1951) identified as essential for change in client-centered therapy have garnered substantial research support: *empathy* (Elliott et al. 2019); *positive regard* in the form of warmth, nonjudgmental acceptance, and validation (Farber et al. 2019); and *genuineness*, including openness and transparency (Kolden et al. 2019). More generally, *emotional engagement* on the part of the patient and the therapist (as contrasted with a detached, intellectual process) also relates to a positive outcome (Peluso and Freund 2019).

The *therapeutic alliance*, a key facet of the patient-therapist relationship, is the most extensively researched of all the common factors. Christoph Flückiger and colleagues' (2019) review encompassed more than 300 studies employing more than 30 different measures and including more than 30,000 participants. As defined by the authors, the alliance is a multifaceted concept, and Edward Bordin's conceptualization has been widely adopted: "a collaborative stance in therapy built on three components: agreement on the therapeutic goals, consensus on the tasks that make up the therapy, and a bond between the client and the therapist" (p. 26). Research on the alliance includes ratings by therapists, patients, and observers. The strength of the alliance is consistently related to treatment outcomes across types of therapy, measures, and raters (i.e., patient, therapist, or observer).

Therapists should take heed: For distrusting patients who struggle with serious problems in close relationships, developing a solid alliance will be challenging, and the strength of the alliance will vary across the treatment and even from session to session or within sessions (Allen et al. 1996; Horwitz et al. 1996). For such patients, as it is with trust, a stable alliance might better be viewed as an optimal *outcome* of therapy than a precondition for effective therapy. Accordingly, researchers have been studying the process of repairing ruptures in the alliance (Eubanks et al. 2019b), although the research is limited in extent. Research to date suggests that repairing ruptures improves the treatment outcome, and there is promising evidence that training therapists in repair of ruptures has a positive effect on the treatment. More generally, I believe that conflict-free, close relationships are less trustworthy than those in which both members have developed confidence that naturally occurring conflicts will be resolved. Conflict-free relationships have not been put to the test. Psychotherapy offers an opportunity to practice conflict resolution in an emotionally fraught context—with a helpful guide.

Given the focus of this book, you might wonder, *is trust a common factor?* I began this book noting what seemed to me a surprising neglect of trust in the psychotherapy literature. I considered the absence of trust among the canonical list of common factors to be one instance of this neglect. Having devoted much attention to the study of trust in the course of writing this book, I can see the logic in thinking of trust as a common factor. At least patients and therapists I have surveyed all consider it important. I discovered the inclusion of trust in a table of common factors, along with 31 others (Cuijpers et al. 2019), but trust is far from having garnered canonical status. I see no reason to believe that decades of research going forward will be devoted to making trust a part of the canon. I speculate that if we had several dozen studies with a few thousand patients in which patients' trusting and therapists' trustworthiness were measured, we would find that trust would fall in line with the canonical group: it would contribute significantly to the outcome, and it would overlap with the other factors. The research on trust also would suffer all the limitations of research on the other common factors.

Alternatively, we might consider trust and trustworthiness an overarching way of thinking about what we want to achieve in psychotherapy. For patients whose problems developed in the context of profound distrust, trust and trustworthiness could be the most valuable gains from psychotherapy. As I implied in the lead-up to this section, these common factors go into comprising a therapist's trustworthiness: being empathic, affirming, and genuine; cultivating a therapeutic alliance; and working to repair ruptures. And there is far more to a therapist's trustworthiness than what these common factors encompass—not least employing specific methods to address the patient's problems and psychiatric disorders, including knowing when to refer to specialists (or, as in my early case, to generalists). Meanwhile, we have yet more ground to cover in developing a comprehensive research perspective on contributors to trustworthiness.

Should Common Factors Replace Specific Treatments?

The decades-long research on common factors has yielded hard-won knowledge, and therapists should be aware of it. Focusing entirely on theories and associated treatment methods and techniques overlooks the entire body of research findings. Compared with the relatively patchy evidence for the superiority of one brand of therapy compared with another, the evidence for the contribution of the patient-therapist relationship is powerful and extensive. In my view, this research on common factors casts a dark shadow over the effort that has gone into developing hundreds of brands of therapy, insofar as the training of therapists and their continuing professional development has greatly overemphasized theories, schools, brand names, and techniques to the neglect of developing therapeutic relationships. I think the pressure from science has led us to putting too much trust into theories, brands, and techniques.

Rogers (1992) proposed that a good relationship is the *necessary and sufficient* condition for effective psychotherapy. This is a tempting conclusion, given the broad comparability in effectiveness among brands coupled with extensive evidence indicating that the quality of the relationship contributes more to the effectiveness of the treatment than the brand of therapy applied. However, relatively small as the contribution of specific treatment methods to outcome may be, we generalists must keep in mind that specialized treatments can have an advantage for targeted symptoms (Marcus et al. 2014).

I have experience with such specialization, working closely with my colleague Tom Ellis, who has specialized in understanding and treating suicidal patients throughout his career. We implemented David Jobes's (2006) approach, collaborative assessment of management of suicidality, which is not a manualized therapy but rather incorporates into psychotherapy a systematic assessment of factors that are known to contribute to suicidality, such as psychological pain, self-hate, and hopelessness. The approach builds a therapeutic alliance in relation to understanding and resolving problems associated with these contributing factors along with assessing weekly progress on rating scales throughout the course of the therapy. I found this approach appealing because it focuses the therapy on key life problems and can be adapted to the therapist's preferred approach (Tom's being cognitive-behavioral, mine psychodynamic). We randomly assigned patients throughout the hospital to therapists who were practicing this suicide-focused approach and to those who were conducting the therapy as usual. We were not optimistic about finding significant differences between these two therapy groups because the twice-weekly therapy sessions were immersed in a plethora of inpatient interventions that we would expect to have an overwhelming influence. Nonetheless, we found significantly greater decreases in suicidality over the course of hospitalization in the suicide-focused therapy group than in the treatment-as-usual group (Ellis et al. 2012). This finding is consistent with potential advantages of specialized methods for target symptoms—suicidality being a particularly crucial target.

More broadly, Bruce Wampold, one of the foremost proponents of common factors, argued persuasively that *the battle between specific methods and common factors cannot be won* (Wampold and Imel 2015). Consider: How could you have a therapeutic alliance without a treatment approach as the basis for an alliance? Could you ignore the patient's problems and symptoms while striving merely to create a therapeutic relationship? Therapeutic for what? Could you ignore the patient's psychiatric disorder—anxiety, depression, psychosis, substance abuse, posttraumatic stress? Not if you work with patients whose functioning is compromised by these disorders. In my experience, all these problems, symptoms, and disorders are typically entangled in relationship problems, and these relationship problems often have developed over much of the patient's lifetime. Accordingly, the common (relational) therapeutic factors are profoundly important—and therapeutic indeed. But the relational problems must be addressed *specifically*, by some means or other. In short, *there is no treatment without a therapeutic relationship and no therapeutic relationship without a treatment.*

Individualizing Psychotherapy

The focus on common factors and therapeutic relationships has taken us one step beyond the more ubiquitous development of methods for treating disorders. But we must take another step. Sir William Osler, the "father of modern medicine," famously wrote in 1906, "It is much more important to know what sort of a patient has a disease than what sort of disease a patient has" (quoted by Norcross and Wampold 2019a, p. 2). Accordingly, researchers have been studying *transdiagnostic* characteristics of patients to which therapies should be adapted, and they have employed meta-analyses showing that such adaptations improve the effectiveness of treatment (Norcross and Wampold 2019a). My cursory review makes no attempt to summarize these huge domains of pertinent knowledge but aims merely to draw attention to their pertinence to therapists' trustworthiness.

Cultural Adaptations

Patient-therapist differences in *cultural, racial, and ethnic background* are liable to pose significant challenges for trusting, and these differences are one of many contexts in which the trustworthiness of the therapist is likely to be on the line. In the context of such differences, patients can have concerns about stereotyping and prejudice along with doubts about the therapist's capacity to understand them. Cultural diversity training is a common requirement in continuing education for professional licensing, but it only scratches the surface and risks perpetuating stereotypes.

Research literature provides some orientation to the challenges, and it falls under two broad categories: cultural adaptations of therapies and cultural competence of therapists (Soto et al. 2019). *Cultural adaptations* include matching patients and therapists for ethnic or racial backgrounds, employing the patient's preferred language, explicitly addressing patients' cultural values, using appropriate rituals and metaphors, and consulting with family members as part of individual therapy. Research has shown a modest relation between the number of such adaptations employed and the treatment outcome.

Perhaps more directly related to trustworthiness is the therapist's *cultural competence*, which includes cultural awareness and knowledge along with skills in engaging diverse patients in treatment while adapting the therapy to their preferences and needs. Patients' perceptions of therapists' cultural competence and *cultural humility* contribute to the therapeutic alliance and treatment outcome (Soto et al. 2019). As Hayes and colleagues (2017) put it, most important is "a humble, respectful, and open approach to addressing culture in therapy" (p. 159). Furthermore, the research evidence suggests that "therapists with cultural expertise acknowledge when they do not have specific knowledge about a culture and have a high tolerance for not knowing" in the context of appreciating the impact of cultural socialization on mental health (p. 163). As with all else, trustworthiness entails learning about patients from the patients themselves. But we need a balance: patients can assist in educating therapists about their culture, but therapists should not put undue burden for their own education on their patients.

Religion and spirituality are prominent aspects of culture that require attention in psychotherapy along with an attitude of cultural humility. My own history is embarrassing, and a confession might be instructive. Several years ago, I worked in long-term therapy with a pastor whose wife's severe psychiatric disorder was a source of his chronic stress and depression. He was devoutly religious; as he doubtlessly inferred, I am not religious. I did not explore the role of his faith in his emotional distress, nor did he bring it up. I think I was apprehensive that our religious differences would lead to a rift in our relationship. In hindsight, I now believe that my failure to address this difference created an unspoken rift that we could have overcome with a more mature attitude of cultural humility on my part. His graciousness made a major contribution to our good relationship; when we ended the therapy, he let me know that he believed that God was working through me. That was high praise indeed. I have not become religious, but I have become far more open in the decades since. I now appreciate that my constriction was a significant limitation in my practice of therapy—likely compromising my trustworthiness in ways I will never know.

Kenneth Pargament and colleagues (2013) made a strong case for psychotherapists to develop attitudes and competence conducive to addressing religion and spirituality in their work when indicated by patients' preferences and needs. As has long been known, spirituality and religious participation are associated strongly with mental and physical health. Less well known is the extent of ill health—mental and physical—associated with what Pargament calls *spiritual struggles* (Exline 2013; Pargament 2007) in three domains: interpersonal (e.g., conflicts with families, friends, and congregations), intrapersonal (e.g., doubt about doctrines and beliefs as well as conflicts about religious prohibitions), and divine (e.g., feelings of alienation and anger toward God or being at war with demonic forces). Also profoundly damaging is *spiritual trauma* associated with sexual abuse by priests and other members of the clergy (Allen 2007; Doyle 2003), which evokes extreme distrust in God or a "higher power," as well as distrust in religious institutions and potentially in authority more generally.

We therapists need not specialize in religious interventions or even be religious to provide spiritually conscious care; we need cultural humility in the form of curiosity and respect for differences along with willingness to plunge into unfamiliar territory. Yet some therapies have been designed to adapt to patients' religious and spiritual needs in the context of treating psychiatric disorders (Hook et al. 2019). Attesting to specificity, controlled studies indicate that integrating religion and spirituality into treatment for interested patients yields similar levels of improvement for psychological symptoms but greater gains in spiritual well-being.

Given the ever-shifting cultural sands, working effectively with *sexual orientation and gender identity* can be challenging for psychotherapists. Stephanie Budge (Budge and Moradi 2019) and Bonnie Moradi (Moradi and Budge 2019) scoured the research literature for studies on the effectiveness of LGBTQ+ affirmative therapies and came up with one major empirical finding: *there are no such studies.* Accordingly, they reviewed the substantive clinical literature and concluded by reiterating the recurring theme: "Clients should be *approached with humility* and curiosity and understood with their full humanity, salient experiences, and identities. This humble approach should be paired with therapists' understanding of the sociopolitical climate for transgender individuals" (Budge and Moradi 2019, p. 152, emphasis added).

Individual differences in race, ethnicity, religion, gender identity, and sexuality commonly have been fraught with tension and conflict, and this conflict is now in full view in our currently superheated political climate. Ideally, the compassion, acceptance, and respect that psychotherapy optimally offers can provide some refuge and a safe space. In this context, however, thinking that becoming trustworthy in conducting psychotherapy is easy or taking trustworthiness for granted—especially in our current political climate—is a failing in cultural humility.

Treatment Preferences and Readiness for Change

There are many pathways to a therapist's office, and the opportunity for patients to express their *treatment preferences* and have them honored will vary. If patients are not offered an opportunity to express preferences, they should make them known. For this purpose, Mick Cooper and John Norcross developed a brief inventory that can be administered to patients prior to assignment to a therapist (Cooper and Norcross 2016). The questionnaire includes a set of rating scales to assess preferences for therapist directiveness, emotional intensity, focus on the patient-therapist relationship, and warm support versus challenge. The instrument also contains open-ended questions to gauge preferences regarding personal characteristics of the therapist, type and frequency of therapy, inclusion of medication, and so forth. Research shows that honoring patients' preferences is associated with better treatment outcomes; moreover, failing to honor preferences nearly doubles the rate of dropout (Swift et al. 2019).

Patients come to therapy suffering and seeking help; naturally, they will work hard and cooperate with therapists in seeking relief. Perhaps this scenario plays out often enough in symptom-oriented treatments. Psychotherapy with patients who struggle with problems in relationships—including distrust—does not go so smoothly, As has been a main concern of psychoanalysis since its inception, patients who are ill may resist the therapist's efforts and even actively fight change. As a therapist, taking a readily developed therapeutic alliance for granted is about as reasonable as taking a trusting attitude and your own trustworthiness for granted.

In contrast to the psychoanalytic concept of resistance, the stages-of-change model was developed to apply to all theoretical approaches and methods of therapy, although it has played an especially prominent role in the treatment of addictions and problematic behaviors more generally (Krebs et al. 2019; Prochaska and DiClemente 2019). Five stages have been distinguished. In the *precontemplation* stage, the patient has no intention of changing and might not even be aware of the problem (e.g., alcohol abuse). Often, persons who are close to the patient (e.g., family members or employers) are keenly aware of the problem, and those who seek treatment are liable to feel coerced (i.e., by an intervention). In the *contemplation* stage, patients are aware of the problem and their conflicts about changing, but they remain uncommitted to taking action. Patients may spend much time in psychotherapy in the precontemplation and contemplation stages; increasing self-awareness and addressing conflicts often calls for an insight-oriented approach in the context of a strong therapeutic relationship. In the *preparation* stage, the patient is committed to changing behavior in the near future and beginning to take small steps in that direction. The *action* stage entails modifying behavior as well as changing the environment or situation (e.g., getting rid of liquor or a stash of pills kept for suicide or terminating an abusive relationship). The *maintenance* stage revolves around consolidating changes and preventing relapse. It is not uncommon (albeit discouraging) for patients to cycle through these stages in the context of relapses. Extensive research shows that adapting the therapeutic approach to the patient's stage of change reduces dropouts and improves outcomes (Krebs et al. 2019).

Personality Traits

In contrast to resistance and readiness for change, *reactance* has been identified as an oppositional or avoidant response to persuasion or pressure to change. Reactance might be perceived (as in a child) to be willfulness or obstreperousness, but it is better understood as being rooted in a fear of losing one's autonomy or independence. Accordingly, reactance lies not in the patient but rather in the therapeutic relationship: reactance is a response to directiveness or, in the extreme, to controlling behavior. Vicious circles can develop quickly as efforts to control abet reactance, which escalates efforts to control, and so on. Accordingly, less directive approaches that give the patient space and emphasize autonomy are best suited to patients who are relatively high in reactance. In contrast, patients who are lower in reactance may benefit from more directiveness. Although the research base is relatively small, substantially better outcomes are associated with matching therapist directiveness to patient reactance (Edwards et al. 2019).

The personality dimension ranging from externalizing to internalizing also has implications for adapting the style of the therapy to the characteristics of the patient. Persons prone to *externalizing* tend to blame their problems or distress on the environment—typically, other persons. In contrast, persons prone to *internalizing* tend to blame their problems and distress on themselves. Externalizers are more prone to action (and anger) and internalizers to introspection (and guilt feelings); correspondingly, externalizers are more extroverted and internalizers more introverted. Although the studies are few, research indicates that externalizers respond better to symptom-oriented approaches that emphasize action, whereas internalizers respond better to insight-oriented approaches that promote introspection (Beutler et al. 2019).

Factors Beyond Psychotherapy That Influence Outcomes

We also must keep in mind that psychotherapy does not take place in a vacuum. Norcross and Lambert (2019a) attribute 40% of the change that takes place to factors *outside* the therapy, prominently including social support and life events. They also include self-change, and, as Amanda Edwards-Stewart and John Norcross point out, we therapists should not lose sight of the fact that "[s]elf-help, not psychotherapy, is the de facto mental health system" (Edwards-Stewart and Norcross 2019, p. 358). The authors noted that 5,000 self-help books are published each year, and there are 25,000 websites devoted to mental health, along with thousands of apps. They cautioned that "less than 5% of commercial self-help books and 1% of web and mobile tools possess any research evidence on their effectiveness or safety" (p. 365). Of course, patients can use self-help resources in conjunction with psychotherapy, and therapists can encourage their use as well as assist with it.

Inside the therapy, we should keep in mind that the patient's characteristics play a far greater role than the therapist's contribution, the therapy relationship, and the treatment method. As in general medicine, the chronicity and severity of the illness strongly influence the outcome. In the field of psychotherapy, patients with severe illnesses respond positively to treatment, but the treatment often must be lengthy and intensive. With some irony, Arthur Bohart and Karen Tallman referred to clients as the "neglected common factor" in psychotherapy (Bohart and Tallman 2010, p. 83) and pointed out that "the client and factors in the client's life account for more variance in the therapeutic outcome than any other factor" (p. 84). Furthermore, they emphasized that the *client* does the work of changing, with help from the therapist.

What Happened to the Therapist?

Decades ago, I went out for my morning jog and crossed paths with Irv Rosen, the director of psychotherapy at the Menninger Clinic. We circled around the park together for a while. I brought up my fraught experience in a research team conducting an intensive study of psychotherapy with patients diagnosed with borderline personality disorder. We were investigating what kinds of interventions would increase (or decrease) the therapeutic alliance within therapy sessions (Horwitz et al. 1996). Some of us had tape-recorded our sessions, which were then transcribed and evaluated by the research group. The group members included a number of psychoanalysts who were senior to me, including my boss, Len Horwitz, the leader of the project and director of psychology. To say the least, this close scrutiny was often painful, as I lamented with Irv while we jogged around the park. The psychotherapy I was conducting was hardly going smoothly (which is par for the course for patients with severe borderline personality disorder). Irv's response: "Now you know why therapists don't do psychotherapy research!" This comment should be restricted to therapists' reluctance to doing research *on themselves*. We are less apprehensive about doing research on our treatment methods. But we cannot exclude ourselves from the research if we want to improve our effectiveness.

Research on treatment methods pertains to trust in an impersonal sense: to what extent can the patient (and therapist) trust that the treatment method will be effective? Starting from the premise that "there is no single right way to conduct psychotherapy" (p. 303), Paul Wachtel (2008) acknowledged that his therapeutic practice "reflects not just my theory but who I am as a person. This is *my* way of working with people. It bears a significant relationship to what my theory is, but it is partly simply me" (pp. 266–267, emphasis in original). Only in the latter part of my career did I fully appreciate the truth and import of Wachtel's stance. Consistent with his view, research on the therapist makes it personal: To what extent can the patient trust *me*? Am I competent? Caring? Able to help? Trustworthy in all these ways? Not necessarily and, under the best of circumstances, not continuously.

To cut to the chase, as editors Louis Castonguay and Clara Hill put it in the preface to their book on therapist effects, "Not all therapists are equal…some therapists are better than others at helping clients…some therapists are substantially less effective, and even more harmful, than the majority of practitioners" (Castonguay and Hill 2017b, p. xiii). Wampold and colleagues (Wampold and Imel 2015; Wampold et al. 2017) conducted extensive analyses of the research literature and concluded that the effect of the person of the therapist "actually is quite large, *much larger*, for example, than the differences between treatments" (Wampold et al. 2017, p. 40, emphasis added). Michael Barkham and colleagues (2017) made the same point more cautiously: "it ap-

---

TABLE 1–3. Notable findings regarding therapists'
effectiveness

A large proportion of therapists are effective (Barkham et al. 2017).

Patients of the top 15%–20% of therapists have twice the recovery rate of the bottom 15%–20% (Barkham et al. 2017).

For severely disturbed patients, the influence of the therapist is four times greater than for the least disturbed patients (Barkham et al. 2017).

Therapists tend to overestimate their effectiveness (Boswell et al. 2017).

Therapists are poor at detecting patients' deterioration (Lambert et al. 2019).

---

pears to be *at least, or maybe more,* important who clients see rather than what specific therapy is offered" (p. 26, emphasis added).

Now I am reiterating the point that therapy researchers largely have been barking up the wrong tree in focusing so much attention on brand comparisons. That line of research, in effect, treats therapists as *interchangeable* with one another. Differences among therapists are canceled out in evaluating the effectiveness of the specific treatment. From a research perspective, like placebo effects in drug trials based on positive expectations, the effect of individual therapists is a nuisance—noise or error variance. In psychotherapy, however, expectations about the effectiveness of the treatment play an important part in the treatment outcome, and these expectations are influenced by the therapist. When we ignore the effect of the individual therapist, we are erroneously attributing the effectiveness—or lack thereof—to the specific treatment. As Barkham and colleagues (2017) commented, favoring research on treatments to the neglect of therapists "is surprising given that they are the most valuable and costly component in the delivery of psychological therapies" (p. 13). But we are not completely in the dark, not least because we now know where we need to shine the light. Research has been illuminating; several notable findings are summarized in Table 1–3.

We need to keep in mind the broader context of the dodo bird verdict: Psychotherapy in general is highly effective. But *no patient receives psychotherapy in general.* Barkham and colleagues (2017) concluded that, compared with the middle 60%–70% of therapists, 15%–20% of therapists have better outcomes and 15%–20% have worse outcomes. Accordingly, "the middle two thirds of therapists cannot be confidently and reliably distinguished from each other with regards to the amount of change they facilitate in their clients" (p. 26). Barkham and colleagues find it reassuring that a large proportion of therapists are doing a good job. Less reassuring, however, is the fact that "the average recovery rate for the more effective therapists is almost twice that of the less effective group" (pp. 22–23); that is a big difference. Also worrying is the finding that "therapists tend to overestimate their own general effectiveness with clients, as well as their effectiveness relative to other therapists" (Boswell et al. 2017). More

specifically, Miller and colleagues (2017) report: "Studies show that the least effective believe that they are as good as the most effective and that average clinicians overestimate their outcomes on the order of 65%" (p. 24). Psychotherapists
are not alone; research shows that physicians also overestimate their effectiveness
(Taylor and Neimeyer 2017).

The broad findings regarding therapist effects need to be qualified. Most
important, differences among therapists come into play most strongly in the
treatment of patients whose problems and disorders are more severe. Barkham
and colleagues (2017) found that the influence of the therapist is *four times
greater* with patients who are severely disturbed than with those who are least
disturbed. Accordingly, they concluded that "if clients present with a low level
of severity, it might be that the required level of clinical skill is more generic to
most practitioners" (p. 25). As severity of disturbance increases, so does the influence of the therapist as an individual.

I have been focusing in this book on psychotherapy as conducted by generalists, who treat patients with diverse problems and disorders (akin to internists
and family practitioners in general medicine). As Michael Constantino and colleagues (2017) reviewed, the magnitude of therapist effects (individual differences) differs for different psychiatric disorders and problems. For example,
therapist effects are more prominent for patients with depression, substance
abuse, or quality of life than for those with psychosis or mania (insofar as psychosis or mania will be more responsive to medication, which could facilitate
psychotherapy). In addition, a given therapist is likely to be more effective in
treating some problems or disorders than others (e.g., more effective with depression than substance abuse or vice versa). Moreover, therapists differ from
one another in the level of consistency in effectiveness. Constantino et al. (2017)
found that "Many therapists demonstrated effectiveness over multiple domains,
yet no therapists demonstrated reliable effectiveness across all domains. A small
but notable 4% of therapists failed to demonstrate positive outcomes on any domain" (p. 56). Finally, therapist effects are more prominent in routine practice
than they are in randomized controlled trials, which require adherence to treatment manuals, wherein therapist differences are deliberately minimized
(Wampold and Imel 2015). In those trials, ideally, therapists could be trained to
be interchangeable. Ironically, therapists vary substantially in their adherence
to the treatment manuals in those trials (Constantino et al. 2017).

I credit the dodo bird verdict for generating a shift in our perspective on psychotherapy insofar as we are witnessing a retreat from the generation of countless
brands of treatment to broadening our purview of myriad contributors to treatment outcomes and their relative magnitude. Over the past few decades, clini-
cian-researchers have developed an alternative way of thinking about the field
under the broad rubric of psychotherapy integration. This approach does not
simplify the life of the therapist; it complicates it. But it provides a platform for
new ways of looking at the psychotherapy literature and going beyond this literature to appreciate the far wider field of knowledge and experience that contribute
to the psychotherapist's personal and professional development.

Psychotherapy Integration

How did we wind up with hundreds of competing brands? Pointing to competitiveness and professional rivalry, Norcross and Alexander (2019) proposed that "professional reputations are made by emphasizing the new and different, not the basic and similar…. [T]here is far too much emphasis on the ownership of ideas" (p. 20). Thus, we have brands, acronyms, jargon, and buzzwords in abundance. But competition and self-promotion are not the whole story. Often, therapists who have been brought up early in their career under one tradition find themselves hamstrung by it and realize that they must be more flexible; they must learn, discover—and sometimes create—something new. I learned in my very first attempt at psychotherapy that I would need to learn something very different. It took me about a decade to get started.

Given that therapists are inundated with an array of brands that they could never learn about—much less master—psychotherapy integration is the only pathway forward that makes sense to me. A concerted effort to overcome professional rivalries and boundaries was launched in 1983 by the formation of the Society for the Exploration of Psychotherapy Integration by therapists united in part in being critical of the wholesale adoption of manualized, empirically supported therapies, which failed to respect the flexibility needed in typical clinical practice. Different approaches to integration include focus on common factors as discussed earlier in this chapter as well as efforts to integrate theories and techniques (Norcross and Alexander 2019). Most appealing to me is the strategy of *assimilative integration* that typically starts with the therapist acquiring a solid grounding in one psychotherapy system and then gradually incorporating theories and combining techniques from other systems. I am partial to the assimilative integration version because it focuses our attention on the *professional development of the therapist*. More broadly, I am partial to the integrative approach because it is the best framework to structure the developmental challenges that all therapists will face—not only in the early years but also throughout their career. Therapists who stand still will be out of step.

I find Wampold's contextual model (Wampold and Imel 2015) especially instructive. As I noted earlier in this chapter, Wampold asserted that the battle between common factors and specific ingredients rests on a false dichotomy: "specific ingredients and common factors are not mutually exclusive but work together to make psychotherapy effective" (Wampold and Ulvenes 2019, p. 69). In the contextual model, psychotherapy begins with the formation of an *initial bond* in which trust plays a prominent role in conjunction with the therapist's understanding and expertise. The fate of the therapy can hinge on this initial bond: "most patients who drop out of therapy prematurely do so after the first session or two" (Wampold and Ulvenes 2019, pp. 72–73). Wampold distinguishes three pathways to change: a *relationship* based on realistic perceptions of the therapist as authentic, warm, empathic, and caring; the creation of positive *expectations* for change by means of an explanation of the treatment that is credible to the patient; and *specific ingredients* that include goals and tasks, therapeutic actions, and the patient's actions that decrease illness and promote health.

I believe that Wampold's way of understanding the relation of the common (relationship) factors to the specific (treatment) factors applies widely to psychotherapy. That is, the relationship "serves as the *foundation* for other therapeutic processes and actions" (Wampold and Ulvenes 2019, p. 73), the "*vehicle* for delivering the specific ingredients" (p. 71), and "*sets the stage* for the client to collaborate" (p. 75). This reasoning is consistent with viewing the therapeutic alliance as valuable insofar as it enables the work of therapy. In effect, a positive relationship and alliance are preconditions for the therapeutic process. Yet *this means-end model can be highly misleading*; it applies best to short-term therapies where cooperation is easily established. Consider patients whose capacity for trusting relationships has been profoundly impaired, for example, those with a history of chronic and severe trauma in attachment relationships. For such patients, the cultivation of trust with an intimate bond is not the foundation for therapy or vehicle of therapy; it is *the work of therapy* and the ideal *outcome* of therapy. Moreover, the therapy will be fully effective only to the extent that the improving quality of the therapeutic relationship generalizes to other relationships beyond the therapy. Furthermore, if profoundly troubled relationships are the fundamental *problem* that therapy must address—as is often the case for severely impaired patients with multiple psychiatric disorders—the specific ingredients will be the way the patient and therapist work together to create a healing relationship and generalize it to other relationships.

Wampold's treatment model is consistent with myriad specific treatment methods as long as the broad components he has identified obtain in the treatment. I find irony in the integrative approach. It is intended to transcend differences, but there are many ways to integrate: a decade after it was created, "psychotherapy integration began to differentiate more clearly into separate paths or subtypes" (Goldfried et al. 2019, p. 44). Different approaches to integration now are being compared for effectiveness in research (Boswell et al. 2019), raising the question "Will more therapists begin to identify as integrative, and will integration become another entry in the theoretical orientation horse race?" (Eubanks et al. 2019a, p. 482). Boswell and colleagues (2019) referred to a "potential blizzard of integrations" and pointed out that "there is a danger that we are recapitulating the very problem integrative therapies were, at least in part, intended to address" (p. 422).

The psychotherapy integration approach will alter neither ambitious competitiveness nor the creative desire to find better ways of thinking and working. I think assimilative integration implies a developmental course for psychotherapists that is the best path to becoming trustworthy over the course of a career. Many will start the journey from a relatively pure form therapy base; others will begin with an orientation to psychotherapy integration (Norcross and Finnerty 2019). Regardless of your starting point (which could be from within the integrative movement), assimilative integration is the natural alternative to developmental stagnation. Given individual differences among therapists and patients, there will be innumerable developmental pathways. But I think the professional literature I have sketched is only one domain of a far greater territory. We have much more knowledge to integrate than the scientific literature on psychotherapy and psychopathology.

Personal Knowledge

William James (1890/1950), a physician and foremost American philosopher, wrote the two-volume founding textbook of psychology. I admire James especially for his broadmindedness, as captured by one of his biographers, Ralph Barton Perry (1996): For James, "psychology meant seeing man in the round—as he presents himself to the physician, the biologist, the traveler, the artist, or the novelist. Hence he was *willing to learn about man from any source*" (p. 193, emphasis added), as we psychotherapists should be.

When I first came across philosopher Michael Polanyi's (1962, 1966) seemingly mundane concept of *personal knowledge*, I found it to be illuminating in relation to my concerns about the intrusion of scientism into the conduct of psychotherapy. Personal knowledge is individual, residing in individual minds. It is the sum total of what you know—not what resides in libraries or on the internet. Personal knowledge puts the knower in the knowledge, highlighting "the personal contribution by which the knower shapes his own knowledge" (Polanyi 1959/2014, p. 13). Keep in mind, as James articulated it, that knowledge of persons is the realm that concerns us. We begin acquiring all this personal knowledge in childhood and continue to do so throughout life; at best, our professional knowledge will enhance it, not replace it.

Thankfully, we professionals are hardly unique in being able to help people with psychological problems; we are newcomers to that ancient endeavor, which has always rested on personal knowledge. I worked with a patient who called me occasionally for many years after we terminated psychotherapy. One time she called me in a crisis; it was late in the evening, and I was unavailable. I talked with her the next morning, by which time she was as calm as could be. She had contacted a psychic who skillfully talked her through the crisis. We psychotherapists may not be psychic, but there is more to our healing than our professional knowledge encompasses.

Hans Strupp conducted a study of psychotherapy offered to male college students suffering from anxiety, depression, and personality problems (Strupp and Hadley 1979). He compared the effectiveness of highly experienced psychotherapists with that of college professors selected for their ability to form understanding relationships with students. On average, patients from both groups showed similar levels of improvement. Emory Cowen (1982), one of my graduate school professors, conducted a study of the personal problems that clients present to divorce lawyers, hairdressers, bartenders, and industrial supervisors. The problems were highly similar to those that patients present to psychotherapists.

I doubt that the professors, lawyers, hairdressers, and supervisors would have comparable success to professionals with persons suffering from serious mental illness; we will not find randomized controlled trials in the literature. But we might ponder these questions: What knowledge do these community providers use? What knowledge did helpers of all sorts use before there were psychotherapists? Consider a parallel set of questions about patients: What knowledge must a patient have to engage in a productive psychotherapy relationship? What knowledge must a patient acquire during the process of effective psychotherapy?

I believe that the primary source of knowledge that psychotherapists bring to bear on their practice is derived from their history of relationships—close relationships most prominently. Here I include the relationship with oneself—personal knowledge at its most personal level. As is true of our patients, our personal knowledge is profoundly shaped by our culture, which, in turn, shapes our upbringing. Most of us are keenly aware of the particularly formative nature of early family relationships, the crucible for learning about ourselves and others. Yet our relational world quickly expands beyond the family, and we learn about relationships through a wealth of interactions throughout our lifetime. Patients bring their personal knowledge of relationships to the process, as do therapists, whose professional knowledge complements their knowledge from personal relationships. All of us learn a great deal about others through gossip—not malicious gossip but rather the ordinary conversations we have about other people, which comprise the greatest proportion of our conversations when we are not working with each other on tasks (Dunbar 1996). We learn from literature, film, theater, and art (Farber 2017). The mainstream media and social media provide a continuous stream of information (and misinformation) about our humanity (and inhumanity).

Apart from their professional knowledge, there is no reason to believe that therapists are better informed or educated than their patients in any of these nonprofessional domains, including personal relationships and interactions. Yet psychotherapists are immensely privileged in one respect: we are privy to a wealth of knowledge gleaned from intimate relationships with a potentially large number of patients who have trusted and confided in us. I have learned a great deal from patients about suffering and psychological problems, but I also have learned a great deal about human goodness, devotion, intelligence, imagination, wisdom, courage, and resilience.

Tacit Knowledge and Unconscious Processes

Polanyi (1966) distinguished two types of personal knowledge, the understanding of which is crucial to understanding the process of psychotherapy: explicit and tacit (implicit). When we think of knowledge, we are most inclined to think of what we express in language. When we engage in psychotherapy—talk therapy—we are concentrating on explication. Could we be overlooking a crucial dimension of the psychotherapy process? As Polanyi put it, "we can know more than we can tell" (p. 4).

Often enough, I think about what I am about to say to a patient. At times I deliberate. Sometimes I plan a strategy of interventions before I meet with the patient. Most of the time, however, we are having a relatively spontaneous conversation. Typically, I don't know what I think until I have said it (at least to myself)—or written it. Invariably, with regard to all that goes into our interventions, we know more than we can tell—far more. In interacting with others, we rely on a wealth of prior experience and knowledge as well as a mass of perceptions and emotional responses to nonverbal cues that we could never explicate except in the most fragmentary way. Therein—in the tacit realm—lies a lot of the therapy. In drawing attention to unconscious processes, I intend primarily to make a humbling point: to a significant degree, *our trustworthiness—and our patients' perceptions of it—will be beyond our conscious control.*

To a large extent, our unconscious knowledge is manifested in performance—dancing, riding a bicycle, playing the piano, catching a fly ball. Literally, we could not put one foot in front of the other without unconscious processes. We could not see, feel, think, speak, or add two numbers. I am partial to philosopher Daniel Dennett's (2017) phrase "competence without comprehension" (p. 51). Such competence abounds, but because it is opaque to our awareness, we fail to appreciate it. Much of our competence develops unconsciously and escapes our notice. But it forms the foundation of trust, as I elaborate in Chapter 3.

Joel Weinberger and his colleague Valentina Stoycheva masterfully synthesized three centuries of literature on unconscious processes, with an emphasis on the burgeoning recent science (Weinberger and Stoycheva 2020). They characterized unconscious processes in the psychoanalytic models as being "affectively charged, nonrational, poorly integrated into the personality, and formed under the crucial impact of early experiences" (p. 50). Now we appreciate the far wider operation of unconscious processes, which are "*normal and ubiquitous*. Rather than being peripheral and unimportant, *they are central and critical to psychological functioning*" (p. 133, emphasis in original). They are central to our unconscious relational competence, in psychotherapy as elsewhere.

A common example of tacit knowledge pertains to the way we read emotional expressions in faces—sometimes unconsciously. For example, subliminal exposure to a threatening face can prime the observer to be more alert to danger, without being aware of the unconscious influence (Armony and LeDoux 1997). Might we become wary and distrusting of another person on the basis of facial expressions, vocal tone, and posture without being conscious of the reasons for our "gut feelings?" Might we quickly feel safe with a person without thinking about it? Will such intuitive responses influence trust in psychotherapy? Yes to all these questions, normally and ubiquitously. Will we be in control of either responding to these nonverbal influences or expressing them? A bit, perhaps. On the whole, however, we know each other, tacitly and implicitly, in ways we do not know.

Unconscious processes unfold automatically; they are relatively efficient, unintentional, and uncontrollable. They are based largely on repeated associations and habits. Much of this implicit learning is guided automatically in conjunction with emotion, most globally as it relates to a good-bad, approach-avoid dimension: "*emotions grab our attention, help us organize our experiences, and play a major role in regulating those experiences*" (p. 224, emphasis in original). We are also unaware of the extent to which our thinking is embedded in bodily experience, as represented in abundant metaphorical language: we "categorize people as warm or cold, feel distant or close to them, feel weighted down by stress, put too much on our plates, and feel our heads spinning" (p. 227). Our discourse in psychotherapy is filled with such metaphors—or should be, if it is to be vivid and evocative. When my colleague Michael Groat and I conducted an educational group to engage patients in understanding others' internal worlds, we asked them to create a visual image of their experience in treatment. "Looking off the edge of a cliff," "Hanging by my fingernails," "Sinking in quicksand," and "In a hole without a ladder" were typical examples. A patient struggling with bipolar disorder gave one of my favorites: "Trying to run up a down escalator." We naturally and unconsciously link our emotional experience to our bodily functioning.

Unconscious processes can be problematic, for example, when we automatically extend relationship patterns from the past to present relationships where they no longer fit—the territory of misapplied distrust. In such instances, making the unconscious conscious to allow for new learning and memory has been a long-standing aim of psychotherapy. Conscious processing enables us to interrupt old patterns and to move into new ways of thinking, feeling, and acting in relationships. With repeated experience of trusting trustworthy persons, trust can become more automatic. We can make the conscious unconscious, as we do in developing skilled performance. To a large extent, the common relationship factors in psychotherapy require such skills, integrating conscious and unconscious processes. Because I am concerned about the complexity of relating in a trusting and trustworthy way, I underscore the balance between deliberation and intuition, with a conscious bias toward the latter.

Reconciling Left and Right (Hemispheres)

In establishing trust in psychotherapy, we should be mindful of lived experience as we endeavor to put so much into words. I find psychiatrist Ian McGilchrist's (2019) distinction between the functions of the right and left cerebral hemispheres instructive—notwithstanding abundant crass popularization in which we are purported to do one sort of thing with our "right brain" and another with our "left brain," as if they are disconnected (which would require neurosurgery). We must understand that "each hemisphere is involved in everything we do.... It's not *what* each hemisphere does but *how* it does it that matters" (p. x, emphasis in original). The two hemispheres "work well together not because they have the same role, but precisely because they have different roles" (p. xv). The distinctive and complementary but potentially conflicting roles played by the right and left hemispheres add "to our understanding of our own minds" and "what it is to be a human being" (p. xxi).

Broadly speaking, the two hemispheres contribute to different takes on the world, based on the pattern of attention being narrow or broad, sustained or fluid: the left hemisphere illuminates a focus (foreground), and the right provides a sense of context (background). For example, when a therapist is conversing with a patient, she might be concentrating on what he is saying but is more subtly influenced by his facial expression and posture. The therapist can shift her attention from the patient's speech to his body language, potentially bringing the body language into the foreground and leaving the speech in the background—perhaps not even listening to what he is saying but hearing the tone.

The following is a list of contrasts, left versus right, that I have drawn from McGilchrist's review. I present some detail only to give you a feel for the pattern of differences, distinguishing throughout the *focus* of attention from the surrounding *context*. We have different relations: independent-interdependent, separate-connected, exclusive-inclusive, individualistic-pluralistic, decontextualized-contextualized. We can take apart or integrate, influence or empathize. We have different versions of knowing: abstract-concrete, general-particular, familiar-new, literal-metaphorical. We shift between categorizing and observing. We can take a physical or biological view: mechanical-organic, lifeless-living, static-dynamic, disembodied-embodied. We can shift between the neat and the messy: clarity-ambiguity, certainty-uncertainty, perfection-imperfection, simple-complicated, resolution-tension.

Having made these broad distinctions, McGilchrist devoted much of his book to making the case that the balance of power in our culture has shifted away from right-left complementarity to the dominance of the left hemisphere in shaping the way we think. Broadly, the right hemisphere serves a more experiential function and the left a more utilitarian function, exerting control over what we experience. McGilchrist titled his book *The Master and the Emissary*, arguing that the left (emissary) hemisphere should be the servant of the right (master), but the roles have become reversed, such that the servant has become the master (McGilchrist 2019). Ideally, he envisioned a process wherein the left hemisphere isolates something particular from its surroundings, illuminating an aspect of the context, thereby *enriching our experience of the whole* as well as allowing us to manipulate aspects of the world to exert control over it. Ironically, "The implicit has, now, to be made explicit. The catch is that in becoming explicit it is no longer the same at all" (p. xxiii).

When I speak and write about psychotherapy, I am focused on my thoughts about it, but these thoughts are continually grounded in my memories of experience with individual patients, and this experience is generally emotional. I speak and write about what I say to patients and what they say to me—it is talk therapy, after all. We need not create another battle in pitting the importance of what we say to each other (explicit, left hemisphere) against the direct experience of being with each other (tacit, right hemisphere)—the figure or the ground. The idea of a contest distracts us from the overall picture: both forms of attention, both ways of knowing, are crucial; they are intertwined continually, and they are best when mutually enhancing. My concern is that with all this talk, we are neglecting the profound importance of the direct experience of being together, the bedrock of implicit learning and the soil in which trust and distrust develop. Underground, this soil remains opaque to us, notwithstanding its being the ground floor of our trusting and trustworthiness.

I have reviewed how the field of psychotherapy is turning from trusting the treatment to trusting the relationship. What I have in mind here, in the psychotherapy relationship and other relationships, is the experience of *presence, living engagement, the sense of the other person, the sense of self in relation to the other, and the feeling of understanding and being understood.* The *feeling of safety* will be the bedrock of healing in the trusting relationship (Sandler 1960). Of course, the living experience can include the *feeling of disengagement, disconnection, and misunderstanding as well as feeling threatened, wary, and unsafe.* These experiences, largely tacit, will determine the fate of the therapy. Although we can never fully capture the experience in words, a crucial part of therapy is verbalizing the distressing experience in the service of overcoming it. Yet, if the talk is to be effective, it must have an impact on the lived experience that should be our greatest treasure. To return to McGilchrist's metaphor, the left hemisphere must continually give back its comprehension to the right hemisphere's experience.

Throughout this book, I keep coming back to problems in *living.* These problems have been the focus of ethical thought for millennia, and I think a crucial domain of the personal knowledge that we therapists bring to our practice is composed of ethical-moral thought. To a great extent, this knowledge has been articulated in the context of diverse religious traditions across the globe, and these traditions will have shaped the ethical thought of therapists and patients—consciously or unconsciously. Religious or not, this cultural heritage is part of our personal knowledge. In the following section, I superimpose ethical thought from philosophy on this broad cultural heritage.

Knowledge of Ethics

In this section, I make the case that a psychotherapist's personal knowledge includes a sense of what constitutes psychological health. At a minimum, this ethical sense is implicit, but I believe that we psychotherapists should make our view of psychological health explicit, not only in our own minds but also in collaboration with our patients, whose views also should be cultivated, articulated, and prioritized in the work. We therapists might not be in accord with our patients about fundamental values, and finding common ground is part of the work. We have venerable professional allies in articulating what constitutes psychological health: philosophers who have developed the field of ethics over the course of more than two millennia in the West (the domain in which I am most knowledgeable).

To be less judicious in my language here, I think the professional literature as I have been reviewing it thus far fails to capture *what I believe to be the essence of psychotherapy: its heart, soul, and spirit.* Heart, soul, and spirit abound in my colleagues' practice as I perceive and hear about it, evident in their devotion and caring, intermingled with their capacity for suffering along with their patients. But this essence tends to be sidelined in our professional discourse.

Accordingly, I have something radically different in mind from psychotherapists' obligatory ethics codes and required events that focus on ethical practice. I am advocating a shift in attitude—a reorientation implied in my more temperate language of science-informed humanism. No doubt, professional ethical principles are compatible with ethical thought in philosophy, for example, including beneficence and nonmaleficence, fidelity and responsibility, integrity, justice, and respect for people's rights and dignity (American Psychological Association 2017; Roberts and Dunn 2019). And conduct consistent with professional ethical codes certainly is essential to psychotherapists' trustworthiness. But I have something broader in mind that relates to the major problem in psychotherapy research that has been the theme of this chapter: The focus on treating psychiatric disorders has overshadowed the need to work with the *problems in living* that play a major role in the development of these disorders. More than that, I think therapists should work from an intuitive and explicit sense of what *a good life* consists of, and they should engage their patients in that quest. In my view, trusting relationships are vital in a good life, especially when—inevitably—that life entails profound suffering.

Highlighting ethics in this section, I am setting the stage for my extensive use of philosophy in discussing trust and trustworthiness along with hope in subsequent chapters. Once we psychotherapists free ourselves from a narrow scientific and technological approach to our work, we need to anchor ourselves in a broader perspective on human life, with a grasp of how it goes well and how it goes badly. We psychotherapists are newcomers to this territory. We have established a foothold in endeavoring to help others with problems in living, but we are a small fraction of those who do so. We have science on our side, but we need much knowledge beyond science. If my experience is any guide, we will never feel that we have enough. Likely, we are not alone in that feeling. The following is a brief introduction to ethics—a small dose. I begin this section by using science to make the case for knowledge of ethics.

From Illness to Health

Sociologist Corey Keyes (2014) reviewed the World Health Organization's advocacy for promoting mental health while giving due attention to the major contribution of mental illness to the global burden of disease. Mental health cannot be equated with the absence of mental illness; recovery from psychiatric disorder is not enough. Mental health must be considered a positive state. With roots in Aristotle (Bartlett and Collins 2011), Keyes used the term *flourishing*, which includes emotional, psychological, and social well-being. He characterized the absence of flourishing as *languishing*. As is true of mental illness, genetic and environmental factors interact in contributing to mental health.

Keyes envisioned mental health and mental illness as two intersecting continua, each ranging from low to moderate to high. He cited 2005 data from the United States indicating that at the high ends, the prevalence of mental illness was 17.5% and the prevalence of mental health was 22.4% (Keyes 2014). These two continua overlap to some extent, but they are relatively independent (sharing 28% of the variability). Accordingly, a person could be free of mental illness yet languishing; alternatively, one could be suffering from mental illness yet flourishing (and everything in between). As Keyes summarized,

> Because there is some genetic overlap of mental illness and health, our findings suggest it may be somewhat more difficult to reach high levels of well-being if one inherits strong genetic risk factors for depression or an anxiety disorder. However, a strong dose of genetic liability to mental illness does not preordain individuals to low levels of well-being and inheriting a low level of genetic risk for mental illness by no means guarantees that an individual will flourish in life. (p. 184)

As ethicists have been advocating all along, flourishing is worthwhile in its own right. However, psychotherapists treating mental illness must be aware of a problem associated with focusing solely on recovery from illness: *flourishing is protective against relapsing after recovering from episodes of mental illness*. As Keyes documented, decreasing from a high (flourishing) level to a moderate level of mental health was associated with four times the likelihood of developing mental illness, and decreasing to a low (languishing) level of mental health was associated with eight times the likelihood of developing mental illness.

Keyes summarized what all psychotherapists should know: "gains in mental health resulted in decreasing odds of mental illness over time," and "losses of mental health resulted in increasing odds of mental illness over time." Accordingly, "If you want better mental health, you must focus on positive mental health—promoting flourishing and protecting against its loss. Public health and organizations cannot promote mental health by solely reducing mental illness, and no amount of wishful thinking will make this fact disappear" (Keyes 2014, p. 189).

From the perspective of ethics, shifting the focus from illness to health takes us back to Socrates. As philosopher Bernard Williams (1985) summarized, "It is not a trivial question, Socrates said: what we are talking about is how one should live." Williams went on to say that "It would be a serious thing if philosophy could answer the question," yet, "it is not true that philosophy, itself, can reasonably hope to answer it" (p. 1). But philosophy can help us think about it, and we should do so as psychotherapists.

I never had a patient entering psychotherapy with the question "How should I live?" Patients' questions relate to more specific problems in living, problems in which troubles with close relationships often play a major part. Yet I have had numerous patients agonizing over the question, in one form or another, "Why should I go on living this life of unending misery?" This *why* question implies the *how* question for psychotherapy: How might life become worth living for me? When the question of suicide is not on the table, the explicit question "How should I live?" is in the (tacit) background. Whether I should live comes before how I should live. But the route to the *whether* is through the *how*. What is the possible path to a life worth living? I think *therapists must have some vision of what makes a life worthwhile* to get any psychotherapy off the ground. Moreover, this question is ethical and moral—the specialty of philosophers who are concerned about the problems of human life.

Ethics and Morals

Ethics and morals overlap, but it is useful to make a broad distinction, as Kwame Anthony Appiah (2008) neatly does: "I'll generally follow Aristotle in using 'ethics' to refer to questions about human flourishing, about what it means for a life to be well lived. I'll use 'morality' to designate something narrower, the constraints that govern how we should and should not treat other people" (p. 37). The entanglement of morals and ethics should be immediately clear: how we treat each other (and are treated by others) plays a major role in how well we live. Appiah puts it succinctly: "doing what is morally right is one of the constituents of human flourishing" (p. 168).

Compared with morals, *ethics* is a relatively neutral term, referring, for example, to a large domain of philosophical discourse about the quality of human life. We need to be able to hear the word *morality* without bracing ourselves for *moralizing*— a kind of judgmental, preachy attitude about right and wrong, good and bad. Here is Appiah's conclusion about how ethics and morality fit together:

> To see each other person not just as someone with preferences, pleasures, and pains, but as a creature engaged in the project of making a life, striving to succeed on the basis of standards that are partly found and partly made, you will see why you should keep promises and respect property, why you should not gratuitously obstruct other people's ambitions or ignore their material, social, or psychological needs. Morality derives from an understanding of what other people are up to; it's not a system of arbitrary demands. And the central thing that people are up to is the central ethical task: each of us is making a life. *That is the human telos: to make a good life.* (p. 203, emphasis added)

I think Appiah's focus on making a good life is right on target as an ethical frame for psychotherapy. In making a life for ourselves, we must respect others as they do the same, and as psychotherapists we should actively promote their effort to do so. In my view, Appiah has articulated the ethical foundation of trustworthiness as it applies to psychotherapy and more broadly to social conduct.

When I taught abnormal psychology to undergraduates, I started by asking them for their ideas about contributors to mental health. I wrote the long list on the board. One semester, after we had generated a particularly long list, a bright woman in the back piped up: "Balance!" At first, I was a bit taken aback. Then her remark reminded me of one of Karl Menninger's book titles, *The Vital Balance*. (Menninger 1963). Making a life for ourselves while attending to the life others are making for themselves is perhaps the most vital balance.

Owen Flanagan (2017) summed up the balance of ethics and morality neatly: we need "an *ethical morality*, a truly good way of living, of being human" (p. 106, emphasis added). To continue this theme, philosopher Christine Korsgaard (2009) penned one of my favorite passages in the ethics literature:

> Your life fits into the general human story and is a part of the general human activity of the creation and pursuit of value. It matters to you both that it is a particular part—your own part—and that it is part of the larger human story. What you want is not merely to be me-in-particular nor of course is it just to be a generic human being—what you want is to be a someone, a particular instance of humanity. So it's like this: in being the author of your own actions, you are also a co-author of the human story, our collective, public, story. As a person, who has to make himself into a particular person, you get to write one of the parts in the general human story, to create the role of one of the people you think it would be good to have in that story. And then—at least if you manage to maintain your integrity—you get to play the part. (p. 212)

A Good Life

If I could inspire you to read one science-informed philosophical book on ethics, it would be Daniel Haybron's (2013) *Happiness: A Short Introduction*. Then you might be inspired to read his more extensive exposition, *The Pursuit of Unhappiness* (Haybron 2008). In what follows, I intend merely to highlight key aspects of his conceptual framework—the big picture that I think therapists would benefit from having in mind as they help their patients grapple with problems in making a life.

For much of his childhood, Haybron spent a few months of the year on "a small, isolated, and relatively undeveloped island, where at the time most residents earned their living from fishing" (Haybron 2008, p. xiii). The rest of the year he spent on the mainland. Life on the island was hard, and, by mainland standards, the islanders were relatively poor. Yet for Haybron, the island "is the only place I've felt at home...like a fully developed human being" (p. xiii). He went on: "fishing was hard work for little pay, and winters could be brutal. But even when working the most unpleasant job I've ever had, my times there were still wonderful" (p. xiv). The islanders were well acquainted with life on the mainland, but Haybron reflected, "I don't believe many of them envied the far wealthier, and allegedly 'freer,' mainlanders at all" (p. xiv). Of the mainland, he observed, "The United States is, by a wide margin, among the most affluent nations in human history, and many Americans enjoy unprecedented freedom to shape their lives.... Yet no one ever accused us of 'knowing how to live'" (p. 23).

These reflections provide the personal context for Haybron's (2008) thinking about a *good life*, which he places at the top of his conceptual hierarchy: "an umbrella concept encompassing the domain of values that matter in a person's life" (pp. 36–37). Living a good life should be one's "ultimate goal in life" (p. 170)— "not just for one's own sake, but period" (p. 171). Then comes the question, "What counts as a good life?" (p. 110).

Capturing what I consider the vital balance, Haybron distinguished two contributors to a good life: 1) well-being, which is more individual, and 2) morality and virtue, which are more social. Both contributors are key concepts in any ethics. Morality and virtue will not be foremost priorities on any psychotherapy patient's mind, and I would consider a patient's desire to become more virtuous worthy of much reflection. Although I have found the broad philosophical school of virtue ethics (Hursthouse 1999) to be of enormous value in thinking about psychotherapy, I will set *virtue* aside here and stick with *morality*—which is sufficiently off-putting to many in its own right.

Rather than morality, of first concern to patients and therapists will be well-being and happiness, and to these Haybron has devoted a great deal of thought. Haybron declares his values regarding the vital balance between well-being and morality: "I want not merely for my children to be well-off or flourish; I want them to be good people and conduct themselves well, *whether or not it benefits them*. In fact this seems more important than their wellbeing" (p. 160, emphasis in original). Well-being, the predominant target of psychotherapy, entails the extent to which your life is "good *for you*" (Haybron 2013, p. 110, emphasis in original). *Subjective* well-being includes your personal experience and how you feel, whereas *objective* well-being fits normative standards, such that others could recognize it—perhaps better than you might. Thus, well-being includes being well, feeling well, and functioning well—what a parent would wish for a child, and what a psychotherapist would wish for a patient. Especially pertinent to psychotherapy is Haybron's (2008) point that an individual's well-being captures what others who provide help are aiming for: "what it is rational to want for someone *insofar as one cares for her*" (p. 40)—we would want the individual to be making a good life.

Haybron (2008) places *self-fulfillment*—"living in a manner that conforms to the sort of person one is" (p. 180)—as the core of well-being. Conversely, an unfulfilling life would be one lived in conflict with one's nature. Consider, for example, an attorney in a chronically high-stress life, hell-bent on achieving status and acquiring wealth, who might be much better off in a more self-fulfilling—if lower-paying—pursuit such as teaching that would be more rewarding and allow for more leisure. What constitutes self-fulfillment depends on the idiosyncratic makeup of the individual, and it is contingent on the individual's success in his or her endeavors, which will always be somewhat chancy.

Haybron (2008) construes *happiness* as a major contributor to well-being, but he ranks it beneath morality in a good life: "to sacrifice the demands of good character in the name of personal happiness—or, I would add, personal welfare—can never be justified. We must, above all, act decently, if not well" (p. 123). More explicitly, morality "is clearly the most important part of the picture, and the most important thing to get right in a good life" (Haybron 2013, p. 111). Moreover, while recognizing the importance of happiness to well-being, Haybron is not content with its popular construal: "the popular 'smiley-face' stereotype of happiness…grossly distorts and oversimplifies the phenomenon: happiness has a much richer, deeper, more complex, and less obvious psychology…. Cheery feelings matter, and do not deserve the abuse so often heaped on them, but they are a relatively uninteresting part of the story" (Haybron 2008, p. 106).

Haybron (2008) construes happiness more broadly as an *emotional condition*, "the aggregate of a person's emotions and moods" (p. 109). From the perspective of your emotional condition, the role of *feeling* happy "is grotesquely exaggerated in the popular imagination, doubtless accounting for much of the scorn heaped on happiness." Consider that "*most happy people don't feel happy most of the time*" (p. 109, emphasis added). Your emotional condition is a relatively enduring disposition to respond to the world, evident in feelings (including at the visceral level), ways of thinking, and behavior (e.g., expressions and tone of voice). On the negative side, your emotional condition might be depressive, anxious, or irritable; on the positive side, you might be characteristically more serene or in good spirits.

Without dismissing it, Haybron ranks feeling happy as least important in one's emotional condition. Second in importance to Haybron is energetic *engagement* with life, "enthusiastically taking up what it has to offer" (p. 114). Here he includes Mihaly Csikszentmihalyi's (1990) concept of *flow*, which refers to your experience when you are actively immersed in activity that optimally balances skill and challenge: too little challenge, and you are bored; too little skill, and you are anxious (or worse, if scaling a mountain).

No reader will be surprised that feeling happy and being actively engaged with life play a significant role in your emotional condition. But Haybron insightfully shifts our perspective to the cardinal value of *attunement* as the core of happiness. Think of attunement as being in tune with your life, a kind of harmony. As a therapist who has specialized in treating trauma, I find Haybron's prioritizing *safety and security* in this context to be right on the mark. He prioritizes tranquility over the more obvious positive emotions: "we might think of tranquility as 'settledness': not merely peace of mind or lack of internal discord but a kind of inner surety or confidence, stability and balance, or imperturbability…. [T]ranquility presents itself in the relaxed, easy posture" (p. 116). Attunement entails feeling at home in your life and, in a relationship, at home and in sync with the other person. Attuned, you have a sense of familiarity and goodness-of-fit in your life, which comes with feelings of confidence and mastery. You can let down your defenses and, in turn, blossom with feelings of openness and expansiveness. Perhaps most importantly, such attunement provides you with a sense of freedom.

We psychotherapists and our patients are all too familiar with lives that fall short of the good life that Haybron so richly describes. We all face myriad potential hazards, which include emotional ignorance. Haybron's (2008) review of recent psychological research shows that we are not particularly good at identifying our past emotional conditions, nor are we adept at anticipating our future emotional states. Worldwide surveys typically show a vast majority of Americans reporting high levels of happiness (e.g., 96% in one large study). Haybron finds these results impossible to believe in light of other studies showing Americans reporting high levels of stress, depression, and loneliness (e.g., half of respondents have no friends in whom they confide and a quarter have no confidants at all). Suicide rates are on the rise (Stone et al. 2018). The American dream might be just that.

With the pursuit of unhappiness in mind, Haybron (2008) proposed the central thesis that "people probably do not enjoy a high degree of authority or competence in matters of personal welfare. We should expect them systematically to make a host of serious mistakes regarding their own well-being. Surprisingly often, people's choices may frustrate their prospects for happiness and well-being rather than improve them" (p. 13). Haybron does not question our right to make such choices; rather, he questions the two pillars of our authority: 1) the *transparency* assumption, that "what's good for a person is relatively easy for that individual to discern," and 2) the *aptitude* assumption, that "people typically have the psychological endowments needed to choose well given the broad ability to live as they wish, with a rich array of options" (pp. 13–14). Consider the odds: to lead a life well "requires more than a numerical majority of good choices, since even one bad choice can ruin one's life" (p. 13). Accordingly, Haybron proposes a systematic imprudence thesis:

> Human beings are systematically prone to make a wide range of serious errors in matters of personal welfare. These errors are weighty enough to substantially compromise the expected lifetime well-being for individuals possessing a high degree of freedom to shape their lives as they wish, even under reasonably favorable conditions (education, etc.). (p. 227, emphasis in original)

Here the potentially pernicious social conditions that have driven all the ethicists over the ages to do their work come into play. An abundance of freedom and an abundance of choice, coupled with potential emotional ignorance, can set us up for failure in the pursuit of happiness. Haybron enumerates the scope of choices we might make: career, life partner, having children, how to raise children, balancing work and relationships, choice of friends, use of leisure time, choice of hobbies, where to live, managing finances, what education to attain, and what talents to develop, just to mention the more obvious ones. I would add the abundance of substances we can ingest, including food and medications. To reiterate, one bad mistake or a series of bad judgments can seriously compromise, ruin, or end your life.

I think Haybron has made a substantial contribution by synthesizing a number of recurring themes in the history of ethics, rehabilitating the concept of happiness in the process. He has drawn our attention to some of the ways that the pursuit of happiness can go wrong, leading to problems in living that can contribute to psychiatric disorders, the common route to a psychotherapist's office. And he provides a remarkably succinct and coherent framework for thinking about what a psychotherapist would need to consider, not only to help patients find their way out of illness but also to help them become well (Keyes 2014). To bring to mind Aristotle's archery metaphor, if we are to achieve our aim, we must have a target (Bartlett and Collins 2011). Haybron has given us a target, albeit not a smiley face that could be drawn on a big sheet of paper.

Positive Psychology

Martin Seligman (2011), who had been well known for his pioneering work on learned helplessness as the basis of depression, took a 180-degree turn:

> I have spent most of my life working on psychology's venerable goal of relieving misery and uprooting the disabling conditions of life. Truth be told, this can be a drag. Taking the psychology of misery to heart—as you must when you work on depression, alcoholism, schizophrenia, trauma, and the panoply of suffering that makes up psychology-as-usual's primary material—can be a vexation to the soul…. If anything changes in the practitioner, it is a personality shift toward depression. (p. 1)

Yet positive psychology represents far more than an emotional preference for the light over the dark. Seligman's widely embraced movement has made a significant contribution to addressing the problems Keyes (2014) identified, with an exclusive focus on illness to the neglect of health: "the absence of ill-being does not equal the presence of well-being" (Seligman 2018, p. 5). Relieving suffering is insufficient: "While not much of a therapist, I sometimes did good work, and in those cases, my patients' negative emotions were normal by termination. Did I get a happy patient? No, I got an empty patient"—not ill, but languishing (p. 206). Positive psychology provides an impetus and some methods for a more balanced psychotherapeutic approach.

Seligman (2011) turned to ethical thought as a guide for promoting health. In line with Appiah and Haybron, he proposed that "psychology could be explicitly about building the *good life*" (Seligman 2018, p. 5, emphasis added), and he proposed that "the goal of positive psychology is to increase flourishing" (Seligman 2011, p. 13). Eschewing the equation of happiness with cheerful feelings, he reframed his thinking as well-being theory, emphasizing eengagement, achievement, and finding meaning in something larger than oneself. He referred to the words of a colleague: "When asked what, in two words or fewer, positive psychology is about, Christopher Peterson, one of its founders, replied, 'Other people'" (p. 20). Seligman's work is particularly pertinent to psychotherapy for its methods designed to actively promote flourishing. Positive psychology employs various self-assessments to guide activities geared to promoting the individual's well-being according to his or her values and strengths. Seligman and his colleagues have developed interventions to enhance well-being and implemented them in diverse settings, including general medical populations, schools, and the military (Seligman 2018).

Philosopher Michael Bishop (2015) criticized positive psychology for proposing lists of contributors to well-being without an organizing theory. Bishop advocated an empirical approach that would study how various contributors to well-being (on positive psychology's list) are related to each other dynamically in networks of connections. From a clinical-developmental perspective, I find Bishop's approach appealing because I aim to identify *cascades* of events and experiences. I am all too familiar with cascades of adversity. For example, early traumatic events, self-destructive behavior, abusive relationships in adulthood, turning to substance abuse as a way of coping, insomnia resulting in an inability to concentrate, profound depression, and loss of livelihood might all end up with a person feeling alone and suicidal. Bishop envisioned positive cascades: for example, extroversion and optimism contribute to social support; social support and hard work contribute to academic success; this success eventuates in occupational attainment and job satisfaction; in turn, this history of positive relationships and success contributes to the development of an enduring relationship, which also stabilizes occupational functioning. Good works are an end result.

My reservations about positive psychology concern not its substance but rather the misguided attitude with which it might be implemented by inexperienced enthusiasts. My concern comes from conducting psychoeducational groups with patients suffering from residual depression associated with childhood trauma. When I enumerated various ways in which they could improve their mood, patients objected that these strategies did not work. They were too depressed to use them. They tuned me out. I learned to start these discussions with what I called the *catch-22s of depression* (Allen 2006): All the things you need to do to recover from depression are made difficult by the symptoms of depression. For example, you should get sufficient sleep, but you suffer from insomnia; you should socialize, but you are withdrawn; you should exercise, but you are fatigued; and you should engage in enjoyable activities, but you lack the capacity for pleasure. When I began with the catch-22s, the patients listened. When patients are in the process of recovery, pep talks and cheerleading will not do; we start with negative psychology. As the research on health and flourishing attests, however, we should not end there.

Mastering the Craft of Psychotherapy

Earlier in this chapter I summarized research showing substantial differences among therapists in treatment outcomes. Moreover, differences among therapists are greater than differences among types of treatments. Knowing about *therapist effects* requires that we turn our attention to *effective therapists*. Accordingly, Castonguay and Hill (2017a) titled their book *How and Why Are Some Therapists Better than Others?* The most prominent research on psychotherapy over the past half-century could be presented under the same title if "Treatments" were substituted for "Therapists." That volume could conclude with a disappointing chapter on the dodo bird verdict, along with the recommendation that the field should have been paying much more attention to therapists.

Here we are squarely in the territory of what constitutes conscientious therapy and what makes us therapists trustworthy providers of treatment. To me, many of the research findings I present in this section are disconcerting if not downright discouraging. Surely, they couldn't apply to me! I am reminded of extensive experience on oral examination committees for graduate students who were defending their master's and Ph.D. theses. All too often, when their results had failed to confirm their cherished hypotheses, they criticized their research methods and held on to their prior beliefs. They ignored the data. True, science advances by self-criticism. Personal knowledge also increases by self-criticism. To be trustworthy, we psychotherapists should not take our trustworthiness for granted. Taking research seriously will help therapists develop reasonable self-trust, relationship by relationship.

Art and Craft

This is the place to amplify a distinction I introduced in the "Introduction." I was invited in 2004 to give a lecture on psychotherapy at Smith College, during which I protested the attempted takeover of psychotherapy by science. At the end of the lecture, a psychologist in the audience, Laurie Pearlman, challenged my protest by pointing out that my lecture was based on findings from science. Afterward, Gerry Schamess, the editor of the college's social work journal, invited me to submit a manuscript based on the lecture, which I titled "Psychotherapy: The Artful Use of Science" (Allen 2008). Subsequently, I came across a different way of thinking, proposed by Jeremy Holmes (2010), who began, "Psychotherapists enjoy debating whether…their discipline is an art or a science." (Apparently, I had been debating myself.) To reiterate, Holmes had a better idea about psychotherapy: "It is perhaps better seen as a *craft*…drawing on both art and science but distinguishable from both" (p. x, emphasis added).

Holmes elaborated several characteristics of crafts: they cannot be learned from books; they require apprenticeship; they are comparatively noncompetitive; and their practitioners form communities or guilds stipulating rites of passage. No doubt, there is art in craft, and psychotherapy should be guided by science but not dominated by it. As I stated initially, I find the word *craft* especially appealing inasmuch as *I consider mastering a craft to be the work of a lifetime.* Now, more than 50 years after I saw my first patient, I would say confidently that I never felt that I had mastered the practice of psychotherapy.

But I think that mastering the craft is the right aspiration, and that aspiration focuses our gaze on the *personal and professional development of the therapist*. I am partial to the psychotherapy integration effort because I think it captures what naturally should be a developmental progression. We might think of *trustworthiness as the most integrative aim of our development as therapists*. We might view becoming locked into a narrow treatment approach as a developmental arrest.

In thinking about how therapists might go about mastering the craft of psychotherapy, we need a criterion for gauging progress. How can therapists improve without knowing if they are improving? The criterion of choice throughout the prior discussion has been treatment outcomes. Research on common factors and individualizing treatment as well as identifying differences among therapists in effectiveness has employed outcomes assessments. As described next, employing such assessments throughout the course of treatment along with providing ongoing feedback to therapists and patients has been shown to improve treatment outcomes. In this context, we might think of therapists' reasonable self-trust as being informed by data.

Outcomes Assessment and Feedback

A number of methods for assessing treatment outcomes have been adapted to track progress on a session-by-session basis and to provide immediate feedback to therapists and patients. Some of these assessments also include patients' perceptions of the therapeutic alliance. Clinicians should be aware that structured questionnaires have been developed for patients to provide feedback to therapists about important events in the session: what was helpful, what they did not like, what they are learning, what actions they are taking, what they want to work on, and so forth (McLeod 2017). But research has focused on quantitative assessments that lend themselves to computerized administration (Chapman et al. 2017; Lambert et al. 2019).

Extensive research shows that feedback over the course of therapy improves treatment outcomes, especially by identifying patients who are at risk for deteriorating in treatment. This finding is extremely important because deterioration in therapy is a significant problem, representing 5%–10% of patient populations (Lambert et al 2019). Moreover, compared with objective assessments, therapists are overly optimistic about patients' progress and notoriously poor at detecting patients who are worsening in therapy (Chapman et al. 2017; Lambert et al. 2019). For such patients, the objective data provide an opportunity for much-needed correction. Of course, the value of the feedback process hinges on its implementation. The major problem is clinicians' reluctance to employ outcomes assessments. Yet it is also problematic when the measures are used perfunctorily, for example, not discussed with patients or not employed to guide the therapy (Maeschalck et al. 2019).

Professional Experience

Is accumulating experience a solid basis for therapists' self-trust! The contribu
tion of therapists' experience to their clinical effectiveness has been a topic of
long-standing research interest. Simon Goldberg and colleagues' (2016) review
of the literature showed somewhat mixed results. Older studies suggested a
moderate positive relationship between experience and effectiveness (i.e., fewer
dropouts and better outcomes). More recent studies, however, have yielded a
more disconcerting finding: they have "generally failed to detect superior outcomes for more experienced clinicians relative to trainees or less experienced
therapists" (p. 2). As the authors noted, all this prior research has been cross-
sectional, comparing groups of more versus less experienced therapists, often
indexed by years since degree. Such studies do not control for such factors as
predegree experience or number of patients seen annually. Preferable would be
a longitudinal design in which therapists could be followed individually over
time, comparing their effectiveness at an earlier point with their later effectiveness. Such a study could directly reveal a developmental progression.

The authors used a longitudinal design to investigate changes in a large set
of psychotherapists' effectiveness over the course of their practice at a university
counseling center (Goldberg et al. 2016). The data, obtained over an 18-year period, included 170 therapists, 6,591 patients, and more than 50,000 sessions.
The results showed an overall *decline* in effectiveness over time (i.e., more clinical experience was associated with poorer outcomes), although greater experience was associated with fewer dropouts. Yet these differences were very slight;
for all practical purposes, there was a minimal relation between experience and
effectiveness. Notably, there were individual differences among therapists:
about 60% showed a decline with experience, whereas about 40% showed improvement. But all these differences were modest in extent.

Goldberg and colleagues (2016) acknowledged several limitations in their
study. All the patients were college students and did not show serious mental illness, for which therapists' experience could play a greater role in effectiveness.
Moreover, the authors studied only the *quantity* of experience (duration of
practice and number of patients seen) and not the *quality* or type of experience.
Perhaps most important from a developmental perspective, the duration of experience between measurements was relatively modest. Before the first assessment, the therapists had an average of 5.15 years of experience since beginning
graduate school. Although the range of experience at the counseling center in
the group of therapists was substantial (from about a half-year to 18 years), the
average level of acquired experience across the study was less than 5 years (and
the median was only about 2.5 years). From my vantage point, that is a drop in
the bucket.

Shifting from the experience of individual therapists to the profession as a
whole, we might wonder about the extent of improvement in psychotherapy
outcomes across time. Is the field of psychotherapy mastering its craft?

Wampold's analyses of decades of meta-analyses showed that the size of treatment effects has been remarkably consistent across time (Wampold and Imel 2015). As Scott Miller and colleagues (2017) summarized, "for close to four decades the outcome of psychotherapy has remained flat" (p. 23). This finding implies that, as a group, we have not improved with experience, despite having developed hundreds of new treatments over recent decades. Remember, however, that this averaging process—homogenizing fruit salads into smoothies—could obscure improvements in the treatment outcomes for some disorders associated with specialized approaches.

Limitations notwithstanding, this research on professional experience should give us therapists pause. Not only have we not mastered the provision of psychotherapy; we are not even on a common developmental course of mastering it—individually or collectively. To be hard-nosed about it (which I rarely am), if we therapists want to believe that our experience practicing psychotherapy has made us more effective, we are relying on faith. I have no objection to faith, but I think the most serious problem lies with the profoundly vague term *experience*. Continuing to conduct mediocre therapy in the same way for several decades will not be of great help. Apparently, we need a different kind of experience. We need to consider this question: what kinds of experience will contribute to developing greater effectiveness over time?

Supervision, Consultation, and Continuing Education

In principle, the course of professional development should be facilitated by supervision, consultation, and continuing education. As Rodney Goodyear and colleagues (Goodyear and Rousmaniere 2017) distinguish the first two of these practices, therapists require *supervision* in their training to be competent for professional licensure, such that the supervisor serves an evaluative and gatekeeping function, whereas qualified therapists seek *consultation* voluntarily to enhance their effectiveness and expertise. Jennifer Taylor and Greg Neimeyer include consultation and *continuing education* as forms of continuing professional development in the service of lifelong learning, defined as "an active, continuous quest for knowledge, growth, and development" (Taylor and Neimeyer 2017, p. 219). Are these methods of promoting professional development demonstrably effective? Are they a sufficient basis for patients' trust and therapists' self-trust?

Gauged by the criterion of improving treatment outcomes, the research literature on the effectiveness of routine supervision is not encouraging, and evidence is lacking that supervisors' level of experience or professional qualifications make a difference (Goodyear and Rousmaniere 2017; Miller et al. 2017). This finding, however, must be considered in light of the fact that supervision commonly relies on unstructured discussion of cases, the value of which depends on supervisees' memory as well as their willingness to disclose problems in the context of being evaluated. As in psychotherapy, the willingness to disclose will be contingent on the quality of the supervisory relationship and the supervisory alliance. To compensate for these problems, reviewers advocate the use of audio and video recordings as well as live supervision.

Although the success of supervision in facilitating professional development is the exception rather than the rule, some research has shown that supervision can be effective. For example, using supervisees' outcomes assessments in supervision has been shown to improve treatment outcomes (Reese et al. 2009). Mark Hilsenroth and Marc Diener developed a model of supervision with the aim of fostering skill in the practice of manual-guided psychodynamic psychotherapy (Hilsenroth and Diener 2017). They employed discussion of videos to foster the skilled use of interventions. Building on their prior research showing that psychodynamic interventions interact with the alliance to improve treatment outcomes (Owen and Hilsenroth 2011), they demonstrated that this theory-guided, systematic supervision enhanced the therapeutic alliance.

As Taylor and Neimeyer (2017) reviewed, the history of continuing education in psychology dates back to the 1940s but began to be widely mandated only in the 1990s. Assessment of the effectiveness of continuing education generally is limited to reports of participant satisfaction; no research shows a relation between satisfaction with continuing education events and improvements in clinical practice. Moreover, "The majority of [continuing education] programs are offered as didactic seminars...even though research indicates that passive learning from didactic presentation does not facilitate long-term learning and registers minimal impact on skill acquisition or client outcomes" (p. 225). Consistent with didactic methods, the authors point out critically that continuing education is "geared toward *knowledge* retention rather than *skill* acquisition" (p. 230, emphasis in original). With McGilchrist (2019) in mind, we might say that knowledge acquired by the left hemisphere (e.g., from the book you are now reading) will be of little value if not put to use by the right hemisphere in living your life.

Where does this leave us psychotherapists who have invested so much in training and continued learning? Miller and colleagues (2017) offered this appraisal:

> When it comes to professional development, two facts are apparent. The first, to the credit of practicing psychotherapists worldwide, is that they want to get better at what they do. This is not only a shared goal; it is a core value. The second is that the traditions and practices informing and comprising professional development do not work. When it comes to improving outcomes, the time, money, and effort expended—even mandated by licensing and certification bodies—are largely wasted. The overall effectiveness of psychotherapy has remained stagnant, and the results of individual clinicians do not improve with time, training, and experience. (pp. 35–36)

We should be grateful for decades of research demonstrating that psychotherapy is effective. But we should not be complacent about improving our work with traditional methods of continuing professional development, much less with the mere accumulation of time in the saddle. We can derive some hope from one agency-wide model of clinical consultation that was integrated with routine outcomes assessments and feedback.

Goldberg and colleagues (2017) conducted an ambitious and instructive study of ways to improve psychotherapists' performance in a community mental health center and training clinic in Calgary, Alberta, Canada. Throughout the project, therapists were assured that their data would not be used in individual performance evaluations. In the 2-year pilot phase, the researchers collected data on two measurement systems to determine the feasibility of data collection. They used objective measures to assess patients' functioning and the therapeutic alliance. Both measures were employed on an agency-wide basis in each session. For the first 4 years, the data were used solely to provide annual statistical reports on outcomes for the agency's purposes.

Although the procedures had been integrated into the agency infrastructure, it became apparent after 4 years that data were being collected for only 40% of the clients (Goldberg et al. 2017). Many therapists objected to the procedure, for example, because of the extra paperwork involved and their assumption that clients would not like to complete the measures and because they already had clinical feedback about the progress of therapy. The agency then stated the policy that therapists could not opt out and would be held accountable for integrating the assessment into their practice. After this new policy was announced, 40% of the therapists resigned. When therapists were hired to replace those who had left, they were informed about the agency culture of feedback.

Along with this agencywide mandate, two monthly consultation groups were implemented, one for students and the other for staff members. These groups were led by an outside consultant, and therapists presented outcome graphs along with their clinical material. After 8 months, the administrators learned that some therapists were presenting only cases that were going well, and they implemented a new policy that therapists must present cases that were not going well according to the outcomes data (Goldberg et al. 2017). Four more staff members resigned (which was relatively few, compared with the previous exodus). The consultation groups then focused systematically on problematic cases. From these group discussions, the therapists developed an understanding of common problems and ways of addressing them. In addition, every 4 months, all of the therapists were provided with summaries of their individually aggregated outcomes data (i.e., number of clients seen, average number of sessions, average outcomes scores at admission and termination, and average extent of improvement). They also were given the agencywide data for the same period so that they could compare their individual outcomes with those for the psychotherapist group as a whole.

This project is especially worthy of attention because it runs counter to the general findings that individual therapists' extent of experience as well as the experience of the field in general (over four decades) are not associated with improved outcomes. As the authors summarized their findings, in this agency, the outcomes were improving from year to year: "clients who came to the [clinic] in 2014 would be predicted to have larger gains over the course of treatment than those who came in 2010." Moreover, "therapists *were* getting better over time…a client seen by a given therapist in the therapist's fifth year at the agency would be expected to show larger drops in reported symptoms over the course of therapy than a client seen by that same therapist in the therapist's first year at the agency" (Goldberg et al. 2017, p. 208, emphasis in original). Contrary to Goldberg and colleagues' earlier study, this project demonstrated that "Therapists *can* improve over time" (Goldberg et al. 2017, p. 209, emphasis in original). This improvement, however, was contingent on a monumental (and costly) agency-wide culture shift that included three key features: 1) detailed and synthesized feedback, 2) a focus on patients who were not doing well in treatment, and 3) an opportunity to learn from peers and a consultant about ways of intervening. With clinical outcomes as a criterion, I view this as a deliberate effort to improve the agency's trustworthiness by means of changing individual clinicians' practice.

Deliberate Practice

A number of psychotherapists interested in professional development have taken cues from the literature on developing expert levels of skill in other domains, such as sports, musical performance, chess, and medicine. The key to improvement is deliberate practice—lots of it. As Miller and colleagues (2017) characterize it, such practice entails a lifelong deliberate effort to improve, which requires seeking out challenges that go beyond one's current abilities. Such practice typically is *not* enjoyable; it is effortful. As measured by treatment outcomes, the top 25% of therapists spend nearly three times more hours per week engaging in deliberate practice than do the bottom 75%. Miller and colleagues advocate a *cycle of excellence* that entails "(a) determining a baseline level of effectiveness; (b) obtaining systematic, ongoing, formal feedback; and (c) repeatedly engaging in activities specifically designed to refine and improve performance" (p. 30). Goldberg and colleagues' (2017) project meets these criteria.

Reviewing the literature on expertise, Franz Caspar (2017) characterized master therapists as voracious learners and asserted that "the best chance of optimally learning from experience exists when therapists have clear, explicit, theoretically driven, individual case conceptualizations serving as a basis for interpreting information emerging in the course of psychotherapy" (p. 208). However, *no single form of deliberate practice has been linked to effectiveness*; rather, a range of activities make a contribution. These include working on case formulations, attending training workshops, thinking about difficult cases, preparing and reflecting on sessions, reviewing recordings of sessions, role-playing, seeking consultation, and collaborating with colleagues in developing skills (Caspar 2017, Miller et al. 2017). More generally, this effort requires a supportive social context in a culture of excellence (as Goldberg and colleagues' mental health center project illustrates).

Compared with other domains of expertise, deliberate practice in psychotherapy is far less straightforward. Psychotherapy does not provide immediate feedback about the effectiveness of our actions. I know immediately (and often) when I hit a wrong note on the piano. In psychotherapy, our main objective criterion for effectiveness is treatment outcome as measured by improvement from admission to termination as well as status at termination (and followup)—delayed feedback indeed. Just as problematic is research reviewed throughout this chapter showing that no specific treatment methods or techniques uniquely relate to treatment outcomes. Skill can be measured by adherence to treatment manuals, but adherence is not enough. For example, a study of cognitive-behavioral therapy that involved 300 hours of intensive training, supervision, and practice found that adherence and competence were unrelated to outcome (Rounsaville et al. 2017). Accordingly, some authors have proposed that *flexibility* in adherence relates more highly to treatment outcomes than does strict adherence (Hilsenroth and Diener 2017).

In sum, we therapists know that we should practice—intentionally and deliberately—but there is no particular method or skill that can be prescribed for practice. We are back to an inherently individual developmental process. The skills we might practice will depend on the treatment methods we have chosen. Given the dodo bird verdict, outcome research cannot guide these choices. If we are to avoid professional developmental arrest, we need to follow a path of psychotherapy integration. Like our patients (when they are fortunate), we follow our treatment preferences. Perforce, we will practice some methods and techniques, more or less deliberately. We cannot take our trustworthiness for granted; we must work at it.

Here I must insert a crucial caveat: for many practitioners who are loaded up with clinical work on top of other personal responsibilities, time for deliberate practice is a luxury beyond reach. If we take Goldberg's work (Goldberg et al. 2017) as a model, a high level of institutional support is required. I have been fortunate to have plenty of it (along with family forbearance).

Interpersonal Skill

If we are to judge from the psychotherapy research literature reviewed early in this chapter, interpersonal skills are more important than any particular technical skills because interpersonal skills influence the effectiveness of any particular methods we might practice. For example, Caspar (2017) summarized research showing that "the ability to communicate in an unambiguous and clear way, empathy, respectful warm contact, the ability to deal with criticism, the ability to cooperate, and interpersonal competence were correlated with fewer

dropouts and better outcomes for patients" (p. 203). Similarly, enumerating fa-
cilitative interpersonal skills, Wampold (2017) listed emotional expression,
persuasiveness, hopefulness, warmth, empathy, alliance-bond capacity, and
problem focus. He also noted the importance of verbal fluency: plainly, communicating clearly and succinctly plays a pervasive role in our talk therapies,
and fluency is "critical for providing a believable, succinct, and adaptive explanation and a cogent rationale for the therapeutic actions" (p. 57). Interpersonal
skill plays a major role in the development of a therapeutic alliance and in repair
of ruptures. William Stiles and Adam Horvath asserted, "A strong alliance is *not
a technique but an achievement,* one that requires doing the right thing over a
period of time" (Stiles and Horvath 2017, p. 78, emphasis added). Interpersonal
skill plays a crucial role in this achievement.

There is an intriguing finding that I believe to be associated with the quality
of the therapeutic relationship. Psychotherapists' reports of *professional self-
doubt* (i.e., doubts about their effectiveness) are associated with *better* therapeutic alliances (Nissen-Lie et al. 2010) and treatment outcomes (Nissen-Lie et al.
2015). As Wampold (2017) understood it, such self-doubt is an indication of re-
flectiveness about one's work. I interpret self-doubt as an indication of humility,
which, to me, is utterly realistic in light of limitations in our knowledge and
skill. Self-doubting therapists apparently have not succumbed to the more common tendency to overestimate their effectiveness (Boswell et al. 2017). They are
self-critical, a basis for trustworthiness. Accordingly, self-doubt likely contributes to greater awareness of problems and mistakes along with motivation to
improve.

Last, we should not neglect the role of self-care in therapists' competence
and trustworthiness (Taylor and Neimeyer 2017). Practicing psychotherapy is
stressful, and it is associated with high rates of burnout, depression, relationship
problems, substance abuse, and suicide. Working for many years in an inpatient
program tailored to professionals in crisis, I saw these problems firsthand in mental health professionals. I particularly enjoyed working with psychologists, but I
was continually struck by their failure to practice what they were preaching, often
in the context of overwork. Ideally, we therapists would be free of illness and high
on the continuum of health—flourishing. Ideally. We need to apply our interpersonal skill to our own personal development and well-being, not least to developing and maintaining stable and supportive relationships that can sustain us in this
demanding work. Practicing what we preach, we should be open to receiving psychotherapy as well as offering it, knowing of its effectiveness.

In the context of treating trauma in attachment relationships, I proposed
that our paramount competence is *skill in being human* (Allen 2013c), the essence of which is our uniquely human capacity for social connection and cooperation. Taking seriously the role of personal knowledge in conducting
psychotherapy—including our implicit (nonverbal) capacity for relating—I
would argue that our developmental trajectory as psychotherapists begins in infancy. Apart from the most highly manualized, technical approaches to symptom reduction, our acquisition of professional knowledge and specialized skills

is of limited value without skill in being human. Mastering that skill is the work of a lifetime, and we will fall short to varying degrees. We best develop the skill of being human in the context of trusting and trustworthy relationships starting early in life.

Summary of Key Points

- Therapists, patients, and students recognize the importance of trust in psychotherapy, but comprehensive thinking about trust is rare in the therapy literature.

- Attention to patients' distrust overshadows what should be the foundation for their trust: therapists' trustworthiness.

- The continuing development of hundreds of brands of therapy runs counter to the long-standing research finding that the quality of the patient-therapist relationship contributes more to the treatment outcome than do the theoretical approach or specific methods employed.

- Psychotherapy is best adapted to more than patients' psychiatric disorders and symptoms, including cultural differences (e.g., race, ethnicity, religion); sexual orientation and gender identity; readiness for change; and treatment preferences.

- Differences among therapists contribute more to treatment outcomes than do differences among treatment methods, such that we should pay less attention to the development of methods and more attention to the development of therapists.

- Conducting therapy requires personal knowledge along with professional knowledge, and personal knowledge includes knowledge of ethics, which is essential to going beyond alleviating illness to promoting health.

- Psychotherapy is best considered a craft, and mastery of a craft is the work of a lifetime. We might think of trustworthiness as the overarching aim of mastering the craft of psychotherapy.

Recommendations for Clinical Practice

- In advocating a shift in attention from patients' problems with trust to your trustworthiness as a therapist, I am recommending that you dislodge yourself from the psychotherapy profession's obsession with perfecting evidence-based treatments for specific disorders. Conscientious practice requires that we therapists be knowledgeable about research but not oppressed by it. As in general medicine, specialization plays a crucial role in developing treatments and generating knowledge that informs generalists. Every therapy requires a treatment and techniques. But the decades-long conflict between researchers and clinicians has been corrosive. The effectiveness of all approaches to psychotherapy hinges on trust and trustworthiness, and the personal qualities of the therapist, including his or her broad personal knowledge, will come first. Specialists are liable to run aground with an exclusive focus on techniques, as I discovered with my first client.

- All therapists must learn theories, treatments, and techniques; however, I recommend prioritizing relationships. Psychotherapy is an interpersonal problem-solving process in which the personal relationship is in the background or foreground to varying degrees. When your relationship with your patient is in the background, as it might be in specialized, symptom-oriented treatments, it is no less important than when it becomes the focus of treatment. Trustworthy psychotherapy of any stripe requires knowledge of the decades-long research on the overriding contribution of common factors that put a premium on the therapist's interpersonal skill, which will provide the foundation for trust. Alongside the plenitude of research on hundreds of therapy brands, we psychotherapists are indebted to Carl Rogers for identifying empathy, positive regard, and genuineness as cornerstones of therapeutic relationships. We are equally indebted to legions of researchers who have studied the therapeutic alliance, the exemplification of a cooperative relationship on which all trust hinges. From decades of experience working with hospitalized patients suffering from serious mental illness, I am convinced that establishing and maintaining empathy, positive regard, and genuineness—along with a therapeutic alliance that requires them—often is a hard-won achievement. Research on short-term therapies can be misleading in implying that you should quickly establish a good therapeutic relationship such that the treatment can proceed smoothly to a successful conclusion. This means-end thinking is simplistic. Relationship problems contribute substantially to the development of serious mental illness, and illness plays a significant role in relationship problems, including the psychotherapy relationship. In this context, creating a trusting therapeutic relationship comprises much of the work of the therapy, and this creation will be one of its main potential benefits.

- Psychotherapy compels a focus on illness, and more than a century of psychiatry has generated a huge body of pertinent knowledge. You need to start with ameliorating illness, but I recommend that you not stop there. We must have a vision of a healthy life, not only for its own sake but also to prevent recurrence of illness. Every therapist will have an intuitive vision of a good life, developed from his or her personal history and cultural background. I believe that we therapists should reflect on our vision and its associated values. Our values shape our practice, and we should encourage our patients to articulate their values—at the very least, to illuminate and explicate differences in values that could hinder treatment. When we aim to persuade, we should do it consciously and acknowledge our intention. I have said things such has "Now I am campaigning for you to appreciate your kindness more and to direct some of it toward yourself."

- As I explicate in the rest of this book, I am recommending that we rethink the problem of trusting in psychotherapy, expanding our view from patients' distrust to the challenges of becoming trustworthy to them. I consider becoming trustworthy in therapy as a patient-by-patient aspiration and, more broadly, as a lifelong project. In a workshop I was conducting about trusting in psychotherapy, a young man just starting out his career anxiously expressed how daunted he was by how much he had to learn and his uncertainty about how to proceed. I sympathized and told him that I hope he continues to feel that way throughout his career. Profound satisfaction is on offer from time to time, but contentment is elusive. Complacency is a sign of trouble: stagnation. We all must keep working at trustworthiness. If you are reading this book, I am now preaching to the choir.

2

Developing Trust and Trustworthiness

I think a developmental perspective best points us to the heart of trust. In this chapter, I place considerable emphasis on early development; however, developmental thinking is apposite to the entire lifetime, and I will be making some links between the early developmental foundations of trust and its continuing development in adulthood. From this perspective, adult psychotherapy provides developmental help.

I start by entering into some technical philosophical territory with the concept of intentionality to set the stage for getting to the essence of trust as it comes to life in social-cognitive and moral development from ages 0 to 6 years. Then I review attachment theory and research as the broader relational context for trust and distrust as they develop throughout life. I introduce Peter Fonagy's pioneering work on mentalizing, which has greatly enriched our understanding of the development of attachments and the nature of trauma in attachment relationships—the bane of trusting. Having embraced mentalizing, I conclude with a disconcerting cultural critique of attachment theory that usefully expands our thinking about trust.

The Intentional Stance

Philosopher Daniel Dennett (1987) mused, "how could anything be more familiar, and at the same time more weird, than a mind?" (p. 2). To understand trust and trustworthiness, we need to understand something even more weird: the *meeting of minds*. Moreover, individual minds develop by means of the meeting of minds. This development requires trustworthiness, and there it can go awry.

Intentionality is the truly weird thing about the mind, if you really think about it. As philosopher John Searle (2010) characterized it, "'Intentionality' is a fancy philosopher's term for that capacity of the mind by which it is directed at, or about, objects and states of affairs in the world, typically independent of itself." He continued, "Intentional states are always *about*, or *refer to*, something" (p. 25, emphasis in original). Mental states *represent* some aspect of the world, not only the outer world (a flower) but also the inner, mental world (a feeling). Thus, the mind can represent itself and the workings of other minds. This quality of being about something external to itself, engaging and relating to something outside itself (including the results of its own mental work!) is quite a trick for "bags of particles," as physicist Brian Greene (2020, p. 237) characterizes us humans. A material object such as a stone cannot be *about* anything; it just *is*. A stone cannot relate to anything else except in *our* intentional minds, where it might be seen as a part of a cairn or stone wall—or, for those who are adept with the intentional stance, an assemblage of stones can be seen to symbolize trust, as in the image on the cover of this book. We bags of particles are *aware* of the world and our parts in it. We see, remember, believe, desire, fear, love, and hate. Ideally, we hope for something and trust someone. Searle also explained that, as part of our intentionality, we can *intend* to do something before we do it and while we are doing it. As we shall see, our full intentionality is a complex developmental achievement.

Dennett (1987) distinguished three stances we can take toward the world in our efforts to understand and predict what will happen in it. We use the *physical stance* to predict the behavior of material objects, including collections of particles. We use the *design stance* to predict the behavior of our technological creations, such as clocks, computers, and cars. We also can use the design stance to understand and predict the behavior of biological phenomena on the basis of their functions (as if designed by evolution)—eyes, hearts, neurons, leaves, and such. Dearest to our psychotherapeutic hearts, however, is the *intentional stance*:

> First you decide to treat the object whose behavior is to be predicted as a rational agent; then you figure out what *beliefs* that agent ought to have, given its place in the world and its purpose. Then you figure out what *desires* it ought to have, on the same considerations, and finally *you predict that this rational agent will act to further its goals in light of its beliefs*. (p. 17, emphasis added)

As Dennett (2017) presents it, the intentional stance we all use to understand ourselves and each other is idealized in an *as if mode*; using only a sketch of what might be in one another's mind, we treat each other as if we are "rational agents guided by *largely* true beliefs and *largely* well-ordered desires" (p. 379, emphasis added). This strategy works insofar as "our expectations are very frequently confirmed, which cements our allegiance to the intentional stance." Here is the critical bit: "when our expectations are confounded, we tend to fall back on 'explanations' of our failure that are at best inspired guesswork and at worst misleading mythology" (p. 380). Now we are in the messy territory of psychotherapy, where we therapists and our patients are liable to find ourselves engaged in inspired guesswork and at risk of creating misleading mythology—especially when striving to reconstruct the distant past, an effort that calls for epistemic humility (Allen 1995).

In the subsection "Attachment Patterns in Infancy and Beyond," I emphasize how human beings learn patterns of relating to our caregivers before we can think and talk; moreover, we can continue using these patterns uncomprehendingly long after we learn to think and talk. However, as we develop greater competence with the intentional stance, we gradually learn in these relationships to comprehend more about our own and others' actions. Then, as Dennett indicated, we learn to tell increasingly elaborate stories about our own and others' actions, often in the context of explaining and justifying these actions to each other and ourselves (Mercier and Sperber 2017). When the need for specialized help arises, patients tell their stories to psychotherapists, and psychotherapists respond with their own stories about the patients' stories. As Jeremy Holmes (1999) astutely observed, psychotherapy goes in cycles of story making and story breaking. We need to create trustworthy stories.

Elasticity in the Intentional Stance

There is something marvelous about the intentional stance that you might not appreciate from what I have said so far: its *elasticity*. We are concerned here with the intentional stance in the way we relate to each other. But we human beings apply the concept far more widely. We apply it to unconscious mental processes—desires, emotions, and motives. We have no trouble applying the intentional stance to many of our fellow mammals—dogs, cats, and horses, to name a few. Ignoring the naysayers, many of us intuitively relate to our domesticated mammalian kin as emotional beings with feelings much like our own (de Waal 2019). And we make far grander extensions. Darwin wrote of evolution: "natural selection is daily and hourly *scrutinizing*, throughout the world, every variation, even the slightest; *rejecting* that which is bad preserving and adding up all that is good; silently and insensibly *working*, whenever and wherever opportunity offers" (cited by Walsh 2015, p. 45, emphasis added). Persons who hold theistic religious beliefs use the intentional stance in developing a relationship with God or a higher power (Allen 2013a; Grandqvist and Kirkpatrick 2013). Yet we can go farther afield, understanding much of the behavior of living agents as being rationally and competently goal directed, in the absence of comprehension. Taking off from the idea that "some species of plants can warn nearby kin of impending predation by wafting distress signals downwind when attacked" (p. 84), Dennett (2017) gives us much license with the intentional stance:

> We are anthropomorphizing the plants and bacteria in order to understand them. This is not an intellectual sin. We are *right* to call their actions behaviors, to attribute these competences to the organisms, to explain their existence by citing the rationales that account for the benefits derived from these competences by the organisms in their 'struggle' for survival. We are right, I am saying, to adopt what I call the intentional stance. The only mistake lies in attributing comprehension to the organism or to its parts. In the case of plants and microbes, fortunately, common sense intervenes to block that attribution. It is easy enough to understand how their competence can be provided by the machinery without any *mentality* intruding at all. (p. 85, emphasis in original)

From what Dennett wrote, I doubt that he talks to his plants. But I can sympathize with an inclination to do so that is rooted in *our* appreciation for their competence and beauty, uncomprehending and unappreciative of themselves as *they* may be.

Minds Need Other Minds

One of the weird things about the mind that we have come to understand from developmental psychology is this: We could not develop a mind on our own. Intuitively, it seems that we must have developed our mind and then realized that others also have a mind like ours, but the reverse is true: as infants, we develop our mind from the outside in, that is, from our caregivers relating to us as minded beings. Using the intentional stance, caregivers also attribute the intentional stance to infants. Our thinking develops through internalizing dialogue (Vygotsky 1978): we speak before we think.

We need other minds not only to create our mind; we continue to need other minds throughout life to maintain and develop our mind. Thinking is no substitute for ongoing dialogue. I do not think we are very good at figuring out our minds by ourselves. To put it baldly, we need other minds to stay sane and anchored in reality, but other minds also can undermine our sanity. We can be subjected to continual misinterpretation, gaslighting, and psychological abuse—at worst, as children, when we are most reliant on other minds for our developing sense of self and relationships.

When development goes seriously awry, a psychotherapist's mind can be required. We need to break up and revise our confusing and pernicious stories, creating stories that are authentically felt as well as being reasonably coherent and accurate. We can best do this story-making through dialogue. The human mind is a social creation, and we need other trustworthy minds to stay anchored in social reality. We are liable to go crazy in solitary confinement. Profound distrust or lack of access to trustworthy confidants can put us in a situation akin to solitary confinement. Short of this extreme, the social isolation imposed by the novel coronavirus pandemic beginning in 2020 has seriously jeopardized mental health. Accordingly, as I describe at more length later in the subsection "Attachment Trauma," I have thought of trauma not simply as resulting from being in emotional pain but rather feeling *alone or invisible* in that pain. We need to care for our intentionality and be mindful of objectifying ourselves and each other. Objectification is my beef with scientism in psychotherapy.

Subjectivity and Personhood

I think it is worth our while to fully appreciate this "fancy philosophers' term," intentionality, for its role in our subjectivity, which we should take as precious in ourselves and others. As the extent of interpersonal trauma attests, *we can and do treat others as objects.* To adopt the physical stance: we *are* physical objects, bags of particles that take the form of human bodies. As bodies, we can be shoved, beaten, raped, and shot. We can be cradled, carried, and healed with medicine, acupuncture, and surgery. Yet, as intentional beings, we are *subjects*, each with a unique and continually changing perspective and experience of being in the world. We subjects are extraordinary objects. In us, nature is not only conscious but also comprehending; through us, the natural world has become self-aware (Morris 2015).

In exalting the mind, as I have been doing here, we must be careful not to think of minds as depersonalized, ethereal inhabitants of the body that relate to other ethereal inhabitants of bodies. We are not minds relating to minds or mental states relating to mental states. We are embodied subjects, thoroughly embedded in the world, engaged in a social life that constitutes our personhood. Without a physical world that includes other persons, subjectivity is inconceivable. Of course, our mental states are in the foreground and are profoundly important when we relate to each other, but mental states are inextricable from the life in which they are embedded and the whole person who is leading the life. *We are persons making a life relating to other persons who are making a life*—ideally, making a *good* life for ourselves and others.

From You and I to We

In a series of books, Michael Tomasello (1999, 2014, 2016, 2019), a developmental psychologist and primatologist, articulated a comprehensive understanding of social-cognitive and moral development that I find extremely helpful in thinking about trust and trustworthiness. Tomasello's account suggests to me that we develop the fundamental *capacities* for trust by the age of 6–7 years. At that age, we have yet to acquire much knowledge about trusting relationships, but we have the basic cognitive-moral skills to acquire it. However, to contend that we have the capacities for trust does not mean that we use them consistently; developmental adversity can impinge on their use, as I discuss later in this chapter in the context of attachment relationships. To add precision to our grasp of uniquely human intentionality, Tomasello begins with evolution.

Evolutionary Perspective

With cooperation in mind, Tomasello distinguishes us humans from our nearest kin, chimpanzees and other primates. Like us, chimpanzees show *individual intentionality*: they are intensely social, and they relate to each other as intentional agents who perceive, remember, and engage in goal-directed actions. In relationships, chimpanzees are affectionate and sympathetic as well as crafty and competitive. Although they are ostensibly cooperative, compared with us humans, chimpanzees are relatively self-centered: "great ape collaborators are basically using their partners, in sophisticated ways, as *social tools*." In hunting, for example, they do not cooperate for mutual benefit; rather, "[t]hey act in parallel when their individual motives happen to coincide." They show a kind of *strategic trust*, "something like relying on the laws of nature," that is, "relying on the fact that the others will continue to pursue their own self-interest." In sum, chimpanzees "*view others mostly instrumentally*: as social obstacles in competition, or as social instruments in collaboration" (Tomasello 2019, p. 194, emphases added).

Reading about chimpanzees here, you might have noticed that we humans have not left that individualistic platform behind; having built much on top of it, we continue to use it—at worst, traumatizing others in so doing. But we have evolved a way of trusting and being trustworthy that hinges on our unique capacities for *shared intentionality*. Caregivers relate to infants as nascent persons from the start, a way of relating that is vital in children becoming persons who relate to other persons as such. But we also can treat others as objects.

I think trust is anchored fundamentally in our cooperativeness, which, in turn, is anchored in intentionality. As Tomasello (2016) notes, "human beings have evolved biologically to value others and to invest in their well-being" (p. 159). Accordingly, we humans are "*ultra*-cooperative" (Tomasello 2019, p. 189, emphasis added) on the basis of intentional capacities. Apes and other primates are sympathetic and cooperative to varying degrees. And we humans can treat each other as objects. Our mixed human proclivities in how we regard and treat each other account for my psychotherapeutic interest in trust. Consider the opposing perspectives in philosophy as Christine Korsgaard (1996) contrasted them: "The primal scene of morality, I will argue, is not one in which I do something to you or you do something to me, but one in which we do something together.

The subject matter of morality is not what we should bring about, but how we should relate to one another" (p. 275).

Turning to cultural evolution, beginning about 400,000 years ago by Tomasello's (2019) reckoning, as hunter-gatherers we became exceptionally cooperative in the context of obligate collective foraging. This development was propelled by ecological challenges: climate was variable, food was scarce, survival was chancy, and the rate of infant mortality was high. This was the context for the emergence of joint intentionality, requiring "collaborative activities…and a system of partner choice and control that made everyone accountable to everyone else for treating collaborative partners with the respect they deserved" (Tomasello 2016, p. 40). Tomasello put the choice starkly: "collaborate or else starve" (p. 63). This collaborative ecological context also called for communal sharing of food and resources, something that chimpanzees do only reluctantly and in limited fashion. We return to cultural contrasts in the discussion of attachment theory and research in the section "Cultural Diversity: How I Mistook Ethics for Science."

Sharing Intentionality

In the context of our ultra-cooperative capacities, here is Tomasello's (2019) passage that anchors my understanding of the developmental origins of trust: "Infants' motivation to align their emotional state with that of their caregiver represents the first instance of the most basic motivational force of shared intentionality: sharing or *aligning psychological states* with others" (p. 307, emphasis added). Making the connection between Tomasello's work and the development of trust, as I am inclined to do, will take a good bit of explaining. I think his phrase "aligning psychological states" is apt for the increasingly sophisticated, cognitive-moral developmental platform on which we build trust throughout life.

Tomasello distinguished three forms of alignment in a developmental progression. *Sharing emotions* in the first year of life sets the stage for two monumental social-cognitive transformations: *joint intentionality,* developing from ages 1 to 3 years, which pertains to dyadic interactions, one mind aligning with another, and in turn sets the stage for *collective intentionality*, consolidated from ages 3 to 6 years. Collective intentionality enables individuals to align with a group and thus to become embedded in a culture. Having developed the capacity for shared intentionality, children move from one world to another: they are inducted into joint intentionality primarily in the world of relationships with adults, and they are prepared for collective intentionality in the world of relationships with peers.

We should not think of these developments as three stages in the sense that each one is superseded by the next. Rather, these are cumulative developments wherein new capacities are added to preceding capacities, with each being a prerequisite for the next. Each level continues to play a crucial role in trusting and trustworthiness throughout life. In discussing each stage, I begin with social-cognitive development, then consider the corresponding moral development, and conclude with implications for trust.

Sharing Emotions

We can put emotional alignment on the ground floor of human relationships, including trusting relationships. As Tomasello (2019) understands it, we humans have an innate "drive toward emotional attunement" (p. 307) that constitutes "the emotional/motivational starting point for all uniquely human psychology" (p. 308) and provides the "underlying emotional substrate for shared intentionality" (p. 55).

Along with imitation, sharing emotion in the form of smiling and laughing promotes emotional bonding. Infants are sensitive to contingent responsiveness—not synchrony but rather caregivers' closely timed and appropriate responses to the infant's signals (Gergely and Watson 1996). Contingent responsiveness characterizes interactions with the physical world: the infant taps a mobile, and the mobile moves. Optimally, in the interpersonal world, contingent responsiveness takes place in the context of aligning psychological states: the infant smiles and the mother smiles. Such contingent responsiveness promotes the infant's sense of agency and self-efficacy, predicated on initiating action that makes something happen in the world. Central to our interest in trust, the infant's sense of agency takes the form of interpersonal influence in the social world. At this first stage of development, the infant exerts influence through emotion, with the extent of influence being contingent on the caregiver's emotional responsiveness: the infant whimpers and the mother soothes. The infant's coordinated turn-taking episodes with the caregiver (e.g., in peekaboo) can be construed as emotion-laden protoconversations. With the coordination of voice and movement, we could imagine the infant and caregiver singing (or perhaps humming wordlessly) and dancing together. Of course, the caregiver's emotional sensitivity also includes soothing responsiveness to the infant's distress, expressed in voice and movement.

For all their emotional coordination, there is a crucial asymmetry between the infant and the caregiver. The caregiver's fully developed intentionality is the foundation for the infant's induction into intentional relating. From the highly developed intentional stance as yet unavailable to the infant, the caregiver treats the infant as a person with needs, desires, feelings, and goals. For example, as Elizabeth Meins (1997) aptly put it, mothers engage in *mind-minded commentary* in their interactions with infants; for example, she might say something such as, "Ahh, you like that!" or "Ouch! That pinched." To continue the proto-conversation metaphor, from the infant's perspective—not understanding the mother's words—we might think of the mother as singing, with appropriate emotional responsiveness to the infant's cues.

Can we think of an incipient moral sense in the first year of life? Tomasello (2016) summarized research on infants' responsiveness to good and bad behavior, cleverly assessed by their attention and responsiveness to animations. For example, one animation showed a red ball seemingly trying to go up an incline. Then a yellow triangle was depicted as nudging the red ball up the hill; alternatively, a blue square was shown pushing down against the red ball's seeming efforts to climb. These and similar experiments showed that, in the second half of their first year, infants expect an intervening figure to be helpful, and they show marked preferences for the helping over the hindering figure. These rudimentary preferences develop very early, in the 3- to 6-month period. As one of the researchers, Paul Bloom (2013), remarked, "the three-month olds clearly preferred to look at the good guys" (p. 28). We might think of these early infants engaging in social evaluation; in so doing, they are showing intuitive glimmers of moral *competence without comprehension*, to bring back Dennett's (2017) useful phrase. They are developing *expectations* that we adults—using the elasticity in our full-fledged intentional stance—might casually label the infants as "trusting" helpers and "distrusting" hinderers. But trusting, in the social-cognitive and moral sense that we rely on in psychotherapy, requires a fundamental transformation of relatedness that goes beyond emotional resonance, taking the form of shared intentionality.

I find it appealing that Tomasello starts his account with sharing emotion because emotional expression and responsiveness continue to play such a vital role in full-fledged trusting and trustworthy relationships, where emotional feelings and expressions become embedded in shared intentionality. In infancy and beyond, we can think of relating on the basis of emotion sharing as competence without comprehension and as something we do unconsciously. But a clarification is in order. In this context, *unconscious* must be qualified to mean *unreflective: felt but not thought about*. As the term *gut feelings* attests, we can feel (consciously) and act on the basis of feelings without understanding the reasons for our feelings and actions (Solms 2021). For example, we might feel safe and come close or feel wary and keep our distance without understanding why we are doing so. To feel emotionally implies a bedrock level of consciousness that is essential to basic trust even if we do not think about it.

When we are well aligned, we continue to engage in emotional protoconversations as adults. In psychotherapy, for example, we carry on two conversations simultaneously—one in words, the other in action. Trusting and perceptions of trustworthiness are influenced by the prominent role emotions play in interpreting mental states, including trying to make sense of the misalignment of words and action (e.g., "You say that you don't mind, but it looks to me like you're tearing up a bit"). This comprehending interpretive process requires a lot of transformative development.

Joint Intentionality

Not generally one for hyperbole, Tomasello (1999) referred to the developing capacity for joint intentionality as *the nine-month revolution*, which begins in the 9- to 12-month period, when the infant starts to join his or her mother in paying attention to an external object. Whereas we could think of sharing emotion as aligning emotional states, joint intentionality entails aligning cognitive states—a meeting of minds in perceiving and thinking about something together.

Here begins the revolution: imagine an infant sharing attention with his mother, the two of them engaging with a third object—a kitten. As Tomasello (1999) described it, "At nine months of age human infants begin engaging in a number of so-called joint attentional behaviors that seem to indicate an emerging understanding of other persons as intentional agents like the self whose relations to outside entities may be followed into, directed, or shared" (p. 61). This capacity for joint attention reflects the confluence of two developmental pathways: sharing emotion and grasping intentional states (Tomasello 2019). Think of the new complexity entailed by a mother and infant enjoying looking at a kitten together. The infant is attending not only to the kitten but also to the mother's attention to the kitten and her enjoyment. Moreover, the infant senses the mother's attention to him—his attention and his enjoyment. The two of them are sharing emotion and attention about a third object and each other. That is a lot of converging intentionality in the context of aligning psychological states. It is revolutionary in inaugurating the infant's entry into the psychological world with expanded awareness and dawning comprehension.

Sharing attention is a cooperative activity that requires coordination and communication; it begins at the nonverbal level, with gesturing and pointing. As they join the revolution, infants are learning to follow the mother's gaze and also her pointing—not looking at her finger but rather toward what her attention is *about* and thereby grasping her intentionality, what is on her mind. The infant also learns to point, directing his mother's attention to his attention and its object—his intentionality. Notice the complexity of intentionality here in its *recursive* quality, wherein one mental state is embedded in another: the infant is aware of his mother's attention to his attention; her intentionality refers to his intentionality. Then think of *social referencing*: wary of the kitten's sudden movement, the infant looks at his mother's emotional reaction to the kitten to see how he should feel about the kitten; in the process, she communicates her awareness of his apprehension and responds in an emotionally reassuring way while expressing her own comfort with the kitten. Then the infant feels safe and free to approach the kitten.

Here I underscore something profoundly important about the 9-month revolution that relates to "learning about me," as Tomasello (1999) framed it:

> As infants begin to follow into and direct the attention of others to outside entities at nine-to-twelve months of age, it happens on occasion that the other person whose attention an infant is monitoring focuses on the infant herself. The infant then monitors that person's attention to *her* in a way that was not possible previously, that is, previous to the nine-month social-cognitive revolution. From this point on the infant's face-to-face interactions with others—which appear on the surface to be continuous with her face-to-face interactions from early infancy—are radically transformed. She now knows that she is interacting with an inten-

tional agent who perceives her and intends things toward her. (p. 89, emphasis in original)

In this scenario, the other person's attention includes emotional attitudes toward the infant, who then develops some understanding of how others feel about her, inaugurating a sense of self, including self-conscious emotions such as shyness and coyness, evident by age 1 year. As Tomasello noted, this is a form of social referencing—gauging how to feel about an object by observing others' emotional reactions to it. Here, the object of the other's emotion is the self. Accordingly, feelings about the self—positive or negative—develop from the outside in. Concomitantly, joint intentionality also entails perspective-taking: the recognition that each individual takes different perspectives on the same object (e.g., viewing the kitten from different angles or distances, responding to it emotionally in different ways). *We are not talking about a mind meld; shared intentionality preserves the individual subjectivity of each who shares in it*, a fundamental basis of trusting relationships.

You can easily appreciate how the development of language during these first few years profoundly enhances communication directed to aligning attention and pursuing joint goals and activities. We tend to think of language as the *sine qua non* of human cognition, and there is no question about the extent to which language enhances joint intentionality: we can communicate about mental states and all else in a way that helps us make our mental states more (or less) transparent to each other in a meeting of minds. But we could not *learn* language without the platform of shared intentionality, first evident in joint attention.

To get to my main concern about trust, I am skipping over a lot of developmental complexity that Tomasello (2014, 2019) detailed in the transition from joint attention to the culmination of joint intentionality in *second-personal relationships* (you and I) around the child's third birthday. Imagine a mother and her daughter taking turns stacking blocks to make a tower. A schematic representation will help you appreciate the complex structure of second-personal relationships. Picture a triangle with mother and daughter at different sides of the base and a *shared goal*—stacking blocks to build a tower—represented by "we" at the apex. Now we have what Tomasello (2016) dubbed a *ménage à trois* (p. 53) with a dual-level structure: two "I"s and a "we"—separate and together, each functioning separately as an individual agent and the two together as a "joint agent" (p. 51). Construed in second-personal terms, one level consists of "I" and "you" (from two perspectives), and the other level consists of "we." Notice how the "we," the shared goal of building the tower, directs the attention and actions of the two individuals, "you" and "I," as they take turns adopting different roles: one builds while the other observes. Each can appreciate the other's different perspective and role in the activity.

Alternatively, imagine the mother and daughter tossing a ball back and forth, which renders the role-reversals and different perspectives more apparent: the mother throws and the daughter catches; then they switch roles. Now consider how the daughter might have learned to switch roles by role-reversal imitation. Imagine the mother beginning by tossing the ball to her daughter, taking the ball back from her daughter, and tossing it to her repeatedly. Then the mother encourages her daughter to imitate what she had been doing, tossing the ball. Then they can toss the ball back and forth. All of this requires co-operation in the context of a shared goal: playing catch as a "we."

The crucial point is this: two interdependent individuals are sharing a goal together while maintaining a sense of the individuality and subjectivity of the other. They are aligning psychological states while maintaining a sense of individuality and recognizing each other's subjective experience and perspective. Tossing the ball back and forth, the mother and daughter are not thinking about trust. But *sharing a goal establishes the basic context for trust*. Think of the daughter wanting to pet a dog they encounter on the sidewalk and needing her mother's encouragement to do so: "It's OK, he won't bite." The daughter hesitates. The mother pets the dog. The daughter joins her mother in the petting. In this scenario, wanting to pet the dog, the daughter depends on her mother's judgment and concern. The daughter has learned to trust her mother, implicitly, in this context. She is trusting competently without comprehending trust as we adults think about it. Not yet.

A second-personal, cooperative relationship rests on a social-cognitive foundation but creates a *moral context*. In pursuit of their cooperative goal, each individual depends on the other to hold up his or her end. Each becomes responsible to the other. Especially as cooperative relationships endure over extended periods of time in increasingly diverse contexts, each partner becomes increasingly dependent on the other in various ways. Concomitantly, they come to *care about* each other, each developing concern for the other's well-being; each wants the other to remain in good shape and provides needed help accordingly. This concern is built on *sympathy* for the other's distress, which Tomasello (2019) referred to as the "*sine qua non* of human morality" (p. 247). But joint intentionality also supports *empathy*, which goes beyond sharing emotion to adopting the other's perspective, understanding the reasons for the other's distress, imagining how the other feels, and experiencing feelings *about* the other's distress.

Tomasello (2016) also envisioned cooperative, second-personal relationships as grounded in *respect*. He sees a self-other equivalence in each having a role in the collaborative activity. Respect for equality includes a mutual recognition of the subjectivity and humanity of the other: "recognition of the other persons as agents or persons just as real as oneself…the recognition of an *inescapable fact that characterizes the human condition*" (p. 56, emphasis added). But cooperation requires respect for the "we" as well as the other "I." Joint intentionality enables social evaluation of others' cooperativeness and thus choice of partners for collaborative activities. Recall the animations: infants prefer helpers. Both infant and adult need to know that they can depend on the other, and they both need to make their dependability known to the other, which is the bedrock of trustworthiness.

Collaboration is cemented by *joint commitment* to a goal, which creates the "we" in the triadic, dual-level structure of second-personal relationships. This commitment might be implicit, by virtue of joining in an activity, such as when the mother joins her daughter in stacking blocks. But it also can be explicit, as in agreeing on the goal (e.g., "Let's build a tower together"). A joint commitment engenders a feeling of responsibility, exemplifying *social self-regulation*, which mitigates the risk of default: each individual is responsive to the joint obligation in a way that calls for staying the course until the two decide together that they have achieved their goal. Failure to fulfill the obligation sets the stage for protests and resentment when the partner quits the activity without any apparent reason, and it establishes a context for guilt and making reparation in the individual who let down his or her partner. As long as cooperation prevails, the "we" regulates each "I," contingent on each individual's self-regulation in relation to the "we."

The context of second-personal relationships established in the first few years of life permits us to use the concept of *trust* without reservations as it applies to dyadic relationships (and, ultimately, psychotherapy relationships). Trusting and trustworthiness require that "we" takes precedence over "you" and "I." *Normative trust* is based on an explicit joint commitment in the context of social norms of trust, that is, an understanding of how we *ought* to act. To be trustworthy, "an individual not only must have certain cognitive and physical competencies but also must have a cooperative identity as a result of treating other second-personal agents with mutual respect" (Tomasello 2016, p. 66). With normative trust in mind, consider Tomasello's summary of cooperation as it developed in early societies:

> The cooperative rationality we are positing here is the ultimate source of the human sense of "ought." Early human cooperative rationality expands human pro-attitudes to include the welfare of others, it presupposes second-personal agents who consider one another as equally deserving of respect and resources, and it focuses on the individual decision making that takes place within the context of the joint agent, "we," formed by a joint commitment. These new elements in the decision making of individuals created a socially normative sense of "ought" that was not just a preference or an emotion, but rather the dynamic force behind their actions. (p. 82)

We might say that, in the very early days, we needed to be trusting and trustworthy to avoid starving. Now we can just drive to the grocery store.

By age 3 years, children have developed a social-cognitive and moral level of development that prepares them for dyadic relationships exemplifying trusting and trustworthiness. Then they are ready for a second profound transformation: the transition from joint intentionality to collective intentionality, going beyond the dyad to the group. This transition reconstitutes the sense of "we" to encompass a dramatically expanded framework for cooperation and trust. Broadly speaking, age 3 is the transitional watershed that ushers in the capacity for collective intentionality, which enables us to become *reasonable* at the social-cognitive level and *responsible* at the moral level. I discuss these aspects

TABLE 2–1.	Distinguishing features of shared intentionality
Joint intentionality	**Collective intentionality**
Develops from ages 1 to 3 years	Develops from ages 3 to 6 years
Dyadic relationships	Relationships with group
Relationships with adults	Relationships with peers
Subjective perspective	Objective perspective
Interpersonal self-regulation	Social-cultural self-regulation
Concern for welfare of partner	Concern for welfare of group and society
Loyalty to individuals	Loyalty to group
Joint commitment	Commitment to norms

of collective intentionality in turn. The distinguishing features of joint intentionality and collective intentionality are displayed in Table 2–1.

Collective Intentionality

The triangular, dual-level structure is crucial to understanding shared intentionality. In joint intentionality, which characterizes second-personal relationships, you and I create a "we" (e.g., a goal) in relation to which we cooperatively coordinate our actions. In collective intentionality, we cooperatively coordinate our actions in relation to increasingly larger groups—ultimately, our society and culture (Figure 2–1). A multitude of "you"s and "I" come under the broad, cultural "we." In our group-minded collective intentionality, the "we" constitutes our cultural common ground, our ways of life and ways of doing things, by which we coordinate our actions with one another. This common ground is normative in providing standards of thought and conduct that govern our activities. A common language is a profoundly important aspect of this common ground. Given this common ground, we can interact with strangers, not only in being able to speak with them but also in adopting customary ways of interacting with them (e.g., greeting by shaking hands, as you might remember having done prior to the coronavirus pandemic).

　　As Tomasello (2016) envisions it, collective intentionality and its common cultural ground evolved in the context of competition between local groups: the "safety in numbers" resulted in "the so-called tribal organization of modern human groups" (p. 88). Accordingly, our collective intentionality comes with an all-too-familiar dark side: "In-group favoritism accompanied by out-group prejudice is one of the best-documented phenomena in all of contemporary social

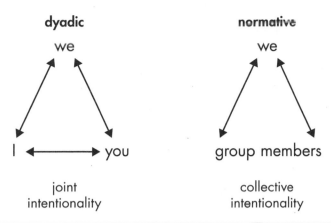

dyadic   **normative**

we   we

I ⟷ you   group members

joint   collective
intentionality   intentionality

FIGURE 2–1. Joint and collective forms of shared intentionality.

psychology" (p. 91). Thus, I want to mention a caveat here that is outside Tomasello's purview. The concept of collective intentionality is complicated by the diverse collectives to which each of us individuals belongs (e.g., gender, ethnicity, religion, political party). On top of this diversity, we have the additional complexities of intersectionality among these collectives. Moreover, the scope of the collective varies dramatically (e.g., from peer group, neighborhood, city, region, and nation to the globe). Our collective intentionality, the "we" to which we belong, is fluid and dynamic. We must trust in the collective, and the diversity and scope of the collective renders trust potentially problematic with the sheer multiplicity of in-groups and out-groups in potential conflict with one another.

The move from joint to collective intentionality coincides with the transition from cooperative interactions with adults to increasingly influential interactions with peers—a move from one world to another, as Tomasello construes it. This transition brings exposure to multiple perspectives along with challenges in coordinating and reconciling them. The child goes from relying on the guidance and authority of adults to working things out with peers who are equal in knowledge and power. In so doing, children are not just following rules but actively creating them, as in play and games. This exposure to multiple perspectives engenders a transition from subjectivity to greater *objectivity*, from what *I* and *you* think to what *anyone ought* to think. Thus, thinking and reasoning take on a normative dimension: the cultural common ground comes to regulate the way individuals think. We become *reasonable*, with varying degrees of objectivity.

The fundamental transition from the dyadic, second-personal "we" to the common ground of the cultural "we" includes *morality*, which bears an especially close relationship to trust. As Tomasello (2019) states, collaborative activities for mutual benefit are the "birthplace of uniquely human sociality and mutuality" (p. 217), and this collaboration applies to both dyads and groups. We show concern for the welfare of our cooperative partners, wanting to keep them in good shape, and the same applies to our wider cultural group; interdependent as we are, we must invest in the social resources on which we depend. If we are to prosper, we have no reasonable choice; as Tomasello (2016) asserts, this "cooperative rationality [is] based on an accurate recognition of social reality" (p. 153). Our engagement with peer groups plays a significant role in our developing broader group-mindedness consistent with our interdependence: "obeying authority is one thing, but being concerned with others and learning to treat them with respect and fairness is another, and it can only come from interactions with peers. Morality is how we work things out with others by means *other* than power and authority" (Tomasello 2016, pp. 156–157, emphasis in original).

Tomasello (2016, 2019) reviewed several aspects of morality that we develop and consolidate with the inaugural period of collective intentionality. The sense of right and wrong acquires more objective, normative force; thus, children enforce moral norms and support punishment of those who violate them, and they are motivated to punish those who harm third parties. Joint commitments are strengthened by explication, which includes making promises. Identification with the group inspires loyalty. A sense of fairness includes ensuring equal and impartial distribution of resources as well as showing respect for ownership. Tomasello underscored the moral-relational basis of such distribution: "we must stress…that the notion of distributive justice is not fundamentally about 'the stuff' but, rather, about being treated fairly and with respect" (Tomasello 2016, p. 117). The cultural "we" also includes shared values, along with consensus on a hierarchy of values according to their relative importance, such as putting life and health above money, as some societies do. A sense of moral responsibility includes feelings of guilt and shame along with motivation to make reparation for transgressions. Crucial to the development of collective intentionality, conventional norms become moralized: "It is thus not the nonconformity per se but, rather, the *harm* that nonconformity may cause or the *disrespect* it may show that evokes negative moral judgments" (Tomasello 2016, p. 126, emphasis added). Of course, when untrustworthy actions are normalized, nonconformity and protest are in order, as has long been the case in relation to civil rights.

As Tomasello (2019) framed it, "children's construction of a moral identity is the capstone of their development in the preschool period" (p. 291). *Moral identity* does not revolve around a desire to be praised but rather the motivation "*to be a praiseworthy person*—a responsible person—in the eyes of the community, including ourselves" (p. 288, emphasis in original). As Tomasello (2016) described it, the moral sense of right and wrong developed by the culture entails balancing four domains of concern: *me*, based on self-interested motives; *you*, related to sympathy and desire to help; *equality*, based on self and others as equally deserving; and *we*, as it pertains to the interests and needs of dyads and the cultural group. Moral decisions require reconciling these four concerns, and Tomasello (2019) made the claim that "human individuals are strongly motivated to preserve their core moral identity as established by their past moral decision-making and judgments" (p. 289). Maintaining one's moral identity requires interpretation and justification of actions, to oneself and others; indeed, our need to justify ourselves to each other could have played a major role in our development of reasoning capacities (Mercier and Sperber 2017). Concomitantly, reasoning with others can promote change and growth in moral identity.

Tomasello (2016) recognized the sheer messiness of human morality, which is "not a monolith but a motley, patched together from a variety of different sources, under different ecological pressures, at different periods during the several million years of human evolution" (p. 128). He quoted Scott Shapiro, who commented that moral disagreements "are entirely sincere. Each of us is willing to do what we morally ought to do—the problem is that none of us knows or can agree about what that is" (p. 130). Acknowledging that morality is difficult, and that we are naturally inclined to be selfish along with being sympathetic and fair, Tomasello concluded his book on morality as follows, with evolution in mind:

> it is a miracle that we are moral, and it did not have to be this way. It just so happens that, on the whole, those of us who made mostly moral decisions most of the time had more babies. And so, again, we should simply marvel and celebrate the fact that...morality appears to be somehow good for our species, our culture, and ourselves—at least so far. (pp. 162)

Competence in Trusting

I have packed into this section of the chapter a wealth of ideas from four of Tomasello's books, and I want to put them into perspective by way of summary before we move on. We humans became an ultra-cooperative species owing to our interdependence. Faced with scarce resources needed for survival, we had a choice: cooperate or else starve. As I think of them, *cooperation and trust are inextricable: if we did not cooperate, we would not need trust; if we did not trust, we could not cooperate.* Tomasello's sweeping synthesis of the developmental literature grounds cooperation in our exceptionally refined intentionality. We not only acquire the capacity to relate to each other through the intentional stance but also become capable of sharing intentionality, aligning psychological states with each other.

From early infancy, sharing emotions comes naturally to us as we resonate with each other and attune to each other; we sing (or hum) and dance together before we learn to talk. On the cusp of our first birthday, we develop the capacity to join with another mind in a revolutionary new way that goes beyond sharing emotions, that is, sharing attention in a triangular way: Two minds attend to a third object and attend to each other doing so. Over the course of the next couple of years, we develop the capacity to form joint goals intentionally and to cooperate in their attainment. You and I become "we" with shared purposes. Each of us has a different perspective and role in our collaborative effort, and each of us recognizes the separateness of the other while we feel, think, and act together—as one, a joint agent. We have become competent in the arena of second-personal relationships, attachment relationships most prominently, which will be a mainstay of our well-being throughout our lifetime.

The evolutionary story I headlined is central to the development of our ultra-cooperative competence in relating to each other. With our primate fore-
bears in mind, it is a genetic story. But with our intentionality in mind, it is a
tale of cultural evolution. Our culture precedes us individuals, but we come to
recognize and appreciate it only after we come together with other individuals—our caregivers first and foremost. From ages 3–6 years, individuals become
embedded in a broader "we" that encompasses groups, society, and a culture. In
striving to make a good life, we become engaged in shared ways of living that
we come to recognize and appreciate as such. We self-regulate our actions in relation not only to other individuals but also in relation to social norms—not
only conventional but also moral and ethical norms.

Although trust is more in the background than the foreground of Tomasello's account, I think he has provided us with a rich conceptual framework
for understanding its essence and early development. Building on his evolutionary perspective, he has attended jointly to social-cognitive and moral development. To understand trust, we need both perspectives: psychology and
ethics, is and ought. To be competent in trusting and in being trustworthy, we
need shared intentionality: aligning emotionally, interpersonally, and collectively under a normative-ethical way of life.

Part of the beauty of Tomasello's way of thinking is his differentiation of joint
and collective intentionality subsumed under the broader category of shared intentionality. I have practiced individual psychotherapy throughout my career, the focus
of which is joint intentionality: the patient's relationships with other individuals, including me. With the theoretical backdrop of psychoanalysis and attachment theory—the professional subculture in which I embedded myself—I focused primarily
on relationships with family members and other close relationships to varying degrees modeled after them. But these individual and family relationships are insepa-
rable from the culture of which they are a product. As a psychotherapist, I consider
myself to have been especially fortunate to have practiced in the context of a therapeutic community, the value of which I appreciated increasingly as I became more
interested in ethical thought. There is no therapeutic community without therapeutic ethics. Joint intentionality is embedded in collective intentionality.

What is the essence of trusting, as we become competent to do it and support it in the first several years of life? I highlight two aspects of trust that stand
out to me. First and foremost, we align psychological states with other individuals, as Tomasello put it. Here I am reminded of philosopher Iris Murdoch's
(1971) words: "I have used the word 'attention'…to express the idea of a just and
loving gaze directed upon an individual reality" (p. 33). She took a stand on the
bedrock of trustworthy joint attention.

Second, as it will concern us in this book, trust has a particular relational context: trust and trustworthiness join hands cooperatively when one person must
depend on another and the other is appropriately dependable. I propose that *in
the case of trust, the shared goal is the well-being of the trusting person, which requires trustworthiness in the trusted person.* As I noted earlier in the subsection
"Joint Intentionality," enduring cooperative relationships entail mutual depen-

dence—interdependence—that encompasses care for the welfare and well-being of both persons. And when we shift to collective intentionality, as it has been from the dawn of human society, the inescapably enduring interdependence of each on all requires concern for the welfare and well-being of all. We should keep in mind Tomasello's (2016) conclusion about the miracle of morality: it "appears to be somehow good for our species, our culture, and ourselves—*at least so far*" (p. 163, emphasis added). Morality hinges on cooperation, and trust is cooperation's partner. Too commonly in the psychotherapy literature, trust has been a relatively silent partner. We cannot have a collaborative therapeutic alliance without trust.

For this interim summary of the nature of trust, I chose to highlight the development of *competence* that Tomasello's account elucidates. Throughout this presentation, I have referred to our developing *capacity* for trusting and being trustworthy. Keep in mind the philosophers' distinction between what is and what ought to be. Genetically and culturally, we humans have evolved the *capacity* to be ultra-cooperative, as long as we are trusting and trustworthy. But we certainly retain the capacities to be neglectfully self-centered as well as exploitative and downright cruel—individually, jointly, and collectively. We can contribute to others' making a good life for themselves and each other. And we can make life miserable for others.

Tomasello's work provides a model for the development of our *capacity* for trusting and becoming trustworthy. *Attachment research crucially expands this model by elucidating the quality of the caregiving relationship that shapes the development and employment of this trusting capacity.* Thus, attachment theory informs us about developmental pathways to distrust—most conspicuously, in the context of attachment trauma. Moreover, attachment theory provides a framework for thinking about trusting and trustworthiness throughout the entire course of life and thus a way of thinking about cultivating trust in the face of a history of well-earned distrust. Accordingly, attachment theory is increasingly becoming integrated into the practice of psychotherapy. Here I will continue to concentrate on the early years, while also making links to adulthood in light of our main interest in trusting in psychotherapy. For the sake of brevity, I am presenting a condensed overview at an abstract level. But we must appreciate the cradle of trust because we never leave it behind.

Secure and Insecure Attachment

I was working in psychotherapy with Michelle, a patient who was chronically suicidal and presented with severe dissociative symptoms (then labeled multiple personality disorder); she was profoundly frightened and distrusting. I was editor of the *Bulletin of the Menninger Clinic* and had first pick of books to be sent out for review. Bowlby's (1988) book on psychotherapy, *A Secure Base*, appeared. In contrast to his three classic tomes on attachment theory (Bowlby 1973, 1980, 1982), this latest book was short, providing an easy opportunity to learn about attachment. I read it and was captivated almost immediately: Michelle desperately needed—and utterly lacked—a secure base. Struggling to understand the bewildering array of problems associated with trauma, I needed a theoretical secure base, solidly grounded in research.

In the previous section of this chapter, I used Tomasello's work to anchor trust in the development of social-cognitive and moral *capacities* needed for *competence* in cooperation, evident in creating a goal-directed sense of "we" in relationships. This competence grows out of emotional connections established in the early months of infancy. Now I turn to the ways in which these capacities and competence are put to use in caregiving relationships and how they are influenced in development by the *quality* of these relationships. Tomasello explicated the normative developmental processes; attachment theory illuminates the ways in which caregiving relationships support these normative processes, fail to support them, or undermine them.

Along with the science reviewed here, the ethical perspective is crucial. I am concerned with our aim of making a good life. Attachment theory and research have illuminated the profound and pervasive role of *emotional well-being* in making a good life. I already have set the stage for attachment in highlighting the relational context for establishing cooperative goals in the form of creating the "we" of interest here. To reiterate my thesis: as I understand it, *trust as it pertains to psychotherapy and close relationships more generally has a specific cooperative aim: ensuring the well-being of the trusting person who is depending on the trustworthiness of the trusted person.* In this context, the quality of the attachment relationship comes front and center. That is how I am now thinking about what I first glimpsed in Bowlby's short book.

We are now approaching a century of attachment research, and the literature is "truly gargantuan" (Mikulincer and Shaver 2016, p. ix). Here I provide the mere gist of this literature as it pertains to trust. I begin by highlighting the primary function of attachment: providing a feeling of security that is fundamental to well-being. Then we consider how different patterns of attachment—secure and insecure—develop in the first year of life and are manifested later in life. The review of common patterns of secure and insecure attachment sets the stage for consideration of trauma in attachment relationships, which is associated with disorganized attachment, a source of profound distrust that can be the bane of psychotherapy: those who most need to trust to establish a sense of security are loath to trust. The section concludes by linking the concept of basic trust to security in early attachment relationships.

Attachment and Emotional Well-Being

Like Tomasello, Bowlby was steeped in evolutionary thinking, viewing the attachment bond between mother and infant as essential to survival, not only in connection with nursing but also in mediating protection from predation: the infant's separation cry draws the mother's attention and thus reunites the infant with the mother. To make a grand evolutionary leap: in us humans, concomitant with its evolutionary origins, this connection in attachment following separation is profoundly rewarding in restoring a *feeling of safety and security* (Sroufe and Waters 1977), what Bowlby construed as the *safe haven* of attachment, physical and emotional. We rely on attachment when we are in danger, threatened, distressed, or ill. Accordingly, separation is a fundamental threat and stressor, and seeking proximity to an attachment figure is our most fundamental response.

Bowlby (1988) was interested primarily in infancy and childhood, our immediate concern in this chapter, yet he was emphatic that our well-being depends on secure attachment relationships throughout life—"from the cradle to the grave" (p. 82). In educating patients about attachment, I make one point above all: *secure attachment is our most powerful means of regulating emotional distress.* This point bears emphasis in part because, in our individualistic culture, you can come to believe that the pinnacle of mental health and maturity is being able to manage emotional distress on your own. On the contrary: from early infancy onward, self-regulation of distress is a backup strategy employed when the connection through attachment is unavailable—momentarily or for longer periods. As we grow older, we become increasingly competent in self-regulation, as we must. But we all are best served by secure attachment connections when we face significant distress. In short, as an ultra-cooperative social species, we are designed for interpersonal regulation of emotional distress by default; the mere presence of trusted companions diminishes distress in a threatening situation (Coan 2016).

Bowlby's collaborator, psychologist Mary Ainsworth, made a major contribution to our understanding of well-being in promulgating a core function of attachment: providing a *secure base* for exploration. Ainsworth observed that securely attached infants were confident in exploring and learning about the world, crawling or toddling off on their own. This confidence was sustained by checking back with the mother to be sure of her availability if needed. Again, this aspect of attachment relationships holds throughout life insofar as we routinely touch base with those to whom we are attached. Accordingly, as I counsel patients, the best way for us all to be independent is to be able to rely on attachment relationships for a feeling of security when we feel threatened or distressed. We are back to the *vital balance* between relatedness and individuality, elegantly integrated by Bowlby and Ainsworth in their appreciation for the complementary nature of the safe haven and secure base. With balance in mind, psychoanalyst Joseph Lichtenberg (1989) instructively construed *self-dependence* as the ability to bridge the gap between separation and reunion. We all leave the nest (we humans most gradually), and our flourishing requires a life of creative exploration. As we become more self-dependent, we can bridge wider gaps in our exploratory activity. But we all need a bridge to a safe haven, from the cradle to the grave.

Attachment Patterns in Infancy and Beyond

Ainsworth devised a laboratory procedure, the Strange Situation, to study attachment security in infants ages 12–18 months (Ainsworth et al. 1978). The infant and mother are brought into a playroom stocked with toys, providing the infant with an opportunity for play; then the mother is instructed to leave the room and return twice, first leaving the infant with a stranger and then leaving the infant alone. As you can imagine, these separations are distressing to infants, albeit to varying degrees. On the basis of the mother-infant interactions in the two reunions, three organized attachment patterns are reliably observed, and they are entirely commonsensical. These attachment patterns, plus the disorganized attachment pattern described by Mary Main and colleagues (see the following subsection), are summarized in Table 2–2. Securely attached infants who have been playing with the toys in the presence of their mother become distressed when she leaves, interrupting their play. They welcome their mother's return; the mother and infant make comforting contact with each other, after which the infant returns to play. The mother's return restores the safe haven and the secure base. The infant's security requires confidence in the mother's availability and *sensitive responsiveness*, as Ainsworth construed it. This confident expectation exemplifies implicit trust. The infant and mother have a cooperative relationship, a goal-corrected partnership, as Bowlby (1982) thought of it. Each depends on the other's responsiveness at the level of emotion sharing and joint intentionality wherein the "we" enables the infant to feel safe and to explore in this strange, novel, and unpredictable situation. So goes much of a good life thereafter, wherein we need a safe haven as a secure base.

Infants who have not developed confidence in the mother's availability and sensitive responsiveness have two basic strategies in managing the distress of separation when they are reunited with their mother: protest her unresponsiveness to command her attention and care or make the best of it on their own. Stick to mother or stick to the toys. Confusingly, in the attachment literature, terminology for these two types of insecure attachment varies widely. I will use the term *anxious attachment* to refer to the protesting variant. Rather than being reliably comforting, the attachment relationship is fraught with distress as well as antagonism associated with the infant's frustration at the mother's inconsistent responsiveness. Thus, infants can demand soothing and resist it, expressing ambivalence in their attachment behavior. Alternatively, in *avoidant attachment*, the infant might seem relatively unresponsive (overtly) to the mother's departure and return, showing more interest in the toys. This avoidant pattern might be mistaken for precocious independence; on the contrary, it is a different strategy for managing distress. The avoidant infant, for example, might have learned that expressing distress leads consistently to rejection ("Don't cry," "Stop fussing") and that the best way to stay peacefully connected to his mother is to keep some emotional distance, managing his distress on his own.

TABLE 2-2. Attachment patterns observed in infancy

Secure: Confident in the safe haven of attachment, the infant reaches out to the caregiver when feeling threatened or distressed; the caregiver's sensitive responsiveness restores a feeling of safety and security that provides a secure base as a foundation for exploration and autonomy.

Anxious: Met with inconsistent caregiver responsiveness, the infant feels frustrated and deprived, protests the limited care, and employs coercive strategies (e.g., tantrums) to elicit attention and responsiveness.

Avoidant: Met with consistent rejection of attachment needs, the infant suppresses expression of distress to maintain a stable connection with the caregiver, relying on self-regulation to manage emotion.

Disorganized: In the face of neglect, abuse, or pervasively disrupted communication, the infant is in a situation of fright without solution; unable to develop a workable strategy for regulating distress, the infant is left feeling afraid, invisible, and alone.

The anxious pattern entails hyperactivation of attachment needs, whereas the avoidant pattern entails deactivation of attachment needs. Both patterns can best be seen as *adaptive strategies* for managing distress in the context of less than optimal responsiveness. *Secure attachment* is the most adaptive way of regulating distress in the context of reliably sensitive responsiveness, and it is the normative attachment pattern (Mesman and van Ijzendoorn 2016): most common, most valued, and associated with optimal functioning in childhood and adulthood. Hence, secure attachment is the primary way of relating to a caregiver, and the two insecure patterns are secondary strategies, adopted when the primary inclination fails.

I marvel at Ainsworth's discoveries in part because of the early age at which infants adapt their way of managing emotional stress to their caregiver's pattern of emotional responsiveness. They have learned how best to manage their distress over the course of their early months, before they can talk and think reflectively. They are displaying remarkably sophisticated *interpersonal competence without comprehension*. Here we see the adaptive unconscious at work (see Chapter 1, "From Trusting Therapies to Trusting Therapists"). Attachment theory is pertinent to psychotherapy because these patterns established in infancy also are evident throughout childhood and adulthood; they can remain adaptive strategies that continue to manifest competence without comprehension. They are employed less competently, however, when they are generalized to relationships in which more effective strategies would fit better with current caregivers' responsiveness. Patients working with relationally trustworthy therapists have an opportunity to learn or solidify a more secure strategy.

As it pertains to trust, Bowlby and Ainsworth's work is complementary to Tomasello's. A great deal of the *capacity* for developing trust in attachment relationships develops remarkably early in life, yet in the context of inconsistent or absent sensitive responsiveness, infants also develop capacities for distrust.

These early patterns serve as templates for trust and distrust in close relationships throughout life (Mikulincer and Shaver 2016). Patients readily understand the adult counterparts of these infant patterns. Trust is exemplified in secure attachment: confidently reaching out to restore a feeling of safety and security when one is threatened or distressed, expecting sensitive responsiveness. Distrust is implicit in the two insecure patterns: anticipating limited responsiveness, feeling ambivalent in reaching out for care, and attempting to coerce care in the anxious pattern; in the avoidant pattern, individuals forgo care and strive to go it alone.

When I educate patients, I need immediately to head off three common misconceptions. First, infant attachment strategies are not carved in stone for life. Although they can be self-perpetuating to a degree, they are adaptable to changes in relationships over the lifetime. Correspondingly, these patterns are relationship-specific to a large degree, even in their inception; in infancy, attachment strategies can vary from one parent to another (Steele et al. 1996). Most important, optimal relating entails *flexibility*. Secure attachment is not a universally adaptive strategy, just as trusting is not uniformly reasonable. Even within a generally secure relationship, you might typically count on responsiveness but sometimes protest and at other times keep your distance.

Attachment Trauma

I use the term *attachment trauma* in two senses: first, to refer to traumatic experiences in attachment relationships and, second, to refer to the traumatizing effects of those relationships—profound distrust most notably. The three typical attachment patterns described in the previous subsection are adaptive insofar as they are adjusted to the caregiver's responsiveness and, in the case of the anxious and avoidant strategies, as they are efforts to make the best of a less than optimal situation. These three patterns also are called the *organized* patterns, as contrasted with what has been called *disorganized attachment*, described by Mary Main and her colleagues (Main and Hesse 1990; Main and Solomon 1990) in their research with the Strange Situation. I begin with an account of disorganized attachment as it appears in infancy, followed by patterns of caregiving associated with disorganization in infancy, and concluding with intergenerational transmission of attachment patterns.

Although a great deal of work went into reliably classifying infants' behavior in the Strange Situation into one of the three organized categories, not all infants fit neatly. Some were recorded as "cannot classify," for example, showing mixed patterns of behavior. Some infants' behavior was markedly unusual and anomalous: "What these infants shared in common was…bouts or sequences of behavior which seemed to lack a readily observable goal, intention, or explanation" (Main and Solomon 1990, p. 122). These atypical behaviors included extremely contradictory behavior (e.g., screaming at the door when the mother left the room and then running away from her when she returned, approaching the mother by backing toward her, reaching toward her with gaze averted) and downright fearful behavior (e.g., frozen and trance like states, wandering in a dazed and confused manner, prolonged rocking, jerking back from the mother with a frightened expression). As Main and colleagues came to understand this behavior, it reflected *fear of the parent* and, more specifically, fright without solution: "an infant who is frightened by the attachment figure is presented with a paradoxical problem—namely, *an attachment figure who is at once the source of and the solution to its alarm*"(Main and Hesse 1990, p. 163, emphasis in original).

Shifts in the expression of disorganization from infancy to early childhood also are worth noting for their failings in cooperative alignment (George and Solomon 2011; Main et al. 2005; Moss et al. 2011). In the Strange Situation, disorganized children engaged in role reversals, having developed controlling strategies of interacting with their mother in the laboratory situation, seen as "desperate attempts by the child to reestablish the protective caregiving-attachment relationship" (George and Solomon 2011, p. 139). These role reversals took two general forms. *Controlling-punitive* child behavior included harsh commands, verbal threats, and physical aggression. *Controlling-caregiving* behavior was expressed, for example, in the child's adopting a cheerful, helpful, attentive demeanor in an effort to engage a passive and deflated mother in play. At this later age, however, some children continue to manifest frankly disorganized behavior.

Main and Solomon (1990) discovered that disorganization is associated with a parent's maltreatment of the child, a link that was supported by extensive research that included home observations and interviews as well as laboratory studies. For example, three broad forms of maltreatment were linked to infant disorganization observed in the Strange Situation (Carlson 1998): physical abuse, physical neglect, and psychological unavailability (e.g., lack of emotional responsiveness, withdrawal, detachment). It is important to appreciate that infant disorganization is associated not only with active abuse but also relatively passive neglect; as Main and Hesse (1990) recognized, infants' fear is associated not only with the mother's *frightening* behavior but also her *frightened* emotional state. It is frightening to have a caregiver who is frightened.

Consistent with Main's observations, Karlyn Lyons-Ruth and colleagues (1999) identified two broad patterns of disrupted caregiving associated with infant disorganization: hostile intrusiveness and helpless withdrawal. Lyons-Ruth also identified a more subtle and pervasive phenomenon beyond frank maltreatment or neglect, namely, *misattunement*, evident in disrupted communication. This disrupted caregiving takes numerous forms: negative-intrusive behavior (e.g., mocking), role confusion (e.g., seeking reassurance), withdrawal (e.g., silence), communication errors (e.g., urging the infant to come close while physically distancing), and disorientation (e.g., abrupt changes in voice). Such disrupted communication could "lead to unmodulated infant fear and contradictory approach-avoidance behavior, whether or not the mother herself is the source of fear" (Lyons-Ruth and Jacobvitz 2008, p. 677). Crucially, disorganized infant attachment was observed even when directly frightening behavior was excluded; psychological unavailability was a sufficient context.

Beatrice Beebe and colleagues' (2010) research on mothers' and infants' interactions most dramatically provided me with a prototype for understanding the relation between lack of emotional alignment and trauma in infancy. Beebe videotaped 150 seconds of mother-infant interactions, meticulously coding second-by-second frames of the film to reveal alignment and misalignment. At the time of the videotaping, the infants were 4 months old. From these recordings, Beebe was able to identify patterns that were associated with disorganized attachment in the Strange Situation when the infants were 12 months old. Imagine predicting attachment patterns at age 1 year from two-and-one-half minutes of interaction in a laboratory at age 4 months. Beebe found two forms of interaction to be predictive of attachment disorganization: 1) inability to "emotionally 'enter' and 'go with' infant facial and vocal distress" (p. 90), as expressed by, for example, closed-up facial expressions, looking away, or failure to provide soothing touch, or, alternatively, 2) striving to override the infant's distress by trying to "ride the negative into positive" through comments such as "No fussing, no fussing, you should be very happy" (p. 94).

Beebe's work poignantly underscored for me what I had earlier concluded: the core of attachment trauma is feeling alone in emotional pain (Allen 2001). A caregiver can leave a child or adult alone in pain either by turning attention away from the pain or by trying to override the pain without recognizing it, insisting on positive feelings instead. We should keep in mind that just as seeking proximity when in pain is natural, so is responding with care. Extensive research also shows what can go wrong with this natural process. Especially informative is the potential intergenerational transmission of trauma, which Main and colleagues brilliantly brought to light.

Main was interested not only in caregivers' behavior in relation to their infant in the Strange Situation as it relates to infant security and insecurity; she was also interested in the ways in which caregivers' attachment history relates to their behavior with their infant. For this purpose, she and her colleagues developed the hour-long Adult Attachment Interview (Hesse 2016), which is akin to a clinical interview in inviting parents to talk about their early attachment history and its impact on them. Main discovered that a parent who had not resolved early experiences of loss and trauma was likely to have an infant who showed disorganization in the Strange Situation (Main et al. 2008). Disorganization in the adult interview was evident in lapses in coherence in narrative that included confusing accounts of early experiences or momentary disorientation such as trance-like dissociative states (also observed in infants showing disorganized attachment). These lapses were associated with the parent's unresolved history of trauma. I have thought of such lapses as a form of posttraumatic reexperiencing in the caregiver that can be evoked by current reminders. These reminders are evoked in the attachment interview by remembering traumatic events and in the Strange Situation by the infant's expression of distress in this attachment context (Allen 2001, 2013b).

Carol George and Judith Solomon identified a *disabled caregiving system* associated with disorganized attachment in childhood (George and Solomon 2008). In addition to a history of unresolved trauma, George and Solomon described a wide range of "assaults to the caregiving system" (p. 848) that can result in an abdication of care: perinatal loss of a previous child; child prematurity or disability; parental psychiatric disorders, including depression, anxiety, and substance abuse; parental divorce; and living in a violent environment, such as in a war zone. We cannot neglect the broader social context within which attachment and caregiving take their form.

Basic Trust in Attachment Relationships

As I have reviewed it early in this chapter, Tomasello's account of social-cognitive and moral development in early childhood is incomplete as it pertains to trust; attachment theory rounds it out with its focus on the feeling of safety and security, which is fundamental to well-being. In discussing trust in more detail in Chapter 3, "Trusting," I make a broad distinction between care and competence. Depending on each other, we are trusting in care and competence; in being trustworthy, we must be caring and competent. To be sure, caring requires its own form of competence (e.g., empathy). Attachment theory puts caring in the forefront of trusting and trustworthiness. I think attachment theory provides a contemporary framework for understanding *basic trust*, as formulated by psychoanalyst Erik Erikson (1963): "The firm establishment of enduring patterns for the solution of the nuclear conflict of basic trust versus basic mistrust in mere existence is the first task of the ego, and thus first of all a task for maternal care" (p. 241). He described the quality of the maternal relationship that creates a sense of trust:

> Mothers create a sense of trust in their children by that kind of administration which in its quality combines sensitive care of the baby's individual needs and a firm sense of personal trustworthiness within the trusted framework of their culture's life style. This forms the basis in the child for a sense of identity which will later combine a sense of being 'all right', of being oneself, and of becoming what other people trust one will become. (p. 241)

Basic indeed. In infancy and to varying degrees beyond, basic trust (or distrust) can be *felt without being understood* or thought about. In his comprehensive formulation, Erikson identified basic trust with sensitive care and embedded it in trustworthiness. He linked trust to a sense of well-being and identity as well as (implicitly) the development of trustworthiness. He also tied basic trust to its cultural context, which provides the link to trusting in the social fabric, which I consider at the end of this chapter and the beginning of the next.

Consistent with thinking about basic trust in the context of attachment, I have construed trusting in psychotherapy as arising in a context where one person who is suffering and feels vulnerable must depend on another for competent caring. This context creates a joint goal (the "we") oriented toward the well-being and welfare of the trusting person. From infancy to adulthood, both persons in their different roles are active in pursuing the joint goal: Although the actions of the trusted person might be in the foreground (e.g., consoling and soothing), the person cared for must actively participate in the uptake of care—receiving and responding appropriately to it (Kittay 2018). Care can be welcomed and appreciated or stonewalled and rejected. Of course, in the context of insecurity, much of the difficult work of psychotherapy revolves around helping the patient be more receptive to care.

Attachment is characterized as an *emotional bond*, in which the caring (trustworthy) person is emotionally engaged, accepting of emotion, protective, concerned, sympathetic, empathic, compassionate—ideally, to use Murdoch's (1971) phrase, guided by loving attention. Could we think of secure attachment in infancy—evidenced in the Strange Situation, for example—as manifesting trust? From the side of the caregiver, of course, we can infer trustworthiness. We might think of the securely attached infant as guided implicitly by trusting expectations—competent in trusting without comprehending it as such.

Attachment research also elucidates the early seeds of distrust. Avoidant attachment is indicative of limitations of trusting in the attachment relationship as a source of emotional well-being. The joint goal of soothing emotional distress is not created or perhaps is contentious. In anxious attachment, the joint goal (the "we") collapses in coercive and controlling behavior and might be reinstituted only grudgingly, perhaps with enduring ambivalence on both sides. Neither of these insecure strategies is an expression of pervasive distrust, implicitly or explicitly. We might see them as expressions of conditional trust, trust with limitations developed in conjunction with deficiencies in caregiving. Or we might see them as trusting (or distrusting) with discernment—impressive relational competence with minimal comprehension, in my opinion, for a 12-month-old.

We psychotherapists are all too familiar with frank distrust that has a basis in failures of trustworthiness in attachment relationships, earlier or later in life, as it is manifested in disorganized attachment: the distrusting person is caught in a plight of fright without solution, desperately needing the security of attachment but fearing closeness and trusting. Providing a safe haven for a secure base, secure attachment supports the dual developmental lines of relatedness and autonomy (Blatt 2008). Maltreatment can fail in both respects: extreme neglect fails to promote relatedness, and abuse fails to respect autonomy. Neither exemplifies a cooperative "we" insofar as neglect fails to establish the "we" and abuse overrides it with control and coercion. The individual who is vulnerable and most needs to depend on the other for care has no workable strategy for obtaining it in that relationship; the most dire scenario is one in which no alternatives for attachment are available, a scenario that can be evident in infancy as well as in later life (e.g., in abusive and possessive relationships).

With trust in mind, I have employed attachment theory to augment To-masello's account of the social-cognitive underpinnings of cooperative relationships. Trusting cooperation requires social-cognitive capacities, but it also hinges on the emotional quality of the relationship: a *caring connection* as exemplified in the emotional bond of attachment in what I have characterized as basic trust. I came to appreciate the nature of the attachment connection more fully when I learned about the concept of *mentalizing* and related research. Moreover, in the context of developing the theory and clinical applications of mentalizing, Fonagy and colleagues (2019a) have homed in on *epistemic trust*, which also bears on the process and effectiveness of psychotherapy.

If the word *mentalizing* is new to you, take heart in what psychoanalyst Jeremy Holmes (2010) wrote: "When I first encountered the term 'mentalising' I found it off-putting, with its abstract pseudo-technical ring.... I have come round to the view that mentalising captures a crucial aspect of psychological health, and psychotherapists' efforts to promote it" (p. 9). I concur.

Mentalizing and Epistemic Trust

To my good fortune, Peter Fonagy was recruited to reshape research at the Menninger Clinic in 1995, initiating what became a 25-year professional collaboration and friendship that also reshaped my thinking about psychotherapy as well as sparking my interest in trust. Based in London, Peter commuted regularly to the clinic and brought many of his colleagues with him over the years. I had discovered attachment theory previously but came to understand it far more deeply in working with Peter and his colleagues. I knew nothing about *mentalization*, a term from the French psychoanalytic literature (Lecours and Bouchard 1997) that Peter introduced into the English lexicon in 1989 (Fonagy 1989) to elucidate a core psychological deficit in patients with borderline personality disorder. Over the course of the next three decades, in close collaboration with his colleague Anthony Bateman, Peter developed a new therapeutic approach for borderline disorder: mentalization-based treatment (Bateman and Fonagy 2016), the effectiveness of which has been established by controlled research (Bateman and Fonagy 1999, 2001, 2009, 2016).

A recent innovation in this treatment approach focuses on the development of trust and advocates that therapists think about trust not only as crucial to the therapeutic process but, more importantly, as a primary outcome of effective psychotherapy. From a developmental perspective, I discuss the concept of mentalizing, its role in attachment and trauma, and its contribution to epistemic trust. As a prelude, however, I use the mentalizing approach to highlight the focus I advocated in Chapter 1: the development of the therapist.

Development of a Psychotherapist and a Psychotherapy

In an episode of the BBC radio podcast *Life Scientific*, Peter Fonagy was interviewed about the role his personal history played in developing the mentalizing approach to psychotherapy (Fonagy 2020). He described his early experience of being a refugee, sent away from his family in France to London at age 15, apparently owing to his father's thought that Peter would be better off in the British culture. Peter's sister remained with the family in Paris. Arriving in London, Peter spoke no English and lived with a family who could not understand his plight. He was sent to school, did not understand the lessons, could not learn much, and failed exams. Getting up each morning, he dreaded going to school, knowing that he would be ridiculed by his peers. Looking back now, he sees that he was bullied in a thoughtless way and has come to appreciate that being abused by peers is more prevalent and more painful than being abused by adults. He knows how it feels to be deprived of trusting social connections. He remembers this adolescent experience as an extremely lonely time that has never left him; he remains able to feel a keen sense of sadness for that socially isolated adolescent boy. This enduring capacity to feel that sadness has helped him enormously in his clinical work; he can reach back to that part of himself and know what it feels like for others to feel alone and despondent.

Peter's path forward was anything but straightforward. During that adolescent period, he became severely depressed and seriously suicidal. A neighbor arranged for him to be seen at what is now the Anna Freud Centre; after the initial interview, he declined to return. Six months later, however, he decided on his own to get help and went back to the Centre, at which point he entered psychoanalysis with Anne Hurry. Although he says he has always wanted to celebrate that 17-year-old boy who was determined to survive under difficult circumstances, he would not have survived without treatment offered in the right way and at the right time. He felt understood "to a T" and described Dr. Hurry as a wonderful mentalizer before he and his colleagues brought the concept of mentalizing into the mainstream of clinical practice. He gave a memorable example of her mentalizing his pride in having purchased his first (old) car. She stopped the session at one point, got up and went to the window, spotted his car, and said admiringly, "Peter, what a wonderful car!" He felt "utterly recognized." He credits Dr. Hurry as well as a mentor who helped him gain admission to University College London; their support established the foundation for the developmental trajectory that ultimately led to his professional contributions.

Peter studied psychology at University College London but had not intended to become a psychotherapist, feeling too close to his depression and finding the prospect of working closely with people too threatening. But he was offered a position teaching psychopathology, which led to his pursuing a doctorate in clinical psychology. He found psychoanalysis appealing in its deep explanation of how the mind works. But when he practiced psychoanalysis as he had been trained, he found the method to be disappointing in effectiveness for the patients he was treating. He found kinship with his colleague George Moran, and the two of them embarked on a project to find a more effective way of working with patients that ultimately led to Peter's formulating the mentalizing approach. From his own analysis, he had come to appreciate how important it is for someone else—another mind—to appreciate how your mind works. To understand your own mind, you need to be understood by another mind, as he came to do with Dr. Hurry's help. The term mentalizing—holding mind in mind—captures the essence of this therapeutic process and its developmental origins in close relationships.

Accordingly, Peter found attachment theory and research to be compatible with the direction of his thinking, and he made a seminal contribution to the attachment literature in his research on the influence of the caregiver's mentalizing on the development of the infant's attachment security. Conversely, in the context of developmental adversity, the lack of a psychologically sensitive mentalizing relationship can be traumatic—as he had learned painfully in his adolescence.

In a remarkable capstone of this personal and professional developmental trajectory, Peter ultimately assumed leadership roles at the two institutions that had been formative in his personal and professional development: he became Chief Executive of the Anna Freud National Centre for Children and Families and Head of the Division of Psychology and Language Sciences at University College London. Although Peter has put a great deal of energy into helping individuals—and helping others do so— I learned from personal conversations that he is convinced that cultivating *institutions'* capacities to support individuals' efforts is essential to sustaining social progress. He was supported by institutions that he now supports. He is keenly aware of the role of trusting in psychotherapy in relation to its broader social context along with the importance of social systems in that context.

Development of Mentalizing

Fonagy and Bateman (2019) introduce the term mentalizing as follows:

> Mentalizing describes a particular facet of the human imagination: an individual's awareness of mental states in himself or herself and in other people, particularly in explaining their actions. It involves perceiving and interpreting the feelings, thoughts, beliefs, and wishes that explain what people do. This entails an awareness of someone else's circumstances, his or her prior patterns of behavior and the experiences to which the individual has been exposed. (p. 3)

This broad conception renders the term mentalizing particularly useful as a way of referring to the psychological connections we make with one another. I reviewed Tomasello's account of the development of joint intentionality with the concept of mentalizing in my mind. Notice that trustworthy mentalizing encompasses not only aligning of psychological states but also appreciating the broader life context in relation to which we understand current mental states. Accordingly, mentalizing entails being able to create narrative, covering everything from stories about current mental states (short stories) to more elaborate developmental stories about a life as a whole (novels).

Although mentalizing is not included in the canon of common factors in psychotherapy, we have thought of it not only as a common factor (Allen and Fonagy 2019) but as *"the most fundamental common factor* among psychotherapeutic treatments" (Allen et al. 2008, p. 1, emphasis in original). Thus, as we understand it, mentalizing is an inherently integrative approach to psychotherapy. No therapy, including behavior therapy, could be conducted without the patient and the therapist understanding what is on each other's mind. The behavior therapist also must understand at least something about the patient's life context (e.g., the history of a symptom). Moreover, in the case of psychotherapies that adopt a developmental perspective (psychoanalysis being prototypical), the therapist must learn a great deal about the patient's life as a whole. Mentalizing is a common factor in our humanity, as Tomasello's evolutionary account attests and everyday experience affirms; when mentalizing is absent we feel dehumanized. Psychotherapy without mentalizing is inconceivable. Trusting and trustworthiness without mentalizing is inconceivable.

As I see it, secure attachment characterizes the quality of relationships conducive to the expression of our developmental capacity for cooperation and trust that I used Tomasello's (2019) work to elucidate. Main's research on the intergenerational transmission of attachment showed that a mother's secure attachment assessed in the Adult Attachment Interview is associated with the infant's secure attachment to her in the Strange Situation (Main 1991). This finding raises some compelling questions: What is the link between the mother's state of mind and the infant's attachment? What is transmitted in intergenerational transmission?

Ainsworth had pointed to an answer by identifying the mother's sensitive responsiveness as influential in infant security. Fonagy and colleagues (1991) designed a study to identify more specifically the means of transmission from maternal to infant security. First, using the Adult Attachment Interview, the researchers assessed mothers' security when they were pregnant with their first child, and then they brought the mothers into the lab when their infant was 1 year old. They found that the mother's mentalizing capacity (in relation to her own attachment history as assessed in the interview) predicted her infant's security in the Strange Situation. I find this correspondence amazing: a 1-hour interview predicted the interaction in separation-reunion interactions in a 20-minute experimental situation more than a year later. In short, the mother's mentalizing (partly) fills the transmission gap between her attachment history and her child's attachment security.

The same holds for fathers (Steele et al. 1996). From this and other supporting research (Arnott and Meins 2007; Meins 1997; Slade et al. 2005), I derive a simple principle: *mentalizing begets mentalizing*—and secure attachment along with it (Allen 2013b). This principle lies at the heart of mentalization-based treatment and, to the extent that it is a common factor, psychotherapy more generally.

There is a corollary to the principle that mentalizing begets mentalizing: nonmentalizing begets nonmentalizing and insecure attachment. At worst, as reviewed earlier in this chapter, nonmentalizing reaches its extreme in neglect and abuse in concert with disorganized attachment. With mentalizing in mind, consider Beebe and colleagues' (2010) analysis of videotaped interactions that predicted disorganized ("D") attachment:

> The future D infant represents *not being sensed and known* by the mother, and *confusion in sensing and knowing himself*, especially at moments of distress. Thus the emerging internal working model of future D infants includes confusion about their own basic emotional organization, their mothers' emotional organization, and their mothers' response to their distress, setting a trajectory in development which may disturb the fundamental integration of the person. (p. 119, emphasis in original)

The mentalizing approach also directs our attention to the personal development of the therapist. If promoting mentalizing is a fundamental goal of therapy, and mentalizing begets mentalizing, the therapist's mentalizing capacity—with its developmental roots in being mentalized—is fundamental to the process: the overarching common factor. The therapist's personal development in attachment relationships—for many of us, including psychotherapy relationships—plays a crucial role in this skill, as Peter Fonagy's account of his professional development illustrates.

As I conceptualize it, Fonagy's recent thinking about trust falls neatly into place with the developmental progression I have outlined. Our social-cognitive and moral capacity to trust is best cultivated by secure attachment relationships, and it is traumatically undermined by relationships that afford no workable path to security. Mentalizing, which requires shared intentionality, plays a prominent role in cultivating secure attachments, which, in turn, are the foundation of basic trust, just as insecure attachments pave the pathway from trust to distrust. Insofar as distrust is associated in its origins and manifestations with impaired mentalizing, mentalization-based treatment provides therapists with methods to identify areas of difficulty and to rectify them. Moreover, Fonagy and colleagues have homed in on another aspect of trust that constitutes the platform for social and cultural learning.

Epistemic Trust

The adjective *epistemic* refers to knowledge; in philosophy, epistemology is the study of the nature and validity of knowledge. Simply put, epistemic trust entails trusting in knowledge being conveyed. As Fonagy and colleagues (2017) defined it, "epistemic trust is an adaptation allowing the infant to receive social knowledge from their better-informed elders...enabling them to benefit from the complex edifice of human knowledge that their immediate culture has available to them" (p. 2). We need epistemic trust to learn from others throughout life, which is the basis for emphasizing epistemic trust in the mentalizing approach.

We should not be misled by the technical term; there is nothing esoteric about epistemic trust. Philosopher Carolyn McLeod (2002), in elucidating prototypes of trust more generally, provided concrete examples of epistemic trust without identifying it as such. Here is her illustration of trust in childhood:

> Kate is a 9-year-old girl who depends on her father, Stefan, to care for her and to explain things about the world. When she does not understand what her class is learning in school, she relies on Stefan to help her. If she does something wrong, she expects him to be able to tell her why. Stefan speaks with authority on many different issues, and Kate usually assumes that what he says is right. (p. 16)

McLeod also gave an example from adulthood pertinent to our concerns with trust in professional contexts:

> For over 8 years Todd has had the same family physician, Dr. Young. He has always depended on Dr. Young to provide him with good medical advice and to perform medical procedures competently. He has kept him as his family physician for so long partly because Dr. Young gives him a lot of information about potential harms and benefits of different procedures or treatments. It is important to Todd that he be informed as much about his health care so that he can be sure he truly wants what he is getting. (p. 16)

To provide a concrete and immediate example of epistemic trust (or perhaps distrust), think about me writing this book and you reading it. I write using the first person deliberately to create a virtual relationship with you—specifically, a second-personal relationship in which trust plays a role. As a reader of books, I like to know something about the author, not only out of sheer curiosity but also to help me understand his or her thinking. In my deliberately conversational style of writing, "I," "you," and "we" appear regularly. Consider *joint intentionality* in writing and reading a book. We share an interest in a topic that we are striving to understand. We are thinking together (I hope) about trust—albeit sequentially rather than simultaneously. We have different roles in this collaborative project: I try to explain, and you try to understand. Mentalizing at an admittedly abstract level, I try to imagine you as trying to understand me, and I try to help you by being as clear as I can about the way I am going about my work (with introductory orientations, headings and subheadings, italics to emphasize concepts, summaries, and so forth). Now I'm going all out in inviting you to think about reading what I've written. Furthermore, I am arguing that psychotherapy—our shared interest—must be considered a personal process that is grounded in the therapist's personal and professional development.

Thus, I am including some personal and professional context for my thinking. You will be more or less aligned with me accordingly (at least remaining somewhat aligned if you have gotten this far in the book). In introducing mentalizing, I also have provided an opportunity for you to align with the personal side of Peter Fonagy's thinking, as I have done.

Thinking of our shared goal of understanding what I think (if not necessarily agreeing with each other), I am firmly convinced that, if I do not try to keep you in mind, I will not communicate well. If I just write what I have in mind, it will be hash to you. (I speak from much experience in having done so.) I hedge my bets by relying on colleagues and others to read rough drafts; they serve as stand-ins for you. Here I am applying Dennett's (2017) elastic use of the intentional stance: Ideally, you are looking at print on a page and engaging in a meeting of minds—yours with mine. You have some reason to want to know what I think. Perhaps more likely, you don't care what *I* think, but you want to know what *someone* with some presumed authority thinks about this particular topic. But you will get to know me in the process. Ideally, I'm earning some degree of your trust—to the extent that what I'm writing makes sense to you and comports with what you know already. You might also be aware of putting trust in the publisher or reviews.

But we also must consider *collective intentionality* in the realm of epistemic trust. Consider how much trust I am placing in authority here: Dennett, Tomasello, Polanyi, Haybron, Bowlby, Ainsworth, Fonagy and his colleagues, among many others. As the number of references and liberal quotations throughout this book attest, I am relying on an abundance of authorities. But the literature is vast, and I am highly selective in my choice of authorities. You are borrowing from my trust in them. I don't trust myself to write a book about trust without putting my trust in many others who have written with a great deal more knowledge than I have. Thus, you are trusting in the trustworthiness of all whom I trust. They, too, rely on the accumulated knowledge of others. If you were wary of trusting me, you could read all my references. In principle, you could read all the sources that have informed me but that I have not cited. But you could not read all the references in all those sources. And you could never share the personal knowledge that informs any one of these writers, much less all of them.

In reading this book, you are placing trust in a large collective of "we" who share an interest in trust and related ideas. And this cascade of trusting is a tiny sliver of cultural knowledge in which you are trusting—or distrusting. Maybe you never thought about the role of the intentional stance in reading a book. Maybe all this sounds kind of nutty. But I think about it when I am reading a book because trust in the author matters a great deal to me, especially when I am reading about matters that are personal—such as trusting in psychotherapy.

Developing Epistemic Trust

Hungarian developmental psychologist George Gergely made a major contribution to our understanding of epistemic trust. Gergely and his colleagues recognized the evolutionary significance of *natural pedagogy*, a uniquely human capacity to teach and learn cultural information efficiently by means of instruction, beginning with primary caregivers early in life (Gergely 2007; Gergely and Csibra 2005; Gergely et al. 2007). As do other species, we humans learn by trial and error as well as by imitation and modeling when we observe others of our kind. In addition, through our receptiveness to deliberate instruction, we have the capacity to quickly learn information that is not intuitive, for example, the use of gadgets such as spoons and, eventually, the use of language. (Often enough, adults need to place epistemic trust in children to help them learn the use of myriad devices and applications.)

Pedagogy requires shared intentionality: establishing joint attention with the shared goal of learning through instruction. The infant's innate proclivities to make eye contact and attend to infant-directed speech ("motherese") prepare the ground for receptivity to ostensive (i.e., demonstrative) communication cues that signal the teacher's intent to convey information to the infant. These cues to pedagogical intentions include making eye contact, raising the eyebrows, widening the eyes, leaning forward, coordinating responses with the infant's actions, taking turns, using the infant's name, and pointing. This stage-setting for teaching implicitly assumes, recognizes, and enhances the infant's feeling of agency and active participation in learning. To speak for the responsive and naturally inquisitive preverbal infant, if the infant could mentalize: "I get it, you want to show me something. I'm ready." As the complex process of cueing attests, the teacher's role in pedagogy requires mentalizing of the infant: knowing what the infant knows and presenting knowledge in a form that the infant can understand and generalize beyond the immediate situation. Such mentalizing is the basis of epistemic trust throughout life, even in its highly indirect form of writing a book that others can comprehend.

We naturally take education and transmission of knowledge as the paradigm of pedagogy, and we think of epistemic trust in relation to the validity and usefulness of the information conveyed. Stretching the concept, Gergely (2007) also identified *emotional pedagogy* as being important for social-emotional development of trust, and he identified the interactive features. This form of pedagogy includes a complex form of mirroring the infant's emotional expressions that requires mentalizing. Consider a mother responding to her frustrated and fussy infant. The mother might respond to the infant's frustration directly with her own matching level of frustration (an experience that should not be unfamiliar to any parent). In this case, her frustration might only compound the infant's distress. Understandable as this maternal reaction might be, it is not pedagogy. Rather, in mentalizing the infant's emotion, the mother imitates the infant's frustration intermingled with her sympathetic concern, using ostensive cues to *express her recognition of what* he *feels, not what* she *feels.* Using ostensive cues, she intends her emotional expression to refer to his feelings.

Emotional pedagogy is a nonverbal form of teaching that entails emotional mirroring alloyed by mentalizing the infant's feelings. This enhanced form of mirroring provides emotional containment and regulation while also promoting subjective understanding of emotions. As Gergely and Watson (1996) aptly characterized it, the mother is providing *social biofeedback*, in effect, "Let me show you what you feel and my awareness of it." Emotional pedagogy is trustworthy to the extent that the caregiver mentalizes the infant's emotional state accurately and models the emotion appropriately. There is ample room for pedagogical failure in the form of confusing emotional miscommunication or downright emotional neglect, as described earlier in the context of attachment trauma.

Epistemic Trust in Psychotherapy

The idea of emotional pedagogy stretches our ordinary academic understanding of pedagogy but identifies a fundamental aspect of emotional learning, namely, a way we learn about our emotional states and feelings, beginning in infancy. Similarly, thinking of this nonverbal form of learning as requiring *epistemic* trust stretches "epistemic" beyond its natural boundaries. Terminology aside, emotional learning at both nonverbal and verbal levels is fundamental to psychotherapy, and this learning both requires and promotes trust.

The therapist's conscious and unconscious emotional responsiveness, evident in nonverbal emotion sharing as discussed earlier in the subsection "Sharing Emotions," will be essential for the emotional engagement intrinsic to effective psychotherapy. The now-outdated stereotype of the stone-faced psychoanalyst has its analogue in still-face experiments with mothers and infants (Tronick 2007), wherein a mother is asked to engage naturally with her infant, who is in a car seat, and then instructed to interrupt the interaction by adopting an immobile and emotionless expression—a highly unnatural occurrence. This nonmentalizing response is distressing to infants (and disconcerting to mothers). With psychotherapy patients, I think it is odd at best.

But the concept of emotional pedagogy usefully goes beyond emotion sharing in pointing to the potential *informativeness* of the therapist's emotional responses to the patient. Empathic reflection of feeling goes beyond mirroring in requiring that the therapist mentalize the patient's emotion, understanding the feelings and their basis; mentalizing entails sharing of emotion coupled with some empathic distance. Achieving the shared goal of emotional understanding requires a combination of togetherness and separateness. I am not averse to becoming tearful with patients when hearing about trauma and loss—I can't help it sometimes. Nonetheless, my feelings must be embedded in attention to my patients' experience and understanding of it in a way that helps them empathize with themselves and understand their emotions. Consciously or not, they are trusting *my* feelings to varying degrees.

Moreover, much of the work revolves around verbalizing, ranging from labeling patients' emotions to creating a more elaborate narrative that encompasses the therapist's knowledge. In this context, *epistemic* trust obviously applies. Furthermore, as psychotherapy attests, epistemic trust pertains to far more than academic knowledge insofar as our primary concern is understanding personal relationships, which includes self-understanding. We acquire ordinary knowledge about individuals, relationships, and human nature from others—including psychotherapists. In addition, as described in Chapter 1, the therapeutic alliance also requires trust in the therapist's professional knowledge about psychiatric disorders, treatment methods, and much else. Effective psychotherapy without epistemic trust is unimaginable.

To return to our starting point in considering the contribution of Fonagy and colleagues' work, you might have inferred that the importance of developing epistemic trust in psychotherapy is to make it possible for the patient to engage productively in the process and to benefit from it. That much is absolutely true, but it misses the main point, which is to enable patients to be more trusting in relationships *beyond* therapy so as to increase their capacity for social learning more generally (Fonagy et al. 2017, 2019b). Psychotherapy does not seek an end point; ideally, it is a catalyst: preparatory in providing help for further development. In short, when psychotherapy goes well, it offers a trusting social connection with lasting benefit. But psychotherapy is one among many interpersonal connections; it should not become an end in itself, and we should not glorify it.

At the end of this chapter, I will come back to epistemic trust to put it in the context of basic trust and social trust more broadly. Before doing so, however, I will address serious challenges to the theory and research on attachment and mentalizing that you have just labored to understand. Having walked up the mountain, we will now jump off a cliff.

Cultural Diversity: How I Mistook Ethics for Science

For the latter half of my career, I advocated using attachment theory as a fundamental scientific framework for psychotherapy not only in my clinical practice but also in teaching and writing. This advocacy was based on what I have construed as the extraordinarily strong scientific foundation of attachment theory, established over several decades of vigorous research efforts. More specifically, I found attachment theory preferable to traditional psychoanalytic thinking because attachment research provided an empirical approach to early development, starting with research on mother-infant observations. I also found Bowlby's thinking fitting for working with attachment trauma insofar as he emphasized the outer reality of traumatic events in contrast to the shift of

---

TABLE 2–3.   Core criticisms of attachment theory from a cross-cultural perspective

Attachment is universal but takes different forms in different cultures.

Attachment theory and research have been overly restricted to WEIRD (Western, Educated, Industrialized, Rich, and Democratic) societies that represent a small proportion of the global population and a tiny fragment of human evolutionary history.

The cultural ideology in relation to which attachment theory first developed was associated with a relatively exclusive focus on the mother in a society that shifted the burden for childcare from the community to the nuclear family, thereby abdicating public responsibility for the welfare of children and their caregivers.

The emphasis on maternal sensitivity in attachment research confounds science and values.

The focus on attentiveness to the child's internal world as a necessary condition for attachment security reflects a cultural bias.

---

psychoanalysis to the inner world in general and to fantasy in particular. Attachment theory appealed to my science-minded side.

In the course of writing this book, I discovered a long history of trenchant criticism of attachment theory and research. Ironically, I now see my attraction to attachment theory as influenced (unknowingly) by my own scientism along with brand loyalty. My problem was culture blindness—incompetence without comprehension. A core thesis of this book is our need to integrate scientific research with an ethical perspective. Compartmentalizing, I relied on attachment theory for scientific grounding and turned to philosophy for scholarly ethical knowledge. But science is not free of ethical influence, and I now appreciate the extent to which our Western cultural ethos shaped attachment research and its interpretation. The critics are articulate, and I will quote them liberally to capture their passionate voices. Table 2–3 highlights the major criticisms discussed in this section.

From its culturally sensitive critics' perspective, attachment theory suffers from two major problems: its claims for universality in attachment processes and its predominant focus on the mother. Marga Vicedo (2013, 2017), specializing in the history and philosophy of science, recounted the early history of attachment theory, focusing on the period from World War II until the 1970s. She explicated the narrowness of Bowlby's evolutionary and ethological thinking and elucidated the cultural ethos in which the preoccupation with mothering took hold. Of course, notwithstanding Bowlby's challenges to mainstream psychoanalysis, he had grown up professionally in a subculture that gave primacy to early mother-child developmental influences. Although attachment theory and research expanded dramatically in the half-century following these early foundations, their legacy warrants reconsideration of the theory's basic premises.

This critical literature is extensive (Hays 1996; Keller and Bard 2017; Meehan and Crittenden 2016; Otto and Keller 2014; Vicedo 2013), and I will present merely the gist of it here by contrasting the prototypical Western culture in which attachment theory developed with an alternative prototype more representative of small-scale, hunter-gatherer societies; these are the kind of societies in which human beings became exceptionally cooperative in the context of obligate collective foraging, as Tomasello (2019) proposed. They are also the kind of societies in which attachment initially evolved and developed. Anthropological research focusing on these societies challenges the universality of attachment security as I have understood it and presented it thus far in this chapter. In the final part of this section, I will consider the implications of this critical perspective for thinking about trust.

One survey of the scientific literature (Röttger-Rössler 2014) indicated that "96% of psychological samples come from countries with only 12% of the world's population" (p. 141). Evolutionary biologist Joseph Henrich (2020) has characterized our cultural perspective as WEIRD: Western, Educated, Industrialized, Rich, and Democratic. Bowlby's thinking, while anchored in evolutionary theory, also was influenced strongly by his own comparatively WEIRD cultural background. More specifically, along with Vicedo (2013), sociologist Sharon Hays (1996) emphasized the postwar context in which Bowlby was working, with heightened social concerns about mental health and its basis in child-rearing. Primarily from the American perspective, Hays elucidated the *ideology of intensive mothering*, based on multiple sources: reviews of the history of mothering and the popular literature on mothering; study of technical manuals developed by prominent experts, including Benjamin Spock, T. Berry Brazelton, and Penelope Leach; and intensive interviews of mothers (including working and nonworking, middle-class and working-class women).

In Hays's words, "the model of intensive mothering tells us that children are innocent and priceless, that their rearing should be carried out primarily by individual mothers and that it should be centered on children's needs, with methods that are informed by experts, labor-intensive, and costly." It is the model of "white, native-born middle class and has long been, and continues to be, the most powerful, visible, and self-consciously articulated" (Hays 1996, p. 21). Hays refers to the child-rearing manuals exemplifying this model as "hesitant moral treatises" (p. 65). *Ideology* is a loaded term, which Hays contrasts with theorizing about "the natural propensities of mothers or the absolute needs of children" (p. x), notwithstanding that "little of what we think of as crucial to appropriate child rearing today is an absolute or biological necessity" (p. 22). She contends that the ideology of intensive mothering "serves the interests not only of men but also of capitalism, the state, the middle class, and whites" (p. xiii). Hence, this critical literature exemplifies a fundamental shift in perspective, from biology to social construction and from science to ethics—moralized, politicized, and gendered. As Hays (1996) describes, considerations of optimal childrearing from the standpoint of working versus nonworking mothers in tandem with controversies about day care loomed large in the context of "mommy wars." The intensive mothering model put mothers in a no-win situation. Those who stayed home felt guilty for not pursuing self-development, whereas those who worked double shifts (inside and outside the home) felt they could not do either fully or adequately.

We should keep in mind that the terms *sensitivity* and *security*, which are used pervasively in the scientific literature, are heavily value-laden. Anthropologist Robert Levine (2014) put this point forcefully, questioning attachment research as "an objective perspective based on empirical evidence" characterizing the human species. In contrast, he argued that Ainsworth's and Bowlby's model "should be seen as part of a twentieth-century moral campaign to change childcare in Britain and America" (p. 51). Moreover, "The basic differentiating concepts of attachment research—*secure versus insecure attachment and maternal sensitivity versus insensitivity* to infant signals—involve moral judgments specific to the Anglo-American cultural ideology of parent-child interaction that became influential in the mid twentieth century and has remained so" (p. 60, emphasis in original). "Mentalizing" is a more value-neutral term than sensitivity, yet we value mentalizing that promotes trust and thus is grounded in care and competence, including psychological and emotional sensitivity.

Ainsworth et al. (1978) put maternal *sensitivity* center stage in attachment theory as it relates to child security. Such sensitivity entails a psychological focus on the child's inner world, aptly described by Elizabeth Meins (1997) as *mind-mindedness*. Is this aspect of intensive mothering universal in child development? With cultural bias in mind, developmental psychologist Heidi Keller (2014) characterized this conception of child-rearing as "based on exclusive dyadic attention between caregiver and child" with a "picture of the baby as an independent agent with its own will and the right to express its own preferences and wishes, and the expectation of their fulfillment." It is "typical of Western middle-class families with a high degree of formal education, affluent life circumstances, and a reproductive style of late parenthood and few children" (p. 10). In Keller's thinking, this Western, middle-class conception of development is exemplified in attachment theory, "where infants experience from their first day the exclusive dyadic attention of one of a few caregivers who try to read the infant's mind in order to be sensitive and responsive interactional partners." This attention includes extensive face-to-face interaction and mutual eye gaze along with sensitive responsiveness to open expressions of emotional distress. In concert with this nonverbal engagement, caregivers engage in "elaborative verbal discourses in which the caregiver explains the inner and outer world" (p. 13). This model is associated with the "pre-eminent goal of psychological autonomy," which is adaptive in Western, middle-class families "representing less than 5% of the world's population" (p. 12). Keller does not deny that *attachment* is universal: "No child would survive infancy without a caring environment and the development of trust in others as well as itself" but argues that "Universality and cultural specificity are profoundly intertwined" (Keller and Chaudhary 2017, p. 134). She asserts that we must "capture what is critical for security and trust in young children under diverse situations" and that what constitutes a positive developmental outcome associated with security "is largely culture specific" (p. 135).

Critics have contrasted the cultural ethos expressed in attachment theory with an ethos evident in small-scale, subsistence-based societies in ecologies with scarce and unpredictable resources. These societies conform more closely to our evolutionary origins in hunter-gatherer groups and characterize "human social organization for more than 99% of the evolutionary history of *Homo sapiens*" (Bogin et al. 2016, p. 62). By this measure, we in contemporary society are extreme outliers in our WEIRDness. I will briefly characterize some common features of these societies that diverge most starkly from our Western prototype, acknowledging that there is much diversity among these societies as well as hybrid intermingling with Western practices. Moreover, American society is far from monocultural, and the cultural humility advocated in Chapter 1 pertains to our thinking about attachment.

We humans are exceptional among primates in requiring a prolonged period of dependence on caregiving that places a great burden on mothers. Human mothers wean infants relatively early and have short birth intervals such that they must care for infants along with older children who remain dependent. Our big human brains are expensive nutritionally to grow and maintain. Mothers depend on others for providing food and other forms of support. Evolutionary anthropologist Sarah Hrdy (2009, 2016) characterized the hunter-gatherer pattern as one of collective and distributed caregiving, wherein kin and non-kin take on what we consider to be parenting (primarily mothering) roles, serving as *alloparents* (other-parents). The range and composition of alloparents vary considerably but often include siblings, grandparents, extended family, and non-kin. The proportion of maternal care in relation to alloparents varies considerably across societies (Keller and Otto 2014), as does the role of fathers (Keller and Chaudhary 2017). Anthropologist Courtney Meehan and colleagues (2016) observed a society in which infants (8–10 months) "interact with approximately twenty caregivers on a daily basis, ten of whom provide intensive investment" (p. 205). They noted that these alloparental attachment relationships "appear to be foundational and influential on the primary attachment relationship" (p. 212); accordingly, "The social network is *not supplementary* to child development and human reproduction but rather serves as *its foundation*" (p. 220, emphasis added).

In these wide social networks, children play an active role in creating their pattern of care; they "attach themselves to those who match them best in terms of temperament and character" (Röttger-Rössler 2014, p. 149), and children as young as 2 years might decide with whom they want to live. Hrdy (2016) emphasized the extent to which children's need to seek care from a range of alloparents bolsters their development of intentionality and other-regarding aptitudes: "social selection would have favored those who grew up more interested in the thoughts, feelings, and needs of others, an emotionally quite distinctive kind of ape prepared to recognize what expressions, vocalizations, or behaviors would appeal to specific others" (p. 28). In sum, the alloparental mode of child-rearing "preadapted apes in the hominin line for greater social coordination" (p. 33) Accordingly, alloparenting is fertile soil for the development of shared intentionality, as Tomasello (2019) described it, and mentalizing, as Fonagy (1989) termed it.

Here I draw several instructive contrasts between contemporary Western middle-class societies ("Western") and small-scale subsistence-based societies with extended caregiving networks ("traditional"). We can contrast the *inward* focus of Western parenting with the *outward* focus of parenting in traditional societies (Keller and Chaudhary 2017; Keller and Otto 2014; Otto 2014). The Western pattern of high levels of face-to-face interaction are not universal: the traditional pattern is characterized by low levels of eye contact and face-to-face interaction; infants are held and carried facing out—toward others. In contrast to the Western emphasis on emotional and psychological care, traditional communities provide more direct physical contact: "babies are fondled, rocked, repeatedly kissed, and caressed during repeated contacts between the caregiver and the child" (Keller and Chaudhary 2017, p. 116). With high levels of body contact, warmth is physical in traditional groups, in contrast with our Western metaphorical variant, emotional warmth (Morelli et al. 2017). In traditional groups, care is expressed in action, such as by ensuring safety and social conformity by controlling what children do. As Otto (2014) writes of the Cameroonian Nso, "Using a mind-minded style when talking to infants is considered *ludicrous*" (p. 222, emphasis added). Rather than providing an opportunity for empathic soothing as in Western culture, expression of negative emotion is actively discouraged by the Nso: "The mothers frequently recite social norms and morals. One mother says to her crying baby: 'Don't cry again!... We don't cry'" (p. 220). As discussed next, what we might consider a precursor of insecure (avoidant) dyadic attachment in Western society might in traditional societies promote security in the community.

A major theme throughout this book has been the need to balance the interests of self and others. This balance is cross-cultural: "In general, two basic human needs are reflected in cultural models everywhere: the need for autonomy and the need for relatedness" (Otto 2014, p. 218). Yet there are striking cultural variations in the tilt as well as the forms that autonomy and relatedness take. Keller (2014) makes the following contrast: the West promotes *psychological autonomy*, which emphasizes "the unique individual and his needs, preferences, intentions, and choices," consistent with the relatively intense focus of attention on "the inner world of the individual" (p. 13). In contrast, traditional societies emphasize *hierarchical relatedness*, with the focus on "the social community of which the individual is a part.... Individuals are born into multiple caregiving networks, with the community being responsible for the well-being of the child" (p. 13). Accordingly, "conversations do not revolve around the child's wishes and intentions but on clear instructions, moral obligations, and social roles and responsibilities. It is not mental-state talk... but the behavior in the here and now" (Keller and Chaudhary 2017, p. 133).

Otto (2014) contrasted psychological autonomy with *action autonomy*, "supported by fostering babies' early motor independence" (p. 221). This autonomy is intended "to put members of the society in the position to perform role-based actions and meet obligations on their own, yet *in the service of the community*" (p. 218, emphasis added). Correspondingly, "mothers believe children to belong to them only as long as they are in the womb. As expressed in African proverbs, "Once born, 'a child belongs not to one parent or home'…instead 'it takes a whole village to raise the child'" (p. 219). When we use the concept of sensitivity, we should consider: sensitive to what? Mothering focused on action autonomy is not insensitive; it is sensitive to the cultural context and community norms.

Having been enamored with mainstream attachment theory for two decades, I find this critical literature fascinating and instructive. I am not only certifiably WEIRD; I grew up in the late 1940s and 1950s when the ethos of attachment theory was developing and the emphasis on intensive mothering was in its heyday. Like a fish living in ignorance of water, I have found attachment theory intuitively compelling and commonsensical—as being *natural*. We champions of attachment theory could respond to the criticism by declaring it irrelevant; we work in a cultural context that mainstream attachment theory fits. I continue to find the science compelling, but I also believe we must be skeptical about its scope—even in our diverse contemporary Western society. And we have much to learn from anthropological research on other cultures. I have long been averse to the extreme and escalating tilt toward individualism in American society; accordingly, I have welcomed attachment theory's emphasis on the lifelong value of relatedness, expressed in the relation between the safe haven and secure base. However, even informed by attachment theory, our Western tilt toward relatedness remains modest.

Hays (1996) made the case that the persistence of the ethos and ideology of intensive mothering derived its power as a counterweight to the cultural championing of self-interest:

> According to mothers, children are emphatically not the individualistic, calculating competitors one encounters in the marketplace…. The seeming innocence and uncorrupted nature of children is what enables them to offer the unconditional love that mothers find so valuable. This is the love that promises to be the grounding for the kind of long-term intimate ties of warmth, understanding, and support that are so difficult to sustain in the larger world. (p. 168)

Accordingly, Hays construed the social contradictions that mothers face—self-development versus devotion to childcare—to be "one central field upon which a much larger struggle is waged" (p. 172). Moreover, "the more the larger world becomes impersonal…the more intensive childrearing becomes," and the social conflict is highly gendered, holding "women responsible for unselfish nurturing while men are responsible for self-interested profit maximization." This division of labor serves to "absolve the public world from responsibility of the values of unselfish care, commitment to the good of others, and willingness to carry out such obligations without direct or material remuneration" (p. 175). But this *abdi-*

*cation of public responsibility came with a high cost: "a tremendous and undue bur-
den on women"* (p. 177, emphasis added). Attachment theory, with the prestige of
science and biology, provided support for this burden. What we might consider a
Western obsession with psychological autonomy and individual development
comes with a high cost: sacrificing concern for the common good (Sandel 2020).

Diving into this social-political history, I might seem to have strayed far
from the territory of psychotherapy and from trust in particular. Not so. As described in Chapter 1, research in psychotherapy supports cultural awareness
and cultural humility. As philosopher Thomas Nagel (1986) famously asserted,
there is no view from nowhere: Each of us therapists comes to the work from a
particular cultural background and perspective—in my case, utterly WEIRD.
Each of us comes from somewhere; our practice of psychotherapy cannot be
dissociated from an ethical and social-political perspective (Cushman 1995;
Prilleltensky 1994). The best we can do is become aware of our individual perspective in the context of other perspectives so as to avoid imposing our own
assumptions unwittingly on others (see Chapter 4, "Becoming Trustworthy").

Fortunately, as described early in this chapter, we develop the capacity for
perspective taking in early childhood. Unfortunately, we do not use our capacities consistently. We cannot be value-free, but we can make our values explicit
without unknowingly justifying them solely by science, as Hays (1996) and
Vicedo (2013, 2017) criticized attachment researchers for doing. We are long
past the postwar period that was Hays's and Vicedo's focus, and American culture is diverse. Nonetheless, we have not left WEIRDness behind. Our trustworthiness as therapists depends on being self-aware and open to diverse
backgrounds, perspectives, and values, including those related to trust—itself
shaped by the cultural contrast we have been considering here.

In the effort to put us on the ground floor of trust by taking a stand on mainstream attachment theory augmented by mentalizing, I might seem to have
painted myself into a corner. To a great extent, as evidenced by this book, I have
invested my career in individual psychotherapy. Moreover, true to my introverted
temperament, I have adopted an introspective approach to psychotherapy; although I am not a psychoanalyst, psychoanalysis is the broad tradition I have adopted (or by which I was adopted). I was startled to read that a mind-minded
orientation toward attachment would be seen as "ludicrous" in other cultures that
are more action oriented. Of course, it has not escaped my attention that many patients in our culturally diverse society prefer more prescriptive, problem-focused
or symptom oriented treatments; they are unenthusiastic or downright averse to
introspective approaches. Concomitantly, they are more likely to place trust in the
methods and procedures of therapy than in the therapist or therapeutic relationship, and I think they are better served by behavioral and cognitive-behavioral approaches. Those of us who are psychoanalytically oriented might interpret a focus
on action as a defense against introspection, and indeed it might be. But an action
orientation also might be viewed as a culturally grounded preference that should
be honored. Conversely, we should be mindful that prolonged introspection can
be a defense against action as well as a culturally grounded preference.

Having painted myself into a corner, I cannot avoid getting some paint on my feet as I continue in the next two chapters to explore the complexities of trust in dyadic relationships. At the same time, the cultural differences just considered will expand our purview.

Basic Trust, Epistemic Trust, and Social Trust

To conclude this chapter and pave the way for the next, I weave together the major facets of trust that I have highlighted thus far and consider them in our broader social context. Table 2–4 summarizes the core distinctions.

Relating Basic and Epistemic Trust

Cognitive scientist Hugo Mercier (2020) succinctly contrasted what I have distinguished as epistemic and basic trust: "Trust takes two main forms: trust that someone knows better...and trust that they have our basic interests at heart" (p. 222). Both require a cooperative connection grounded in shared intentionality. Consistent with Erikson's construal, I associate basic trust with attachment, a feeling of safety and security, and a context of care. When we therapists use the word *trust*, unqualified by adjectives, I think we generally have basic trust in mind.

In contrast to basic trust, epistemic trust pertains to the acquisition of cultural knowledge that is essential for social functioning as well as vital for the evolution of culture. Basic and epistemic trust are similar in requiring an ethical-moral context of trustworthiness exemplified in benevolence and goodwill. In my way of thinking, basic trustworthiness puts a premium on caring, and epistemic trustworthiness puts a premium on competence—that is, knowledge. Prominent in the ethics of epistemic trustworthiness is honesty, along with helpful intent. As with cooperation and trust, we can pull apart basic and epistemic trust conceptually, but they are best in partnership. Consistent with Fonagy and colleagues' view, I see basic trust as the ideal context for the early development of epistemic trust and for its ongoing manifestations. Mentalizing plays a key role throughout development: "*If I feel that I am understood, I will be disposed to learn from the person who understands me*" (Fonagy et al. 2019b, p. 176, emphasis in original).

The confluence of epistemic trust with basic trust in a mentalizing context is consistent with emphasizing the role of epistemic trust in psychotherapy and in early attachment relationships. Yet, as noted earlier in this chapter, epistemic trust extends far beyond close relationships (e.g., even in reading a book). Whenever we seek knowledge from others—ranging from experts to political

---

TABLE 2–4. Three types of trust

Basic trust: Trusting in care for well-being, with caregiving in infancy and secure attachment as a prototype

Epistemic trust: Trusting in knowledge conveyed by means of pedagogy that is perceived as personally relevant and generalizable; conducive to rapid acquisition of cultural knowledge

Social trust: Trusting in the community as contrasted with dyadic relationships, best exemplified and developed in small-scale societies wherein alloparenting (distributed caregiving) plays a prominent role

---

leaders—we are in the territory of epistemic trust (or distrust). Hence, in diverse contexts, basic trust, a mentalizing connection, and epistemic trust come apart. We place epistemic trust in many persons whom we would not confide in or depend on for caring.

I might seem to have left us on a cultural battlefield with the mainstream attachment literature at odds with the vast span of human history and its ongoing cultural diversity. The same discord applies to mentalizing and epistemic trust insofar as they are concordant with attachment theory. Mentalizing engagement certainly comports with the ideology of intensive mothering as Hays (1996) characterized it. Thus, I confess that I was disconcerted to read Otto (2014) asserting that engaging in mind-minded commentary with infants would be considered "ludicrous" among the Cameroonian Nso. This is not to say that mentalizing per se is culture-specific; on the contrary, as a form of social cognition, mentalizing is a human universal. Like other human universals (e.g., running, using language), mentalizing can be done more or less skillfully. Indeed, as Hrdy (2009) argues, extensive alloparenting promotes the development of mentalizing by increasing the breadth of social interactions early in life. The cross-cultural comparisons show, however, that mentalizing as it is manifested in intensive mothering is not universal in the development of culturally adaptive attachment relationships.

Similarly, I was surprised to read anthropologist David Lancy (2016) reporting that instructed learning through teaching (pedagogy), our dominant view of cultural transmission, "is, in fact, quite rare in the ethnographic record." More pointedly, "in numerous cases, direct instruction would be considered an infringement of the child's autonomy" (p. 173). Accordingly, epistemic trust as we think of it in the context of pedagogy would not be a prominent form of social learning. In small-scale societies, culture is learned through the agency of the children more than adults' pedagogical efforts; children are expected to learn more from participation in activities than from adult instruction—to a great extent in activities with peers, such as play and games.

To summarize, Lancy makes a case for "children learning their culture via informal processes, largely at their own pace and initiative" (p. 193). In contrast to

Western culture, in small-scale societies, "intensive, direct verbal instruction is quite rare and the construction of lessons where the practice is reorganized completely to optimize learning rather than production is almost unheard of" (p. 194) Anthropologist Alyssa Crittenden (2016) introduced the concept of "work play" to emphasize how children in small-scale societies learn to become productive in foraging in the context of play with peers: "play is the foundation of hunter-gatherer social life and may be integral to the development of egalitarianism" (p. 163); furthermore, "[t]he utility of this activity cannot be disputed: children are, indeed, feeding themselves and providing substantial caloric investment by way of self-provisioning and food sharing" (p. 168). The capacity for this nonpedagogical cultural learning develops naturally in the context of shared intentionality—and collective intentionality in particular—as Tomasello (2019) explicated, although this learning is not embedded in attachment, mentalizing, and epistemic trust as we construe them.

Despite the stark cultural differences that I have sketched in the context of criticism of attachment theory, I do not feel embattled but rather feel appreciative of the potential for a more inclusive perspective. Attachment theory, augmented by understanding of mentalizing, is extraordinarily well supported by research; in my view, this account of development needs no defense, although routine scientific debate always is in order. But its purview is limited to the extent that we remain under the sway of attachment theory's own developmental origins—developmentally arrested, as it were. Cross-cultural perspectives are instructive.

In educating patients about (mainstream) attachment theory and research, I talk about the caregiver's contribution to the child's security and insecurity—typically, using the mother-infant interaction as the prototype. Then I raise the question "What does the mother need to provide caregiving (including mentalizing) that is conducive to security?" The response: "Security." But her security and mentalizing capacity depend not only on her dyadic attachments (e.g., her partner) but also on social support more generally. Hrdy's (2009, 2016) concept of allomothering and alloparenting more generally—*allocaregiving* might be best—is a compelling model for social support. More generally, we should expand our purview beyond basic trust and epistemic trust to think about social trust, in the sense of trusting in a community. Imagine this: "The communal responsibility for children puts [Cameroonian] Nso parents at ease. They can allow their infants to explore the whole village area without knowing their whereabouts, because they rely on the caregiving and watchfulness of the community" (Otto 2014, p. 220). Not where I live.

Social Trust

The potential advantage of alloparenting, shared care, and attachment networks exemplified in small-scale, non-Western societies should be obvious. The development of collective intentionality, the capacity to relate to an expanded "we" in the sense of a shared way of life, provides a platform for *social trust*, which "emphasizes the distributed relationship across a *community*" (Gaskins et al. 2017, p 330, emphasis added). To reiterate. to be trustworthy in providing security through care, mothers need security, which can be grounded in social trust. Keep in mind Meehan and colleagues' (2016) assertion that alloparental care is not supplementary; it is foundational. Extremely stressful circumstances that undermine community cohesion perforce will undermine caregiving.

In contrasting Western and non-Western societies, Keller (Keller and Otto 2014) asserted that "both models aim at describing and explaining children's development of trust in others as well as trust in their own agency" (p. 309). In the communal model, however, "the sense of security is based on trust in the availability and reliability of a caregiving environment rather than in individual attachment relationships" (Keller 2014, p. 14). Expanding on this point, she explained that "[t]he development of trust to a larger social network extends the range of trusting relationships and thus promotes *security as a contextual/environmental dimension and not a personality characteristic or an interactive process between two individuals*" (Keller and Chaudhary 2017, p. 132, emphasis added). Hence, we can think of trust and the associated sense of security as associated with a group as a whole as well as the secure base provided by a network: "If a child has trustworthy experiences with many people in her group, the child may extend these feelings of trust to others whom she knows less well but is willing to 'test out'" (Morelli et al. 2017, p. 168).

Writing about the socialization of trust, anthropologist Thomas Weisner (2014) also took a broad view: "The universal socialization task for cultures regarding attachment concerns the learning of trust, not ensuring the 'secure' attachment of an individual child to a single caregiver in dyadic relationships." The cultural task is to foster the development of "trust in *appropriate other people*" (p. 263, emphasis added). Sensitive caregiving is "only one part of a nurturing ecocultural *environment*" (p. 267, emphasis in original). Moreover, sensitive and trust-promoting parenting is not only attentive to the child but also "attuned to the cultural expectations and cultural world as well" (p. 272). In a community-oriented network, "Children become adults with relational and attachment security different from, but no less competent and healthy than, what might be a working model of a single secure base, which is then to be generalized to others" (p. 273).

From the perspective of social trust, we who treat attachment trauma that originated in an isolated dyadic context by relying on another isolated dyadic relationship—individual psychotherapy—are going about it the hard way: we must generalize from the dyadic context of psychotherapy to the broader social context. For all its seeming advantages, we in the WEIRD world where intensive mothering takes pride of place in the relatively isolated, nuclear-family context of an industrialized and individualist society pay a significant price: we must develop social trust in a network belatedly rather than from the ground floor of infancy and early childhood. This challenge is especially daunting when the early attachment was traumatic and the ground floor is a foundation of distrust.

A couple of decades ago, I made the point in a patient-education group about trauma that psychotherapy must be a bridge to other relationships, and it can be hard to get on the bridge. A patient responded wisely, "It is even harder to get off the bridge." Fonagy and colleagues' (Fonagy et al. 2019b) advocacy of trusting beyond therapy as the optimal treatment outcome points us in the right direction: off the bridge. Moreover, as it has expanded (Bateman and Fonagy 2019), the mentalizing approach goes far beyond individual psychotherapy to incorporate group therapy, couples therapy, and family therapy as well as community and institutional interventions (e.g., working with school systems and the justice system, including courts and prisons). As I see it, by bringing others onto the psychotherapeutic bridge, these broader interventions pave the way off the bridge. Of course, not only epistemic trust but also—more fundamentally—basic trust must be cultivated in psychotherapy and generalized beyond it. Moreover, basic and epistemic trust are best generalized with social trust in mind. A caveat: social trust must be adapted to the level of trustworthiness of the society.

A Good Society

As a psychologist practicing individual psychotherapy, I can imagine my social worker friends reading the foregoing and saying, "Now you're starting to get it." Fuzzy as it may be from my psychological orientation, I think we need a concept of social trust, and I will expand on it in the next chapter. I am writing these words in the midst of a pandemic coupled with political and racial division; we are in the midst of profound and pervasive social distrust. As the cross-cultural literature attests, we cannot divorce caregiving and its developmental aims from its social context. WEIRD societies such as the contemporary United States are WEIRD more in a persistently dominant ideology than in actual composition, where diversity reigns—even if the WEIRDest among us are blind or even antagonistic to it.

To be most expansive about it, security and trust depend on a trustworthy society—a Good Society, for example, as Robert Bellah and colleagues (1991) envisioned it. Those authors quoted theologian John Snow as follows: "the absence of generational rootedness in a certain place with a long term commitment to its community and economic life makes money—cashflow—the primary source of security" (p. 261). This broad social territory takes us beyond joint intentionality to collective intentionality, as Tomasello (2019) distinguished them. And it takes us beyond the collective intentionality of science: "a really 'professional social scientist' could never be only a specialist" but rather "would also see social science as, in part, public *philosophy*" (Bellah et al. 2008, p. 300, emphasis added).

I lack the expertise to know how much the small-scale societies are idealized in what I have written or in the sources I have cited. In my view, idealizing our contemporary WEIRD society would be tantamount to delusional thinking. Hays appreciated the need for ideals, but she criticized the tremendous burden those ideals placed on American mothers to whom the *public responsibility* for caring and welfare have been delegated. We psychotherapists rightly aspire to create a safe space in which trust and trustworthiness can grow—often enough, in fits and starts. But this safe and psychologically protective space cannot be divorced from its broader social context; in all societies, attachment must take a form adapted to its social context.

I once spoke with a group of patients about trusting in hospital treatment, after which a woman approached me expressing dismay about her difficulty overcoming her distrust. I responded with an idea that was obvious to me but reassuringly novel to her: learning to distrust is reasonable and adaptive in the absence of trustworthiness; the problem to be overcome is distrusting people who are trustworthy. Conversely, practicing on the bridge of psychotherapy, if we promote trusting with the anticipation that patients should merely generalize their newfound trust to other relationships when they get off the bridge, we will be doing them a disservice. As noted earlier in relation to secure and insecure attachment, *flexibility* is most adaptive. So it is with trust and distrust: each is adaptive, contingent on trustworthiness. Discerning the extent of trustworthiness requires mentalizing, and it is no small challenge. I am not inexperienced in being deceived.

With early development in mind, I have started by distinguishing basic, epistemic, and social trust; with the help of philosophers' ethical thinking, I elaborate these and make more distinctions, teasing out the complexities of trusting and trustworthiness, in Chapters 3 and 4, starting with trusting. In the end, I hope you will appreciate how much we gloss over when we casually use the word *trust* in passing.

Summary of Key Points

- Trusting and trustworthiness require the uniquely human capacity for shared intentionality, that is, the mutual recognition of subjectivity associated with mental states conjoined with the proclivity to come together in a meeting of minds that enables us to participate in joint attention, joint commitments, and cooperative activities. Shared intentionality integrates the sense of separateness with an experience of togetherness: you and I can establish a "we" that regulates our actions.

- Trust and cooperation are interdependent. In the context of psychotherapy and close relationships more generally, trust has a cooperative aim in relation to a shared goal: ensuring the well-being of the trusting person who is depending on the trustworthiness of the trusting person.

- Our evolved capacities to form trusting partnerships are shaped in infancy and beyond by the quality of our attachment relationships: secure attachment is conducive to trust, and in secure attachment—attachment trauma most conspicuously—is conducive to distrust.

- Evidence of insecurity by age 12 months and its precursors early in the first year of life show that trust and distrust begin to develop at the unconscious, implicit level; this early learning can continue to influence trust over the subsequent course of development.

- Mentalizing contributes to the development of secure attachment and trusting relationships. Mentalizing in psychotherapy has the potential to restore and promote trust and, most importantly, to promote trust in relationships outside and beyond psychotherapy.

- Attachment theory has been criticized as being culture bound, more specifically, as based on the WEIRD (Western, Educated, Industrialized, Rich, and Democratic) social prototype. This criticism points to the need to shift the balance from focusing on dyadic (e.g., mother-child) relationships to greater attention to trusting in the community.

- Although all three types of trust are intertwined, we can make broad distinctions between basic trust (in care), epistemic trust (in knowledge being conveyed), and social trust (in the community).

Recommendations for Clinical Practice

- You might not need to think about trust when treating patients who have a history of reasonably trustworthy relationships who are cooperating in seeking practical help for circumscribed symptoms. By no means is all serious mental illness associated with a long developmental history of trauma in relationships, but much of it is—albeit in association with other contributors (Allen 2001). You should think about your patient's distrust in you and its foundations in his or her prior relationships and social contexts, often beginning in childhood and continuing into adulthood. I advocate this stance: your patient's distrust is reasonable, and you must develop your trustworthiness in the course of your relationship. When you have come to know your patient's history of untrustworthy relationships and problems with trust come to the fore, tell your patient how you are thinking about his or her distrust. You might elaborate that you will need to learn both to trust each other and to be trustworthy to each other, and it will take time—perhaps a long time. You also might frame the development of trust in the psychotherapy as a treatment goal, with two caveats in mind: First, although trust is crucial for the therapy process itself, developing more trusting relationships beyond the therapy is the ultimate goal. Psychotherapy can become an isolated refuge of trust; if it remains so over a long period, it can become an obstacle to developing trust where it is most needed—in other relationships. Second, as it has been in the patient's past, distrust will continue to be reasonable in the future to the extent that other persons are not trustworthy.

- As implied in this chapter, I recommend that you adopt attachment theory as a developmental framework for understanding trust and distrust. I had the good fortune to work in a hospital setting where I was able to create psychoeducational groups using attachment theory and mentalizing to orient patients to treatment (Allen et al. 2012; Groat and Allen 2011). Short of systematic instruction in groups, I used attachment theory in clinical formulations that I wrote for patients in individual therapy (see Chapter 4). In educational groups, I emphasized the most remarkable research finding: we learn to adapt our ways of seeking care to specific relationships before we can think and talk about how we do it (competence without comprehension). We naturally generalize what we have learned from previous relationships to new relationships, often unconsciously. Attachment research also shows our potential for new learning in infancy and beyond, associated with the flexibility of attachment strategies. Over the course of development, flexibility is abetted by awareness and reflection about ways of relating—for which we use the concept of mentalizing. As framed in this chapter, research on attachment and mentalizing gives us ways of understanding trust and distrust as well as trustworthiness and untrustworthiness.
- Those of us who practice talk therapy—plain old therapy, as I came to call it—must be mindful that, to a large extent, our

trustworthiness will develop on the nonverbal level on the basis of unconscious skill in emotional responsiveness: sharing
emotion, as Tomasello described it; responding emotionally in
a way that reflects how your patient feels rather than becoming completely caught up in your own feelings, as Fonagy and
colleagues articulated it. You will have some control over your
emotional responsiveness, but too much deliberate effort at
such control will backfire and likely abet distrust. As the still-
face experiments show, too much restraint over emotional expression will be disconcerting at best. I found that much of my
psychotherapy supervision revolved around encouraging
therapists to be more natural in relating to their patients—
genuineness, as Rogers construed it.

- Developing trust requires attention to patients' nonverbal expression of emotions and attitudes as well as your own—after
the fact—and reflecting on them. And your patient is liable to
be more aware of your emotional expressions than you are, in
which instance your trustworthiness will entail openness to
learning from these expressions. For example, in the session
following one in which a patient had thrown a piece of furni-
ture across the room, we talked about how we both felt. I emphasized how frightened I had felt; she had perceived me as
angry. Of course I was angry, but I was much more aware of
my alarm. I have commended the developmental principle
"minds need other minds," and this need goes both ways in
therapy.

- Immersing myself in the literature critical of attachment theory
taught me a lesson about cultural humility—embarrassingly belatedly. Our current cultural context of social-political strife
has brought multiple cultural divides to the forefront. Although some of us are more WEIRD than others, none of us is
exempt from the need for cultural humility. We all come from
somewhere, and—no matter how experienced and well educated we might be—our ignorance is vast. I was taken by the
metaphor in the title of a book by Marcelo Gleiser (2014), a
physicist: *The Island of Knowledge*. The larger the island, the
greater its perimeter of ignorance. Awareness of the limitations of your knowledge is a mark of wisdom (Sternberg
2019), which—if my experience in conducting psychotherapy
is any guide—always seems in limited supply.

3

Trusting

The preceding chapters have addressed several aspects of trust: trusting in psychotherapy as a form of treatment, basic and epistemic trust in dyadic relationships, and social trust more generally. In this chapter, I rely substantially on the work of philosophers to address several additional permutations of trust. I consider the relation between trusting and merely relying on someone, trusting a person versus trusting in the person's actions, and the distinction between trusting in care and trusting in competence. I also review aspects of distrust, with emphasis on discernment in distrust—just as we need to trust well, we need to distrust well. The discussion of distrust leads into John Gottman's work illuminating trust and distrust in couples as well as various means of repairing betrayals of trust. I then address the complexities of trusting and distrusting oneself and conclude by elucidating the close connections between hope and trust. We will not leave science entirely behind, but ethics will come into the foreground.

The Ethical-Moral Basis of Trusting

As I noted in the "Introduction," the words trust and trustworthiness are prototypical of *thick* terms that combine facts and values, being descriptive and evaluative at the same time (Williams 1985). "You can't trust him" is a morally freighted description. I agree with Katherine Hawley (2012) that trustworthiness is "thought of as a moral virtue" (p. 45). Being trusted and accepting of that trust entails a moral obligation (Lagerspetz 2015; Potter 2002)—or, more strongly put, an ethical demand (Løgstrup 1997) Conversely, to be distrusted is to feel wronged (Faulkner 2011). When I urge you to reflect on your trustworthiness as a therapist—at least not to take it for granted—I risk moralizing and offending you. I aim instead to highlight the complexities and challenges of being a trustworthy therapist. As therapists, we all will fail to varying degrees, as we do in life more generally. I am advocating awareness, not condemnation.

Our dependency puts trust squarely in ethical-moral territory. As Olli Lagerspetz (2015) put it, "If one were to briefly describe the life of the human being as a species, one characteristic would easily spring to mind: our dependence on other people. It is the very fabric of our lives" (p. 1). Alasdair MacIntyre (1999) elaborated the same point in his book *Dependent Rational Animals*:

> We human beings are vulnerable to many kinds of affliction and most of us are at some time afflicted by serious ills. How we cope is only in small part up to us. It is most often to others that we owe our survival, let alone our flourishing, as we encounter bodily illness and injury, inadequate nutrition, mental defect and disturbance, and human aggression and neglect. This dependence on particular others for protection and sustenance is most obvious in early childhood and in old age. But between these first and last stages our lives are characteristically marked by longer or shorter periods of injury, illness, or other disablement and some among us are disabled for their entire lives. (p. 1)

MacIntyre explained that to depend on others we must trust them. And we must depend not only for basic care—in young and old age as well as in between—but also for help with practical reasoning in many domains, such as in evaluating what is good for us, imagining alternative possible futures, developing self-knowledge, and becoming dependable to others.

Depending on others—trusting—entails making yourself vulnerable to disappointment, betrayal, or exploitation. Yet, if precarious dependency and vulnerability were the only concomitants of trusting, distrusting would be the more reasonable strategy. Sadly, many persons who have not been able to depend on others adopt this strategy to avoid vulnerability. Abetting this attitude, our culture prizes individualism and autonomy. Of course we need to manage on our own—until we must depend on others.

Lagerspetz (2015) made the crucial point that I emphasize in talking about trust with distrusting patients: "In a relationship involving trust I am likely to *feel less, not more, vulnerable* than with people whom I do not trust" (p. 56, emphasis added). In the context of trustworthiness, dependence is a solution, not a problem. Lagerspetz urged his readers to imagine switching roles from trusting to being trusted. Would you think of the person trusting you as being more vulnerable for doing so? In his words,

All things considered, the concept of vulnerability may be an avenue to understanding the ethical significance of trust. But the relation between trust and vulnerability may be construed in different ways. On one level of understanding, speaking of trust as accepted vulnerability naturally induces us to look for ways to reduce such vulnerability, because vulnerability counts prima facie as something to avoid.... We can understand the issue in a different way if we think instead of how to face the vulnerability of the other, a fellow mortal who approaches us with trust. (p. 67)

The ethical context I have sketched here provides the justification for promoting trust *in* psychotherapy with an eye toward fostering trust *beyond* psychotherapy. Consistent with an ethical framework, anthropologists' critiques of attachment theory directed our attention beyond dyadic relationships to consider social trust more broadly. Next I bring in philosophers' perspectives with an eye toward illuminating the high costs of pervasive social distrust that often originates in dyadic relationships.

Trusting in Community

Even in our highly individualistic WEIRD (Western, Educated, Industrialized, Rich, and Democratic) culture, we rely unconsciously and pervasively on generalized social trust. We take trust in community for granted—until it is disrupted by social upheaval and oppression or by trauma in individual relationships so severe as to render a person fearful of almost any social contact. After considering how trust is—or should be—woven into our social life, I focus on a more specific communal domain, that is, trust in communication.

Trusting in the Social Fabric

In the context of our cooperativeness, Paul Faulkner (2017) commented, "thankfully, trust is part of *the fabric* of our society" (p. 111, emphasis added). I like this metaphor. Similarly, Lagerspetz (2015) referred to trust as "a pattern in the weave of life" (p. 95). I am inclined to stretch the metaphor, considering that trust *is* the social fabric of our life—not just part of it. In this sense, trust is not only a state of mind; it is a way of life. We live in trust before we understand it.

Taking trust as our default position, Onora O'Neill (2002) commented on its pervasiveness: "For all of us trust is the most everyday thing. Every day and in hundreds of ways we trust others to do what they say, to play by the rules and to behave reasonably" (p. 23). Annette Baier (1986), whose work catalyzed much of the contemporary philosophical interest in trust, elaborated this point:

Trust, the phenomenon we are so familiar with that we scarcely notice its presence and its variety.... We do in fact, wisely or stupidly, virtuously or viciously, show trust in a great variety of forms, and manifest a great variety of versions of trustworthiness, both with intimates and with strangers. We trust those we encounter in lonely library stacks to be searching for books, not victims. We sometimes let ourselves fall asleep on trains or planes, trusting neighboring strangers not to take advantage of our defenselessness. We put our bodily safety into the hands of pilots, drivers, doctors, with scarcely any sense of recklessness. (pp. 233–234)

The pattern of trust becomes visible in the fabric when trust comes into question. As Knud Løgstrup (1997) put it, "Trust and distrust are not two parallel ways of life. Trust is basic; distrust is the absence of trust...distrust is a 'deficient' form of trust" (p. 18). Lagerspetz (2015) expanded this point: "the positions of trust and distrust are not symmetrical. Trust must be assumed as the default stance and distrust as a subsequent challenge to it. Speaking temporally, the personal development of the individual proceeds from the initial stance of unconditional trust toward greater distrust and discernment" (p. 135). My social fabric analogy is tame compared with Baier's (1986) metaphor: "We inhabit a climate of trust as we inhabit an atmosphere and notice it as we notice air, only when it becomes scarce or polluted" (p. 234). As Lagerspetz (2015) commented pointedly, we are liable to recognize trust *posthumously*—after it has died: "If I start to look for reasons for trusting, the game is already over" (p. 134).

As social fabric, trust is a necessity—for example, if you want to fly on an airplane, sleep on the train, and then find out how to get to the restaurant where you are planning to eat without being poisoned. But when the fabric is torn—or shredded—trust might seem like a luxury. Planes and trains have been blown up by terrorists. Children are shot in schools. With widespread domestic violence and child abuse, the home can be a dangerous place. Trusting what you see and read on the internet is becoming increasingly perilous. All such assaults on trust are pernicious: "*Where we cannot trust and be trusted*, we are shut out of society at large—not only because our contacts with others turn difficult and unpredictable in a practical sense, but because *we are divested of our very capacity as a social agent*" (Lagerspetz 2015, p. 1, emphasis added).

Trusting in Communication

Trusting in communication is woven into the social fabric: Løgstrup (1997) asserted that all speech takes place in the context of fundamental trust, and Faulkner (2011) pointed out that our folk psychology includes the assumption that people generally try to tell the truth. The fact that we are profoundly and pervasively dependent on others for our knowledge puts communication in ethical-moral territory.

Williams (2002) linked trusting in communication to the value of truth and the *virtues of truth*, namely, "qualities of people that are displayed in wanting to know the truth, in finding it out, and in telling it to other people." He distinguished two virtues of truth that bear on trustworthiness, *accuracy* and *sincerity*:

"you do the best you can to acquire true beliefs, and what you say reveals what you believe" (p. 11). He made a strong claim: "to the extent that we lose a sense of the value of truth, we shall certainly lose something and may well lose everything" (p. 7). No doubt, learning the truth and counting on the trustworthiness of those who convey it has a great deal of *instrumental* value; knowledge is a means to an end. But Williams also put a great deal of weight on the *intrinsic* value of truth and truthfulness; we value them for their own sake. Scientists seek the truth in part for its potential technological benefits, yet many also pursue truth for its own sake—often with a passion. What if people told the truth only because they did not want to put their reputation at risk? Could we count on that?

Faulkner (2011) proposed that we hold to a "paired *norm of trust*" (p. 148, emphasis in original): We expect others to tell us the truth, and we expect others to presume that we are telling them the truth. Moreover, in speaking, we implicitly assume responsibility for what our listeners thereby come to believe, and we can be held accountable for it. This sense of responsibility is part of the moral territory of communication. Faulkner presented his views as a *trust theory* regarding our warrant for believing what we are told. We cannot routinely rely on evidence: imagine trying to verify on your own the massive evidence for climate change. In believing what we are told, we implicitly believe the speaker to be trustworthy. We trust *the person* and, accordingly, believe what the person says.

Trusting in the truth of what someone says can be complicated in its own right, but as Faulkner (2011) reminded his readers, our warrant for believing a speaker also depends on our warrant for believing all the others by whom the speaker was informed. Here we are back in the territory of epistemic trust. Faulkner used the analogy of a *bucket brigade* in the passing along of information and knowledge, a fitting analogy for the way I characterize readers of this book trusting in what I have written. We rely on a chain of knowledge transmission and implicit trust; distrust separates the links.

Recall from Chapter 2, "Developing Trust and Trustworthiness," Fonagy and colleagues' contribution in drawing our attention to an ultimate aim of psychotherapy: helping patients become more trusting in the wider community for the sake of ongoing social learning. Potentially, communication with the psychotherapist opens the door to broader social communication beyond the therapist's office and, in conjunction with enhanced epistemic trust, serves the ultimate goal of "*reintegrating the patient into the large, complex, ever-moving stream of human social communication*" (Fonagy et al. 2019b, p. 172, emphasis added). Yet these authors acknowledged "the inherent limitations of clinical interventions in cases where the patient's wider social environment does not support mentalizing" (p. 176). Trusting is adaptive only to the extent that it is matched by trustworthiness. As family therapists are likely to appreciate most keenly, "the consolidation of therapeutic gains—and indeed any meaningful improvement in quality of life for the patient—is contingent on the patient's social environment tolerating and supporting these changes" (p. 177). Alarmingly, many political communities are now riven by distrust. Many people feel downright disoriented in the face of ostensibly alternative realities. I do.

No one in their right mind would claim that the norm of truth telling requires that we be naively credulous. As Williams (2002) declared, people "know that they can tell a lie, as every day millions of people do, and the heavens will not fall; if the heavens were going to fall, they would have fallen already" (p. 85). Faulkner readily acknowledged that acceptance of what we are told must be *reasonable*. It makes no sense to accept what we do not understand, and we rightly question what contradicts other beliefs we hold with conviction, yet we must remain open to persuasive argument (Mercier 2020). Short of reasons to the contrary, Faulkner advocated an *attitude of charity*, giving the speaker the benefit of the doubt and making an effort to understand the speaker's point of view as potentially credible. This trusting attitude is certainly good advice for psychotherapists. Of course, we always can rescind our charitable attitudes.

To sum up, trust and trustworthiness are normative, valued for their own sake, and unthinkingly taken for granted in our relationship to the community as our default stance. The word *normative* refers to a standard; we would have no use for the word if standards were met invariably. I like what O'Neill (2002) wrote: "I think that deception is the real enemy of trust"; furthermore, "the most common wrong done in communicating is deception, which undermines and damages others' capacities to judge and communicate, to act and to place trust with good judgment" (p. 70). Pointedly, she explicated, "Obligations to reject deception are obligations for everyone: for individuals and for governments and for institutions—including the media and journalists" (p. 97). She did not give up on trust, nor should we:

> The risk of disappointment, even of betrayal, cannot be written out of our lives. As Samuel Johnson put it "it is happier to be sometimes cheated than not to trust." *Trust is needed* not because everything is wholly predictable, let alone wholly guaranteed, but on the contrary *because life has to be led without guarantees.* (p. 24, emphasis added)

Trusting Beyond Reliance

Being able to rely on someone is a necessary condition for trusting him or her. I worked with a suicidal patient who had all but given up on humanity. In the context of extensive early trauma, he described growing up with his mother as extremely confusing because she was highly caring and empathic but totally unreliable; she couldn't be counted on to show up on time or to follow through with commitments or promises. My patient became so disillusioned and frustrated with his mother that he gave up confiding in her, and this was a huge loss because her caring had been his only refuge throughout a long siege of adversity. His father consistently minimized his suffering. His peers bullied him, and some of his friends betrayed him. For these reasons, he lamented being unable to depend on his mother. Reliance entails confidence in predictability and availability, a cornerstone of secure attachment. But reliance is not enough for trust in its rich psychological sense.

TABLE 3–1. Contributors to trustworthiness

Being motivated by goodwill toward the trusting person

Being motivated by the fact that the trusting person is counting on you

Moral competence and integrity

A noncoercive context; willingness to be trusted

Think about widely varying senses of the word *trust*. You will understand me if I say I trust my wife but I don't trust my car. You won't blink if I say I trust my dog. As philosopher Carolyn McLeod (2002) poignantly remarked, "for some people it may feel more natural to trust a dog than to trust a human; an example is a child who has been neglected or physically abused" (p. 167). You can trust your car (or not) in the sense of relying on it to start. Similarly, if you need to see someone, you could rely on that person to show up at a certain time and place if you knew his or her habits and could predict his or her behavior. Trust in the sense that matters most in this book adds something to reliance. In trusting a person, we rely on more than behavior; we rely on shared intentionality—a meeting of minds. Table 3–1 summarizes the main psychological contributors to trustworthiness to be discussed next.

Counting on One Another

Annette Baier (1986) highlighted the territory of interest to us: "What is the difference between trusting others and merely relying on them? It seems to be reliance on *their good will* toward one, as distinct from their dependable habits" (p. 234, emphasis added). Karen Jones (2012) considered "good will" to be too vague as a basis for trustworthiness and asserted more pointedly that trust entails *counting on* another person—a masterful application of common language that I will adopt. Think back to trusting your car to get you to work. You also could trust a colleague to pick you up on her way to work. Your car doesn't care if you are relying on it, but, presumably, knowing that you are counting on her matters to your colleague. Going back to development, think of the "we" here. You and your colleague created a joint goal of getting you to work, with different roles: she shows up in her car, and you are there waiting for her.

More specifically, Jones (1996) construed trusting as going beyond cognitive expectations in incorporating an *affective attitude* of confidence and optimism that the trusted person will be "directly and favorably *moved* by the thought that someone is counting on her" (p. 9, emphasis added). Consistent with a mentalizing framework for thinking about reliance, Jones (2012) referred to our need to make decisions about trusting by "taking into account *the mental life* of the other, including their beliefs, intentions, desires, and expectations" (pp. 63–64, emphasis added). Correspondingly, being trustworthy entails "taking into account the fact that others are counting on you" (p. 64). Accordingly, going beyond reliance and reliability by taking mental life into account is the "distinctive work for which we need our concepts of trust and trustworthiness" (p. 65). We might need to think carefully about trusting our car when the battery is on the way out, but we will not be relying on our capacity for shared intentionality.

With vulnerability in mind, Jones (2017) subsequently elaborated her understanding of "counting on" as follows: "To count on something or someone is to embed in your plans and goals an expectation that, if false, means you risk being left worse off than you otherwise would have been" (p. 91). To use the language I have adopted, shared intentionality affords those who are trusted "a distinctive way of responding to the fact of other agents' dependency *through recognizing that very dependency*" (pp. 99–100, emphasis in original). I think Jones has articulated the most succinct and straightforward confluence of trusting and trustworthiness as follows: "*this dual structure of dependency—counting on the other in a domain, and counting on them to respond to the fact that we [are] counting on them—is the heart of trust*" (p. 100, emphasis added). Here we also have the heart of trustworthiness: it matters to you that the other person is counting on you. We have built this foundation for the heart of trust by early childhood in our capacity for joint intentionality: children protest breaches of joint commitments, for example, when a partner walks away from a cooperative activity without explanation.

When you are in the position of being trusted, your trustworthy appreciation of being counted on motivates your commitment to coming through. For example, you are less likely to allow competing interests to interfere with your plans to meet the trusting person's needs. If Charlene calls and you make plans to meet with her to talk about an urgent and painful decision she must make, you will not let a subsequent invitation to go to an appealing event stand in the way ("Sorry, I'd love to go with you, but a friend is counting on me..."). Your steadfast commitment to Charlene requires recognizing her plight and her depending on you for care and help.

The Moral Context of Reliance

As Jones (1996) put it, "when we trust a friend, the competence we expect them to display is a kind of *moral* competence" (p. 7, emphasis in original). Hence, we rightly resent the lack of reliability when trust comes into the relationship. As Lagerspetz (2015) stated, "Trust has a moral aspect that is absent in reliance" (p. 15). For example, if you seek someone out at a time and place they normally appear, you do not feel betrayed if they do not show up; they had no idea you were counting on them to be there. If they knew your need to see them was urgent and promised they would be there, you would feel let down and resentful.

Prioritizing the moral aspect of trusting relationships, McLeod (2002) took issue with the view that we count on the trusted person to be motivated primarily by goodwill toward us: "trust is a moral attitude, which is what distinguishes it ultimately from reliance" (p. 37). In her view, we trust in *moral integrity*. Moral integrity entails commitment to doing the right thing, along with integrating your actions with what you stand for morally. Integrity also entails accountability: if the trusted person fails to come through as anticipated, she will explain, apologize, and make amends. Furthermore, such integrity is not only personal; it is also embedded in social norms: "Those who act with moral integrity act on what they take to be the best moral reasons for everyone to act" (p. 26). To refer back to development, here we have the combination of joint intentionality (the apology) and collective intentionality (the normative expectations) operative by age 6 years.

In my view, being motivated by goodwill and being motivated by moral integrity are not mutually exclusive; they are mutually reinforcing. But McLeod pointed out that they can come apart: "Surely, I can trust what motivates some people to act respectfully toward me is their own moral sense rather than my trust in them" (p. 32). Consider Mark, a patient who wants help with a pressing decision and is trusting his psychotherapist, Dr. Rey, to show up on time for his appointment. At the end of their last session, they talked about this impending decision and agreed to consider it in their next session. To Mark's chagrin, just before the appointment, the receptionist called to let him know that Dr. Rey needed to reschedule. When Mark protested, the receptionist let him know that Dr. Rey had to see another patient who was in an "emergency situation" and that they would fit him into her schedule as soon as possible. Mark felt disappointed and frustrated, thinking that his welfare was taking a back seat. Intuitively, however, he recognized the justification for rescheduling. When Mark and Dr. Rey met again, Dr. Rey apologized for having to reschedule, especially in light of Mark's need to discuss his difficult decision. Mark accepted the apology and said he understood. Would he consider his therapist more trustworthy if, on the basis of her concern for him, she had seen him instead of the patient who was in a more dire situation? Her moral integrity should bolster his sense of confidence. If he learned that she rescheduled his appointment because she didn't want to miss a sale and went shopping instead, that would be a different matter. To reiterate, we have an intuitive appreciation that trust is embedded in joint and collective intentionality: the "we" goes beyond you and I.

Another ethical-moral aspect of trust is its noncoercive quality; we enter into genuinely trusting relationships voluntarily. Jones (1996) gave an example of entrusting without trusting, based on coercing reliance:

> If I can rely on another's fear, my ability to control the purse strings, or the foolishness of another, I might be fully justified in entrusting them with something I care about, for I can know that they will not dare harm it or that it won't occur to them to do so. In such cases, confidence in some other aspect of a person's psychology has replaced confidence in her goodwill, but where this other thing is sufficient to ensure adequate performance, I need not also depend on her goodwill. This is not to say that relationships of reliance aren't sometimes *mixed* or can't depend on both kinds of elements. (p. 19, emphasis added)

If your patient reveals that he "trusts" you not to reveal what he has told you because "confidentiality is a legal requirement of your job," you will not feel trusted.

Coercing reliance entails a failure of shared intentionality, a loss of the "we" on which trust depends. Creating alarm in another person is a common coercive strategy when trust in ordinary responsiveness is lacking. A child who needs attention and care might frighten his mother by climbing a tree within her sight, or a patient who feels neglected might alarm his therapist by displaying fresh cuts on his arms or talking about options for suicide. To respond to such dependency with "They're just trying to get attention" is to fail in mentalizing by minimizing the need. The child or patient *warrants attention* but seeks it in an ineffective way—one that is liable to backfire by evoking anxiety, frustration, and resentment, thereby undermining trust (Allen 2001).

I agree with McLeod (2002) that moral integrity and competence are fundamental in trusting relationships, although they often are in the background. But I think Jones (2017) brought us to the most prominent psychological ballpark with her idea of reciprocity: *counting on and being counted on*. As I have been construing it, concern for the trusting person's well-being plays a predominant role in trustworthiness. But the challenges of trusting—taking account of the mental life of the trusted person, as Jones aptly put it—do not end with that person's assurance of concern for your welfare; they begin. In what sense—and for what—do we count on others when we are trusting them? In what are we placing trust? Here, the process gets complicated.

Degrees of Trust

I think a patient would be naïve to be uncritically trusting of a therapist at the outset, and I think therapists would be naïve to take their trustworthiness for granted. Having discussed the gradual development of the *capacities* to trust, we can think of the gradual *employment* of these capacities—selectively.

Placing Your Trust

As I noted in discussing trusting in communication, we can place trust in a speaker or we can place trust in what was spoken. To introduce a bit of technical jargon that I have come to find indispensable, philosophers refer to this difference as two-place versus three-place trust, that is, trusting the *person* versus trusting the *action* (Baier 1986; Domenicucci and Holton 2017; Faulkner 2017; Jones 2012). I am interested mainly in the two- and three-place senses of trust, but for context, here is the whole four-place list:

1. Kayla trusts.
2. Kayla trusts Caleb.

3. Kayla trusts Caleb to take care of her cats while she is away.
4. Kayla trusts Caleb to take care of her cats because she knows he likes cats.

One-place trust indicates a general *disposition to be trusting*. This optimistic attitude characterizes what I described previously in the context of trust in community. When we move to four-place trust, we are edging into doubt if not outright distrust. Kayla trusts Caleb to take care of her cats because she knows he likes to play with them. Perhaps she feels a need to bolster her trust in Caleb's actions by mentalizing some self-interest on his part. She would feel more trusting if she believed he would take good care of her cats because he appreciates how much she loves them.

Hawley (2012) gave us an account of optimal two-place trust, contrasting it with the three-place alternative: "If you are lucky, there are one or two people you can *trust absolutely*. But not everyone is as lucky as you, and for the most part we trust different people, to different degrees, to do different things" (p. 6, emphasis added). Ideally, two-place trust entails trusting without qualification, unreservedly. When I was discussing this chapter with my wife, Susan, she remarked, "I trust you absolutely," as I do her. We are lucky indeed. But I need to qualify my statement about trusting "without qualifications." Susan would not trust me to fix her car. (She more or less trusts me to drive it.) So "absolute trust" does not entail trusting the other person in every possible domain; that is a matter for three-place trust. No one is competent in everything. To put it vaguely, two-person trust implies trusting the trusted person to be responsive in all respects that might come to matter in the particular relationship, without thinking about potential restrictions. "I trust you absolutely." *Enough said*. "Absolutely?" When we start to query the limitations, doubt about trust has come into play.

Three-place trust entails trusting another person to *do* something or to *know* something (the latter being epistemic trust). The boundaries of three-place trust can be fuzzy. Rarely is the trust we care about limited to some specific action (e.g., picking up a child from school). Rather, as already implied, we trust people with whom we have enduring relationships in one or more broad *domains* and roles (e.g., for help with childcare, as confidants, for financial support). You might think that if you extend the domains widely enough, three-place trust merges into two-place trust. Perhaps. But I would not make that reduction; I think trusting a *person* is different from trusting in *actions*, no matter how broadly construed. No doubt, both kinds of trusting relationships are extremely valuable. Three-place trust leans fairly heavily on reliance, and it is noteworthy that you can trust in a specific action without trusting the person: Even if you don't trust a speaker, you can count on that person for the truth if he or she is testifying under oath and penalty of perjury. Or you can entrust someone with something (e.g., your money) on the basis of a contract or legal sanctions without trusting him or her personally. In these instances, *trust* collapses into mere reliance; the fact that you are depending and counting on the "trusted" person does not motivate him or her.

In my way of thinking, two-place trust (in a person) has obvious *intrinsic value*. Such trust has many benefits, but a trusting relationship is valuable in itself, for its own sake. Recall Hawley's point: "If you are lucky, there are one or two people you can trust absolutely." Useful? Of course. But such a relationship is good in itself, arguably, among the highest goods. In contrast, three-place trust (relying on actions and knowledge) has more obvious *instrumental value*, as a means to an end. As Faulkner (2017) stated, "This [instrumental] form of trust, its *contractual* form one might call it, cannot be fundamental; or at least it cannot be so if trust is something that is intrinsically valued" (p. 118, emphasis in original).

Here is a chicken-and-egg question: Which comes first, trusting in a person or trusting in the person's actions? Lagerspetz (2015) put two-place trust first: "Some tendency to trust must be presumed as a given already before strategic relations develop" (p. 41). Thus, he advocated starting with "simple trust…[because] we are unlikely to trust people *with* anything unless we trust *them*" (p. 51). Recall that we trust what a speaker says when we trust the speaker. But consider this: How do we learn to trust a person as a person? Wouldn't a history of his or her actions play a cardinal role in the development of such trust? Also recall the idea that reliance is a precondition for trust and that trusting anchors reliance in perceived trustworthiness. As we rely successfully on a person's actions, we are likely to broaden the scope of that reliance and then to come to trust the person. In this scenario, three-place trust evolves into two-place trust. We should think in terms of *synergy rather than sequence*: ideally, two- and three-place trust build on each other over time. We would hope for this synergy as psychotherapy relationships develop. Conversely, being let down on occasion will erode trust in the people who let you down, and you will be less inclined to rely on their actions—or on *them*.

Deciding to Trust

Ordinarily, we do not think about trusting, and we do not decide to trust. Sometimes, however, we do need to make decisions because we must take action that requires depending on someone when we are hesitant to do so. Lagerspetz (2015) argued against the idea that trusting typically entails voluntary decisions, but he gave an example of an exception:

> Consider what might look like a quintessential "decision to trust": stepping down from a quay into a tiny boat in moderately rough weather. The decision may further involve small momentary, as it were, sub-decisions such as grasping the boatman's outstretched hand and taking the cue from him for when to make the leap. Perhaps there is a moment of hesitation, an inquiring look into the man's eyes and then the decisive step. On the whole the case might be described in the terms that many studies of trust would favour: as a case of weighing a risk against the perceived trustworthiness of those whom we rely on. (p. 69)

Alternatively, imagine someone who, already afraid of flying, has seized on well-publicized evidence of untrustworthy airlines, airplanes, and pilots. His distrust reinforces his fears. His plight. His father is acutely ill in a hospital across the country, and the illness could prove fatal. He must decide whether to get on a plane.

Our patients likely will be deliberating and deciding about how much to trust us therapists and others. Walking into our office will not be a one-off event, like stepping into a boat or getting on a plane. If there are decisions to be made—in how much to confide, for example—there will be a multitude. None of us makes a decision without context. Trusting is a way of thinking about a relationship and thus is a lens for perception. Lagerspetz (2015) asserted that trust is not as much a matter of deciding as it is *interpreting*. In evaluating a person's trustworthiness, we face a paradox: "we are adducing evidence in support of trust or distrust, but trust and distrust are in turn used to interpret evidence" (p. 80).

The way we construe our interactions and relationships influences our trusting. The therapist looks at her watch, and the patient exclaims, "I saw that! You can't wait 'til this session is over and you don't have to deal with me anymore. I've been thinking that you'd like me to quit this therapy." The therapist replies, "I'm concerned that you saw it that way. Let me tell you what I was thinking. I wanted to see if we had enough time left to talk about something I've been wondering about that could be painful and complicated. Now I'm glad that we do have some time left to talk about your feeling that I'd like to be rid of you."

Some of the difficulty in thinking about deciding to trust relates to the distinction between trusting as an attitude and trusting as an action. We cannot simply decide to adopt an attitude toward a person, but we can decide to ask for help. I am in accord with Faulkner (2011), who wants it both ways: "trust is both an attitude and an action" and they interact inasmuch as "an act of trust follows a decision to trust" (p. 151). The *attitude* of trust that grounds trusting actions develops—more unconsciously than consciously—from trusting *actions*; actions and attitudes are synergistic, a synergy that we promote in psychotherapy.

Jones (1996) took this way of thinking one step further in a path I find appealing. Here is her reasoning: "Because trust involves an affective attitude, it is not something that one can adopt at will…. [T]rust cannot be demanded." But she allows that there can be "an element of decision" in adopting an attitude. Her final point is the one I adopt: "While trust cannot be willed, it can be *cultivated*" (p. 16, emphasis added). In the service of cultivating trust, Jones referred to attention: "We cultivate trust by a selective focus of attention toward the grounds for trust and away from the grounds for distrust" (p. 16). Cultivation implies nurturing and growth, befitting psychotherapy. Decisions will come into play in the gradual process of growing trust. I advocate using another word that bridges the gap between action and attitude: *allowing* yourself to trust, gradually and cautiously. With psychotherapy in mind, I draw a broad distinction between care and competence. Ideally, our patients will allow themselves to trust us in both domains, to the extent that we are caring and competent.

Trusting in Care and Competence

Toward the end of his life, philosopher Ludwig Wittgenstein wrote to his friend Norman Malcom to inform him that he had been diagnosed with prostate cancer. Referring to the prospects for treatment, he wrote, "I have an immensely kind doctor who isn't a fool either" (Malcom 1958, p. 95). There we have the ideal combination of care and competence. You can think of a two-by-two matrix with the less than ideal forms, caring without competence or competence without caring. And this matrix also would include the worst case: neither care nor competence. Notably, caring well requires its own interpersonal competence.

Trusting in Care

We come into life prepared to trust in care; in much of social life thereafter, we have the luxury of trusting unthinkingly—if our basic trust has not been assaulted traumatically by neglect, abuse, social oppression, or political upheaval. Maybe we need a concept of *basic trauma* for assaults on this expansive concept of basic trust; such assaults are by no means rare.

With trusting in care as a backdrop, I am allowing for blurring the boundaries between basic trust and social trust to encompass a more expansive sense of trust as primordial, unconscious, and a precondition for social life more generally—as in the metaphor of trust as the social fabric. Lagerspetz (2015) expressed this overarching conception fully in a way that encompasses Erikson's (1963) usage and my own focus on caring relationships as the wellspring of trust:

> The notion of *basic trust* plays an important role in the philosophical trust debate. The idea is, in brief, that some form of generalized trust is necessary for human life and even sanity to prevail. We need to believe in the essential continuity of the social life around us, and we must act on the assumption that people generally are not hostile or out to deceive us. The idea of basic trust also implies that this attitude is essentially groundless; basic trust must be innate or primordial. Initially, we encounter the world with a self-evident sense of trust, a natural substratum for the subsequent growth of more reflexive approaches to the world of human and physical relations. (p. 131, emphasis added)

In the same vein, Baier (1986) elaborated this unreflective nature of infant trust, allowing for an elastic use of the word: "My account of trust has been designed to allow for unconscious trust…as well as for conscious trust the truster has chosen to endorse and cultivate" (p. 244). Hence, Baier found it plausible to suppose that "infants emerge from the womb already equipped with some *ur-confidence in what supports them*" (p. 244, emphasis added), and she put this ur-confidence on the ground floor of trusting:

> Infant trust that normally does not need to be won but is there unless and until it is destroyed is important for an understanding of the possibility of trust. Trust is much easier to maintain than it is to get started and is never hard to destroy. Unless some form of it were innate, and unless that form could pave the way for new forms, it would appear a miracle that trust ever occurs. (p. 242)

Infants' natural confidence is best safeguarded by love, as Baier understood it: "The best reason for confidence in another's good care of what one cares about is that it is a common good, and the best reason for thinking that one's own good is also a common good is being loved" (Baier 1986, p. 243). Love exemplifies the "we" in the relationship. Loving *entails* care for the well-being of the loved.

Primordial trust is innate; distrust is learned, but it also is learned unconsciously. As we have seen, insecurely attached infants have learned to reserve their trust unconsciously, being competent if not comprehending. In light of these nonconscious strategies in infancy, Lagerspetz (2015) rightly stated, "In the small child, the opposite of trust is typically not called doubt, distrust or suspicion but, perhaps, *fear*" (p. 146, emphasis added). If not outright fear, I would opt for aversion or wariness—none mentalized explicitly. Indeed, understanding problems with trust as such can be a long time in coming, as psychotherapeutic work on elucidating poorly comprehended patterns of distrust attests.

Baier (1986) could have been writing about psychotherapy here:

> there is no strain whatever in the concept of automatic and unconscious trust, and of unchosen but mutual trust. Trust between infant and parent, at its best, exhibits such primitive and *basic trust*. Once it is present, the story of how trust becomes self-conscious, controlled, monitored, critical, pretended, and eventually either cautious and distrustful of itself, or discriminatory and reflexive, so that we come to trust ourselves as trusters, is relatively easy to tell. What will need explanation will be the ceasings to trust, the transfers of trust, the restriction or enlargements in the fields of what is trusted, when, and to whom. (p. 245, emphasis added)

To set the stage for turning to trusting in competence in the next subsection, I want to underscore the distinction between basic trust and instrumental trust—trust in the *person* as caring, contrasted with trust in the person's *doing something* for which you are counting on them. Critical of philosophers' emphasis on the instrumental value of trust, Lagerspetz (2015) proposed the metaphor of starting with an empty shopping cart and a shopping list, looking for profitable opportunities for placing trust—"a rather sad comment if philosophy is assumed to reflect central concerns of the culture in which it is produced" (p. 156). In contrast, basic trust in care pertains to the quality of a relationship, as Faulkner (2017) put it, "a basic *attitude* that one can take *towards a person,* which involves making positive presumptions about their goodwill toward oneself" (p. 121, emphasis added). Construing trusting as an *attitude of the heart,* Stephen Darwall (2017) proposed, "When we trust…we invite the person we are trusting to accept our trust and trust in it, to trust that we are indeed trusting him." He added, "When we trust someone, we implicitly invite him to trust himself also. We regard him as trustworthy and bid for him to see himself this way as well" (p. 35). Ideally, in psychotherapy as well as in the rest of life, trusting and trustworthiness go both ways, and all these reciprocal relations are mutually enhancing.

As I think of it, basic trust in care entails trusting the other person with your feelings, your well-being, and—at the fullest extension—your life. You entrust the other person not with something concrete but rather with *your person,* that is, *you.* I also find appealing a complementary way of thinking about a mutual relationship of basic trust. In an interchange with Lagerspetz (2015), Baier proposed that the "entrusted 'goods' may…consist of the *trustful relation itself"* (p. 52, emphasis added). I think Baier showed profound insight here: we should think of absolute trust (Hawley 2012) as *mutual commitment to the trusting relationship,* which includes confidence that inevitable ruptures will be healed in a cooperatively caring partnership. I cannot think of any more valuable contributor to making a good life.

Trusting in Competence

Karen Jones (1996) explicated the importance of combining trusting in care with trusting in competence: "At the center of trust is an attitude of optimism about the other person's *goodwill.* But optimism about goodwill is not sufficient, for some people have very good wills but very little *competence,* and the incompetent deserve our trust almost as little as the malicious." She went on to say that "When we trust professionals, from plumbers to physicians, we expect of them a technical competence (and *minimal decency)"*—words especially pertinent to our agenda (pp. 6–7, emphases added). Regarding minimal decency, I agree about plumbers, I want more from physicians, and I think a good measure of basic trust in care beyond minimal decency is essential in psychotherapy. As Jones fully appreciated, trust in competence pertains to all our trusting relationships, although it is highlighted in professional relationships. In this subsection, I focus directly on our main interest, psychotherapy relationships.

What constitutes competence in conducting psychotherapy? The answer is nearly unfathomably complex. As described in Chapter 1, "From Trusting Therapies to Trusting Therapists," to benefit from experience, therapists are advised to engage in deliberate practice. Yet, given the diversity of treatment approaches, we cannot make specific prescriptions for *what* to practice. In what sort of competence will the patient trust? We could come back to common factors: competence in caring and in developing a collaborative therapeutic alliance. From the perspective of trust, I would advocate skill in creating and maintaining an experience of "we," including skill in reinstating it when it is lost—as it frequently will be. Therapists, take heart: we develop the capacity to create the sense of "we" by age 3.

As I discussed in connection with placing trust, repeated experience of trustworthy actions (including mentalizing) might ultimately develop into a feeling of trust for the person. This development is more prominent in longer-term therapies; to the extent that such trust develops in any therapy, the trusting relationship takes on *intrinsic* value, being valuable as such. Yet patients seek psychotherapy for practical help with problems ranging from specific symptoms (e.g., a phobia) to more pervasive problems in living (predominantly in relationships). The more specialized treatments (cognitive-behavioral therapies, generally) entail patients trusting in procedures and the therapist's skills in implementing them. To that extent, patients' trust has *instrumental* value.

Even as an undergraduate student, I had the skill to conduct systematic desensitization, a form of exposure therapy, because the procedures (teaching relaxation and creating a graded series of imagined challenges) were simple to follow for me and my patient. However, when it came to helping him with more general problems in living, I was in over my head—not competent and not trustworthy in that domain. Appropriately, I did not trust myself to help. Although it was a stretch that would not be done these days, I could be trusted to do systematic desensitization because it was a simple procedure. Ironically, I was performing the one genre of therapy (for problems with anxiety) that Jerome Frank concluded late in his career required a particular brand of therapy: exposure therapy (Frank and Frank 1991). But it is instructive to think about the other end of the continuum from systematic desensitization for a public-speaking phobia: exposure therapy for the treatment of trauma. In that case, implementing the procedures becomes far more daunting and requires far more skill, including a blending of care and competence. Moreover, especially in the context of attachment trauma, the patient needs to trust not only in the therapist's skill in the procedures but also in the therapist as a person.

Edna Foa's (Foa and Rothbaum 1998) extensively researched prolonged-exposure treatment for posttraumatic stress disorder illustrates the need to trust the therapist as a person as well as the procedure. The therapist engages the patient in recounting traumatic experiences in full detail, repeatedly, in the presence of the therapist. The sessions are audiotaped, and the patient plays the recordings at home for additional exposures. The treatment also can be enhanced with in vivo exposure (e.g., if the patient was sexually assaulted in a parking garage, going back into parking garages—in a safe context). On paper, the skill required to conduct this treatment seems modest. The procedures and the thinking behind the treatment can easily be explained to the patient.

Yet, when you take into account the potential terror that remembering details of trauma might evoke, attachment needs come to the fore: a feeling of safety in the relationship with the therapist is crucial to enable the patient to engage in the treatment. Then consider that a history of attachment trauma will evoke distrust, especially in the fraught context of remembering and reliving past attachment trauma. In this context, the conduct of the treatment requires an exceptional level of interpersonal skill. Foa's cognitive theory (Foa and Rothbaum 1998) does not take into account that care and competence (including competence in care) must be blended in prolonged-exposure treatment for trauma, and the patient must trust in both: the caring, compassionate, calming engagement of the therapist contributes a great deal to making this painful experience bearable, manageable, and ultimately therapeutic (Morrison 2011).

In addition to trusting in the therapist's skill, patients also must trust in the therapist's knowledge, the domain of epistemic trust, which consists of knowledge conveyed by the therapist to the patient. Yet trusting in the therapist's knowledge goes beyond epistemic trust, encompassing an extraordinarily wide range of knowledge—personal and professional—that informs the practice of therapy, consciously and unconsciously. And personal knowledge includes ethical knowledge, albeit rarely based on reading philosophy.

To sum up, I have drawn attention to various strands of trust in therapeutic work, but we need to weave the whole fabric together in practice. I have distinguished between trusting in care and competence and have delineated various features of each of these. In our various relationships, we interweave these facets in a variety of textures and blends—focusing our attention more on care or competence. We use the loom of mentalizing to do much of the weaving. Fortunately, we generally do this inherently complex interweaving intuitively—when all goes well. As we consider next, all the strands in the intuitively woven fabric of trusting can come apart in the process of distrusting. Then we need to create a safe relationship to focus on the source of trouble and figure out how we might rectify it.

Distrusting Well

We should trust the trustworthy and distrust the untrustworthy—to the extent that they are trustworthy and untrustworthy. Baier (1986) proposed that we need to "trust not only our trust but, even more vitally, our distrust" (p. 260). We need to get distrust right, distrusting well, and it is not easy, especially for individuals whose capacity for developing trust has been damaged.

Following Jones (1996), we should distinguish the *absence of trust* from active *distrust*:

> Given that trust and distrust both involve attitudes…they do not exhaust the possible stances we can take toward another's goodwill and competence…[and] the absence of trust is not to be equated with distrust, for one may fail to trust without actively distrusting—one may simply not adapt any attitude at all toward the goodwill and competence of another. (p. 16)

In the course of cultivating a trusting relationship in psychotherapy, we might hope to move from active distrust to absence of trust, a more neutral stance that implies openness to trusting, perhaps contingent on the therapist's passing the patient's tests. As a therapist, I am not averse to being tested if the tests are not unreasonably difficult.

In short, we all *trust selectively*—at least we should—with respect to persons and domains. To reiterate, such selectivity does not necessarily imply distrust, but rather implies good sense. We also must think in terms of degrees. I think of a graded scale of limitation ranging from vigilance to suspicion to distrust. *Vigilance* entails being alert to difficulty, problems, and danger—being watchful, paying close attention, and monitoring. Imagine, as a patient, your first sessions with a psychotherapist, when you are not taking anything for granted. Is she paying attention? Listening? Understanding? Remembering? Responding emotionally? Letting you know what she's hearing and thinking? How are you feeling as the session progresses? After you have left the office? Over time, if all goes well, such vigilance will lessen, but it will wax and wane—likely waxing when you address problems or experiences that entail a deeper level of trust (e.g., revealing a shameful secret).

Vigilance is sensible. We use the term *hyper*vigilance to refer to what seems to be an excessive level; with hypervigilance, we are on the road to suspicion. With *suspicion*, you enter the realm of heightened uncertainty, imagining without clear evidence that something undesirable, wrong, or dangerous is in the offing. When you are vigilant, you are paying attention; when you are suspicious, something does not feel right. Imagine a therapist in the following scenario in which Jones (1996) considered suspicion regarding a salesperson recommended by a reliable friend:

> On the basis of the recommendation, I believe that the salesman is trustworthy, yet I find myself unable to help viewing him with suspicion. I continue to see him as untrustworthy, although I am not yet prepared to abandon my belief that he is trustworthy. I cannot articulate why I view him with suspicion, except to say that there is *something creepy* about him, something in his manner that I don't like. (p. 24, emphasis added)

In this example, lacking justification for a belief that the salesman is truly untrustworthy, Jones concluded that her distrust could not be justified. Yet, if the stakes were high (as they would be in psychotherapy), she would be inclined to act on her feelings: "This is because emotions and other affective states often do represent the world in the way it is: those we are suspicious of often are untrustworthy" (p. 24).

Running counter to the current climate of social distrust, Hugo Mercier (2020) argued that our proclivity toward epistemic vigilance should allow more space for *open vigilance*, that is, alertness to valuable information provided by social communication, which is vital to our development and well-being and for which we have evolved sophisticated social-cognitive capacities. Ideally, we can assess plausibility of information (consistency with prior beliefs), use our reasoning capacities to be responsive to good arguments, identify people who know better (e.g., on the basis of past performance), gauge the extent to which the incentives of those who communicate are aligned with our own, and judge whether others are diligent in obtaining and providing information that is useful to us. We could construe Fonagy and colleagues' (2019a) efforts to promote epistemic trust as cultivating *open* vigilance: looking for opportunities to acquire knowledge rather than shutting ourselves off to them.

I am generally in favor of "trusting your gut." Feelings can be a lot more discerning than beliefs. But there is also something to be said for open-mindedness in the midst of imaginatively suspicious uncertainty, especially if you have an exceptional inclination toward distrust. As Jones noted, you can cultivate either trust or distrust through selective attention and interpretation—starting down a path, fixing your attitude, and blinding yourself to contrary evidence. You could feel, for example, so desperately in need of closeness and caring that you imagine people to be more trustworthy than they are; in so doing, you blind yourself to what others would see as red flags. Ultimately, you are blindsided, reinforcing distrust. Not uncommonly, on this roller coaster individuals oscillate between the extremes of trusting and distrusting. Regarding the latter, at its apex, suspicion becomes paranoia, flagrantly unwarranted distrust. Excessive suspiciousness can turn into a self-fulfilling prophecy: in any relationship, looking for signs of betrayal and making accusations of untrustworthiness generate defensiveness and ill will, which can lead to withholding at best and retaliation at worst. Psychotherapists are expected to be sturdy in the face of unreasonable suspiciousness, especially when they appreciate its origins in earlier relationships. But therapists are human, and their effectiveness can be undermined by relentless suspiciousness along with continual unreasonable tests they are bound to fail. I witnessed many escalating crises in hospital treatment: As a paranoid patient became angrier and threatening, the staff became more controlling and restrictive, continually escalating the patient's paranoia. Someone needed to back off. I once recommended "unilateral disarmament" to a threateningly provocative patient who continually felt threatened.

The absence of trust lies in an emotionally neutral zone, whereas distrust implies a negative judgment about the person distrusted. As Hawley (2012) put it, "To distrust someone is to think less of them, to think of them as doing something wrong, however minor" (p. 9). Here, the domain of distrust makes a difference in judgment: in most relationships, we are likely to be more forgiving of failures of competence than failures of goodwill, the latter being associated with more moralized criticism. In a recent conversation, Len Horwitz put it this way: patients forgive mistakes of the mind but not of the heart. But we want both care and competence, especially in relationships with professionals in which we are specifically seeking implicitly professed competence and are likely to resent incompetence.

We also need to think about limiting our willingness to be trusted along with limiting our trust. Being trusted can be an unwelcome burden. And trusting can be presumptuous in failing to consider the trusted person's willingness to be trusted. Hawley (2012) explained:

Calling someone "untrustworthy" is a moral criticism, and it's not something I'd like to hear about myself. But that doesn't mean I'd prefer to be drowning in others' trust, constantly expected to do as others prefer. *Sometimes I want to be left alone with my own choices without having others rely on me.* (p. 9, emphasis added)

Clarifying the extent to which a trusted person is willing to be relied on is an important matter, especially in psychotherapy relationships. Therapists' failure to be clear about these limits can lead to unwarranted imputations of untrustworthiness, when the absence of trust would be more fitting. Here we come back to being trustworthy in limited domains. Accepting phone calls, for example (especially at 3 A.M.), is a matter for discussion and negotiation. Explicitly limiting domains of trust—setting clear boundaries—is an aspect of trustworthiness that can prevent distrust.

Trust and Distrust in Couples

Looking back on his decades of research and treatment with couples, Gottman (2011) construed his earlier approach as "essentially a 'cookbook' with practical recipes" (p. 37) for building relationships. He concluded, "It all felt too mechanistic," and "something fundamental, mysterious, and basic was apparently missing from our analysis" (p. 38). He came to appreciate how, from the beginning years of their relationship, "couples work to see if they can trust each other in various areas of their lives. They are setting up a secure relationship as a base for building up a life together" (pp. 76–77). He discovered in his study of newlyweds that all their conflicts revolved around trust. He enumerated typical concerns that dominated their discussions: "'Can I trust you to be there for me when I am upset?' 'Can I trust you to help me with the housework?' Can I trust you to back me up even if it's against your mother?' Can I trust you to keep your promises?'" (p. 107). The overriding question is this: "Are you there for me?" (p. 176), which I construe as basic trust. As my colleague Michael Groat reiterated in the patient-education groups we led: "I need to know that you have my back."

Gottman is rare among developers of therapies in putting trust front and center in the treatment, and his approach is compatible with the ground we have covered in this book. He explicitly links his work on trust to the attachment literature, describing trust as "the mysterious quality that somehow created safety, security, and openness for both of them" (p. 39). As Fonagy has done, Gottman construes trusting as central to the *outcome* of treatment inasmuch as it promotes resilience to future challenges and problems that could otherwise undermine the relationship. Although he does not use the term *mentalizing*, Gottman implicitly promotes this concept in the moment-to-moment interactions between partners as well as in helping them develop a coherent narrative of their relationship. Finally, he grounds his thinking in research with couples that includes meticulous coding of videotaped interactions as well as structured interviews to assess aspects of their family history, their attitudes to ward emotion, and their narrative of their relationship: their oral history, the "story of us," which is perfect language to capture the shared intentionality of the "we" in their relationship. Here I focus on his illuminating work on the development of distrust and its extreme form in the context of betrayal, which starkly illustrates the loss of the "we" and its restoration in efforts to rehabilitate trust in the wake of betrayal.

From Distrust to Betrayal

Through his research on interactions and narratives in couple relationships, Gottman systematically traced the antecedents of distrust and their progression into the worst-case scenario of distrust: betrayal. He validated his theory in part by relating the hallmarks of distrust to the likelihood of divorce. Here I summarize his understanding of distrust in relation to attachment theory, the markers of distrust in interactions and narratives, and the turn from distrusting to betraying.

Recall that depending on someone in the context of a plight brings trust to the fore. Gottman applies the concept of *attachment injuries* from the literature on couples therapy: "incidents in which one partner responds or fails to respond at times of urgent need," including "perceived abandonment, betrayal, or breach of trust in a *critical moment of need* for support expected of attachment figures" (Brassard and Johnson 2016, p. 815, emphasis added). Thinking in terms of attachment injuries prompted Gottman (2011) to conclude that "the atom of eroding trust is the unavailability or the unresponsiveness (or turning against) of a partner when the other is in need of understanding, comfort, or love—that is, not *'being there'* for our partner when he or she needs us" (p. 344, emphasis added). To use Jones's language, we could say that the partner could not be *counted on*. Using Fonagy's language, we could construe the injury as linked to *mentalizing failures*. Using my understanding of the crux of attachment trauma, we could think of the trusting partner feeling left *alone in pain, feeling invisible.*

Gottman identified four recurrent patterns of interaction during discussions of conflict that are highly predictive of divorce: *criticism* related to a perceived personality flaw in the partner, with "selfishness" being a prototypical accusation; *defensiveness* evident, for example, in proclaiming one's innocence or meeting attack with counterattack; *stonewalling*, in the failure to engage with the partner nonverbally and verbally; and *contempt*, expressing an attitude of superiority, evident in name calling and put-downs, such as correcting the partner's grammar. Among these "four horsemen of the apocalypse" (Gottman 2011, p. 121), one stands out: Contempt is the "most corrosive" of the four (p. 325); more specifically, "Contempt is our single best predictor of divorce. We also found that a husband's contempt predicts the number of a wife's infectious illness in the next 4 years. It is interesting to note that the frequency of contempt among happy couples is nearly zero" (p. 123). All these damaging patterns exemplify failures of attunement and mentalizing.

The development of distrust also is evident in relationship narratives obtained in the oral history interviews conducted with couples. As distrust evolves in the context of attachment injuries and conflicts, the dynamic story-of-us shifts from being positive to a negative reframing of the relationship history. Unresolved conflicts haunt memory. Negative sentiments override and obscure whatever positive attributes or actions might be present. Hypervigilance abets distrust. The sense of "we-ness" in the story-of-us is undermined by a transition to "me-ness," heralded by

> deciding that one's partner has lasting negative traits that 'explain' the continual negativity. Empirically, the most common negative attribution is 'my partner is selfish.' This fact shows that it is precisely trust that erodes. People stop believing that their partner is thinking about their best interests. (Gottman 2011, p. 203)

The pathway from trust to distrust to betrayal is marked by a fundamental shift in the balance of interests in the relationship. Gottman described this shift with elegant simplicity. *Trustworthiness* entails looking out for your partner's interests (as well as your own); *untrustworthiness* entails no longer looking out for the partner's interests but rather focusing exclusively on your own interests; and *betrayal* entails looking out for your own interests at the *expense* of your partner's interests, that is, when pursuing your own interests is detrimental to your partner.

Furthermore, the shift from distrust to betrayal is marked by a fundamental shift in mentalizing the benefits and costs of the relationship. The couple's relationship becomes devalued; then imagined alternative relationships become more valued by comparison—and, ultimately, pursued. Loyalty shifts to disloyalty. Addressing conflicts in the relationship shifts to confiding about problems in the relationship to a new partner. Secrets and deception come into play, and untrustworthiness dominates. Over time and often insidiously, the accumulation of relatively common and reciprocal attachment *injuries* and associated emotional withdrawal potentially evolve into an attachment *trauma* as a result of betrayal.

Restoring Trust

Gottman (2011) described three contexts in which trust becomes salient, with the potential for erosion or cultivation. The first consists of *everyday interactions* that entail bids for connection and comprise "micro trust tests" (p. 178), such as simple requests, sharing events, problem-solving, affection, empathy, and sexual intimacy (p. 198). Turning away from or against the partner in these everyday situations will erode trust, whereas turning toward the partner will re-

store trust. The second context consists of *regrettable incidents*, fights being prototypical. Gottman said he frequently is asked, "What do couples fight about
mostly?" He answers, "Absolutely nothing," explaining, "they usually hurt each
other's feelings in very ordinary, seemingly meaningless, small moments that
seem to arise from about absolutely nothing" (p. 202). For example,

> a couple is watching television and he has the remote control. He is channel surf-
> ing when she says, "Leave it on that channel." He says, "Okay, but let me first see
> what else is on...." She responds by saying, "No! Just leave it. I hate it when you
> channel surf." He throws down the remote and angrily says, "fine!" She responds
> by saying, "I don't like the way you said 'fine.' That hurt my feelings." He says, "I
> said 'fine' because you are always going to get your way, so fine, have it your way.
> I don't want to argue." She says, "I don't even want to watch TV with you any-
> more." He responds by saying, "I don't want to talk about it," and leaves the
> room. (pp. 202–203)

In such incidents, trust is eroded by dismissing attitudes toward emotion, emotional flooding, building resentment, and developing a pessimistic narrative
about the partner (e.g., in the TV example, he or she is "selfish"). This cascade
prepares the path to hopelessness about the relationship. Such incidents become resolved and hope is restored when the events are processed in the context of mutuality, which includes attunement to feelings, acceptance of
responsibility, expressing needs, and planning for future incidents.

Gottman's third context for trust becoming salient is *discussions of conflict*,
which he has studied in detail. The stage is set for cultivation or erosion of trust
in the *first three minutes* of the discussion: if negativity is not interrupted
quickly, the couple becomes absorbed in it and potentially emotionally flooded.
Strikingly, earlier research (Gottman 1994) showed that "only 4% of couples
were able to turn around a conversation that started negatively" (Gottman 2011,
p. 283). These discussions of conflict exemplify and cultivate hope and trust
when they begin with a predominance of positive feelings, evident in affection,
humor, and agreement. They also entail empathy, acceptance of responsibility,
and positive perceptions of the relationship.

We might also think of the ways of cultivating trust that Gottman discovered in the contexts of everyday interactions, regrettable incidents, and discussions of conflict as *distrust prevention*. Cultivating trust builds hope in the
relationship. Without such skillful responsiveness and conflict resolution, distrust is liable to harden and runs the risk of betrayal. Cultivating trust in the aftermath of betrayal requires a major effort. Gottman views restoring trust after
betrayal as tantamount to creating a new relationship. This creation requires
hope, which entails the daunting challenge of recovering from hopelessness
about the relationship.

Trust begets trust: Trusting the betraying partner—courageously, in a state
of heightened vulnerability—has the potential to increase the partner's trustworthiness (responsiveness to being counted on). Ongoing distrust is liable to

undermine the development of trustworthiness. Suspiciousness is likely in the context of betrayal, but Gottman advocates vigilance. Trusting and trustworthiness develop together, as do distrusting and untrustworthiness.

Gottman (2011) laid out a set of prescriptions for restoring trust after betrayal. These prescriptions are self-explanatory, and I will merely enumerate them: without defensiveness, the betrayer listens nondefensively to the partner's feelings; the betrayer expresses remorse; the couple creates transparency (vigilance) and refrains from behavior that could rock the boat; the couple comes to understand how the distrust and betrayal developed in the relationship; the couple establishes mutual cooperation; and the hurt partner accepts an apology and begins a complex process of forgiveness. All these prescriptions offer pathways to hope in the relationship.

I cannot read Gottman's work without thinking about mentalizing, and the mentalizing approach to couples therapy, explicated by Efrain Bleiberg and Ellen Safier, bears mention in this context. They advocate "a systematic effort to stimulate and restore mentalizing and trust" in the couple's relationship (Bleiberg and Safier 2019). The mentalizing treatment begins by educating the couple about mentalizing and trust as well as conducting individual and joint interviews to assess mentalizing capacities in the context of the relationship. These interviews elucidate each individual's manner of mentalizing the self, the partner, and the relationship, including the early development of the relationship. Throughout the treatment, the therapist strives to maintain an inquisitive, not-knowing stance and purposefully interrupts nonmentalizing while highlighting effective mentalizing. As I interpret Bleiberg and Safier's thinking, basic and epistemic trust are intertwined: "Promoting mentalizing serves to signal the possibility of trust, which in turn opens the relationship to joint learning and exploration, mutual soothing, and the effective reciprocity that sustains in each partner a sense of coherence, hope, joy, and meaning" (Bleiberg and Safier 2019, p. 153).

Trusting and Distrusting Yourself

In patient education groups about attachment and trauma, I always included a session about "your relationship with yourself," using secure attachment as the ideal model (Allen 2005). I started the group by asking how you know you have a relationship with yourself, and someone would quickly identify the internal dialogue or "self-talk." In all the years I conducted these sessions, I can recall only one patient saying that she was unaware of talking to herself in her mind (and most acknowledged talking to themselves sometimes out loud, as I also do).

Psychologist Charles Fernyhough (2016) studied inner speech thoroughly and pointed to "a separation between myself as speaker and myself as listener," adding, "If we really do talk to ourselves, then the language that ensues must have some of the properties of a conversation between different parts of who we are" (p. 33). This conversation is highly variable in form, ranging from "condensed and telegraphic at one moment to a full-blown internal conversation at the next" (p. 107). Moreover, "the 'speaking-hearing' distinction [is] not always clear cut," and the experience can "often be placed along a continuum between these two extremes" (p. 176). The crucial point for us is that this dialogue is social: "our consciousness is peopled by social agents…internal self-talk has its origins in interactions between people, and…it represents the different perspectives of the social agents that constitute it." Thus, "the voices give us plenty of clues to the social identities behind them. Where there are people, there is the possibility of attachments and even sympathy" (p. 222). Here is something to ponder regarding the voice in your head: "Is it *you* speaking to *you*, or are *you* the thing that is endlessly spun by that conversation?" (p. 246, emphasis in original). How you talk to yourself has its origins in how others talked to you about yourself, and your self-talk influences who you are. If sympathetic attachments were the only origins of the relationship with yourself, I would not be writing about trusting yourself.

In teaching and writing, I advocate a secure attachment relationship with yourself because this relationship provides a safe haven (self-protection, comforting, soothing) and a secure base (encouragement for exploration and autonomy with confidence in the safe haven in times of trouble). Holmes (2001) proposed the term *internal secure base* to refer to our capacity to evoke secure internal working models of attachment that provide a feeling of security during episodes of distress. Consistent with the attachment literature as a whole, I did not view the relationship with oneself through the lens of trust. I am now advocating the idea of being trustworthy to yourself.

To use Jones's (2017) language, you should count on yourself to be caring toward yourself and competent in your decisions and actions. To use McLeod's (2002) moralized language, you can count on your moral integrity—acting in a way that is consistent with your values. In self-trust, McLeod also included moral responsibility to yourself: caring for your welfare, following through with your plans and projects, and being accountable to yourself. She gave a straightforward account of such self-trust:

> Some people seem to be able to trust themselves well throughout a variety of domains. When they face difficult life choices they can usually trust that what they will decide to do is right for them and that they will live up to whatever commitment they make to follow through with their decisions. These are not people who are arrogant necessarily or overly confident. They are people who know themselves well, know what they have to do to be happy or comfortable in their lives and what they are capable of achieving. Although they must have knowledge of the external world that allows them to identify what it is that makes them happy or comfortable, self-knowledge is probably the main factor in their justified optimism toward themselves. (p. 59)

In the following subsections, I begin with the problem of distrusting your-self, elaborate on trusting yourself for care and competence, discuss ways of promoting self-trust in therapy, and explicate the value of balancing self-trust and self-distrust. Remember that we generally trust without thinking about trust; perhaps we should think and talk about it more in psychotherapy.

Distrusting Yourself

If we accept the principle that trusting should match trustworthiness, you should trust yourself only to the extent that you are trustworthy. Just as you must be able to trust yourself, you must learn when to distrust yourself—perhaps being vigilant, if not downright suspicious—when you might not be able to count on yourself. Distrusting yourself can be profoundly undermining, such that we must learn to distrust ourselves effectively. We are all prone to self-deception, which should make us cautious (e.g., realizing that we put ourselves at risk by keeping fattening foods in the cupboard when we embark on a diet). Excessive self-confidence can get us into trouble. Thus, you cannot be fully trustworthy to yourself without also trusting others, relying on their help and judgment when you are uncertain of yourself. Accordingly, depending on others is essential to being trustworthy to yourself. And self-trust is social in another sense: As Darwall (2017) pointed out, others knowing that you do not trust yourself could make them reluctant to trust you. *If you cannot count on yourself, you cannot count on yourself to be counted on, and others cannot count on you.*

To bring to mind the feeling of being unable to count on yourself, think of the all-too-common plight of struggling with acute episodes of a chronic ill-ness. Although general medical analogues abound, we can take psychiatric dis-orders as examples. Imagine the following: vulnerability to panic attacks that ultimately prevent you from leaving your house; not feeling able to make plans with a friend for fear that you'll be too depressed to go; contending with poorly controlled manic episodes in which you go on spending sprees that could bank-rupt you; or dissociative episodes that render you unable to remember where you left your car in a parking garage—or worse, suddenly realizing you are in bed with a stranger. All these experiences are painful, and being unable to count on yourself can be the most painful part. What if you could not count on your-self to care enough or know enough to get the competent help you need to put you in a better position to count on yourself? To take the extreme, what if you were actively endangering yourself through deliberate self-harm and suicide at-tempts?

I talked with patients in trauma education groups about the quality of their relationships with themselves and, more specifically, how they talked to them-selves. Self-hate was common, and harsh self-criticism was ubiquitous. After some discussion, I stated flatly that the terms *abuse* and *neglect* are apt for this kind of relationship with yourself, having been internalized from earlier traumatic relationships. Abuse can be physical as well as psychological (e.g., self-injury as well as self-criticism and contempt born of self-hate). We know all too well that it can be extremely difficult to extricate oneself from an abusive relationship, as the experience of traumatic bonding (Allen 2001; Dutton and Painter 1981) attests: the abuse heightens fear and the associated attachment needs, and the absence of other protective relationships cements reliance on the abusive person (e.g., a child depending on a parent or a spouse dependent on and controlled by a possessive partner). Similarly, neglect can be physical as well as psychological (e.g., neglecting health or safety as well as minimizing, dismissing, or ignoring painful feelings). None of these traumatic experiences in the relationship with oneself was foreign to patients in these trauma education groups.

In principle, if not easily in practice, you can leave an abusive and neglectful relationship with another person. Extricating yourself from a traumatic attachment relationship with yourself is another matter. You can escape temporarily (or more continuously) by drug and alcohol abuse. You can escape permanently by suicide, which is commonly fueled by a damaged sense of self, including self-hate (Jobes 2006; Orbach 2011). To put it starkly, if you cannot stand being with yourself, killing yourself is one obvious solution.

Abusing and neglecting yourself are extreme forms of basic untrustworthiness to yourself. Abusive relationships often include criticism and psychological assaults that can undermine self-trust in competence generally and epistemic self-trust more specifically: "You're stupid." "You're worthless." "You'll never amount to anything." "You don't know anything." "You're crazy." "You can't do anything right." This sort of barrage undermines self-worth (Allen 2001), but it might be even more damaging in undermining self-trust, especially early in life, when the foundations of self-trust must be developed. Hawley (2012) commented on the impact of verbal abuse and insults later in life: "domestic abuse can reduce the victim's self-trust to the extent that it becomes difficult for victims to trust themselves either to judge the reality of the situation, or to find a way out" (p. 77). Commonly, such later abuse is preceded by a lack of self-trust stemming from trauma in earlier relationships (Allen 2001).

Gaslighting bears mention as a profoundly disorienting experience in undermining a person's sense of reality and trust in his or her perceptions. I served as the therapist for Brenda, a despondent and perplexed woman whose psychiatrist husband attributed their marital problems to her "severe personality disorder," for which she sought hospital treatment. Brenda did not describe her husband as harsh or mean but rather considered him to be sympathetic to her personal failings, albeit in a "pitying" way. Along with a number of professionals who worked with her, I was unable to discern any personality disorder. A social worker found Brenda's husband to be elusive, and he declined to be involved in her treatment. Brenda was able gradually to get her bearings in a treatment program that provided a lot of opportunity to develop trusting relationships with her peers as well as members of the clinical staff. Although feeling shocked and disillusioned, she also was profoundly relieved when her hospital psychiatrist identified the process of gaslighting and explained it to her. In the process, she began to extricate herself from the relationship and to regain her self-trust.

Basic and Epistemic Self-Trust

Imagine trusting yourself absolutely. With a bit of conceptual strain, we might employ the model of two-place trust, that is, trusting yourself as a person in relation to yourself—not just regarding various ways you might behave toward yourself. You would, relatively unthinkingly, trust in your goodwill and compassion, counting on yourself to look out for your welfare and best interests. When you are feeling distressed, guilty, or apprehensive, you might calm yourself, forgive yourself, and encourage yourself. You might even say that you love yourself. If all that were generally so, we could say you have *basic self-trust*. Lacking such basic trust in yourself would be hugely problematic. And it is for many of our traumatized patients.

Turning from care to competence, we move to three-place trust, trusting yourself in various domains and actions, with room for much variability. We can think of *epistemic self-trust* as one important domain. You generally trust your senses and well-established skills, unthinkingly, which Linda Zagzebski (2012) referred to "the natural trust in one's epistemic faculties" (p. 38). Yet we have room for doubt. How much do you trust your reasoning? Ample research provides grounds for doubt (Kahneman 2011). How well can you trust your memory? How much do you trust your memories from early childhood? More specifically, the extent to which memories of childhood trauma can be trusted has generated extremely contentious debate as well as much scholarly research (Allen 1995). How much do you trust your feelings? Emotions are informative, and we need to rely on them, but they also can be misleading (e.g., feeling anxious and perceiving harmless events as threatening). How much do you trust your judgment of others' trustworthiness? Research on lie detection warrants caution: gut feelings are responsive to nonverbal cues, and these cues are unreliable indicators of lying, such that we must gauge trustworthiness by more sophisticated social-cognitive means (Mercier 2020).

Also in the realm of competence, Zagzebski (2012) made the case for rational, *epistemic* self-trust. She distinguished two levels of epistemic self-trust: first, "the general trust in our faculties" and, second, "the particular trust we have in our faculties when we are *conscientious*—exercising our truth-seeking faculties in the best way we can" (pp. 49–50, emphasis added). Epistemic conscientiousness includes "intellectual attentiveness, carefulness, thoroughness, and openness to new evidence" (p. 49). As Zagzebski observed, "once a person becomes reflective, she thinks that her trustworthiness is greater if she summons her powers in a fully conscious and careful way, and exercises them to the best of her ability" (p. 48). Conscientiousness comes in degrees, and "higher degrees of conscientiousness require considerable self-awareness and self-monitoring" (p. 49). Zagzebski summarized, "It is in virtue of self-trust that I believe everything I believe" (pp. 50–51). We cannot always be marshaling evidence for our beliefs. Self-trust gives us a legitimate reason to believe what we believe: "either self-trust is in the category of reasons [for belief] or there are no reasons. That is why it is rational to have self-trust. Self-trust is the foundation of what we take rationality to be" (p. 51). Self-doubt can be downright paralyzing (e.g., checking and rechecking as in obsessive-compulsive disorder).

Developing Self-Trust From the Outside In

Many patients in my trauma education groups were striving consciously to improve their relationship with themselves. Invariably, in the course of these conversations, a patient would assert that you cannot love others until you love yourself, implying that self-love is the condition for loving relationships. I offered a different perspective: Your relationship with yourself develops from the outside in. For better or for worse, relationships with others provide the models for your relationship with yourself. So is it with trusting yourself. As McLeod (2002) pointed out, "Self-trust and distrust are relational in being socially constituted. They are molded to a significant degree by the responses of others and by societal norms" (p. 37). Concomitantly, "A supportive environment for good self-trusting and self-distrusting is one in which people receive truthful and constructive feedback about themselves" (p. 77).

Albeit without focusing on trust, Marsha Linehan (1993) provided therapists with a pertinent dialectic: engaging patients through a *balance of validation and challenge.* Adopting patients' perspective and validating the reasonableness and understandability of their feelings, beliefs, and actions promotes their self-trust. Commonplace validating responses include "What you're saying makes sense to me." "I can understand why you're feeling that way." "I imagine I'd feel that way if someone said that to me." I am especially partial to Bateman and Fonagy's (2006) idea of a mind influencing a mind as an expression of validation:

> The patient has to find himself in the mind of the therapist and, equally, the therapist has to understand himself in the mind of the patient if the two together are to develop a mentalizing process. Both have to experience *a mind being changed by a mind.* (p. 93, emphasis added)

When the therapist questions the seeming unreasonableness of a patient's anger and the patient provides the therapist with the series of events that led up to it, the therapist is in a position to empathize with the patient's outrage, and the patient will feel empowered by having created a meeting of minds.

Conversely, Linehan (1993) also drew our attention to the damaging effects of *invalidation.* I associate invalidation at the extreme with mentalizing failures (Allen 2013b) as evident in abuse (being torn down and degraded) and neglect (being ignored, unseen, unheard, and invisible). *You can't feel counted on—*trusted and trustworthy—*if you don't count.* Beginning early in life and continuing throughout, mentalizing is the crux of validating, through which the individual feels attentively and accurately seen, heard, felt, and understood. Feeling that you as a person and your point of view are taken seriously is to be trusted and to feel trustworthy at the most basic level. From this perspective, psychothera-pists are in a potentially crucial position to provide such validation. Validation is indicative of trusting; validating yourself is a sign of trusting yourself. Con-versely, to invalidate yourself is to distrust yourself (e.g., "I was stupid to think that way"; "I'm too sensitive"). When patients sided with those who accused them of making mountains out of molehills, I countered that the molehill in the present must be viewed in the context of the mountain in the past.

Psychotherapy would be of limited value if it only provided validation; as Linehan (1993) fully appreciated, change requires considering different perspec-tives, provided by challenging points of view. Nonetheless, validation remains crucial in establishing a foundation for effective challenge: "Only when authentic validation occurs will the patient feel that the clinician understands; it is from here that the patient and clinician can diverge and start considering different per-spectives" (Bateman and Fonagy 2016, p. 236). Validation coupled with chal-lenge is a recipe for growth.

I have a memorable experience of challenging a patient, which was tolerable by virtue of her experience of feeling validated in much of the therapy. Jasmine talked about extreme (potentially heart-stopping) use of cocaine in a way that was shockingly casual. When I looked horrified, on the basis of my facial ex-pression alone, she protested that I was being "judgmental." I countered that my expression was a "reasonable reaction" to her self-endangering behavior and ac-knowledged the contribution of my parental feelings of protectiveness. Later in treatment, Jasmine revealed being frightened of her cocaine abuse, and she made a point of arranging for solid follow-up treatment for substance abuse.

Balancing Self-Trust and Self-Distrust

The example of Jasmine underscores the fact that trusting yourself can be a pre-carious and risky endeavor. As Katherine Hawley (2012) proposed, "sometimes I really ought to distrust myself, whether or not I can bring myself to do so." She gave the example of addiction:

> Sometimes, self-trust seems to involve a divided self, a contrast between the "me" who must decide whether to trust, and the "me" who is the target of the trust—often in the past or the future. The current me is not tempted to smoke, but can I trust the later version of me who has had a glass of wine, or should I instead take precautions to remove any temptations from later me? This divided self picture prods us towards treating self-trust as a special case of trusting oth-ers, thinking of our earlier and later selves as especially intimate "others." (p. 76)

In this passage, Hawley's perspective is relevant to a notorious flaw in no-suicide contracts made in the psychotherapist's office (Lineberry 2011): While in a rela-tively calm state of mind, the patient vows to contact the therapist or a suicide hotline before acting on suicidal thoughts. However, when the patient is in the emotional state of being overwhelmed and despairing, the contract or the therapist does not enter his or her mind. Taking precautions—getting rid of the gun, the rope, or the stash of pills—could provide some mental space for considering alternatives to suicide. In high-risk contexts such as drug addiction and suicidal states coupled with impaired capacity for emotion regulation, some self-distrust is fitting, and hope enters the scene. Ideally, hope will motivate and sustain efforts to make use of help, the prospect of which is increased by getting rid of ready means for self-harm.

McLeod (2002) underscored the relation between trusting in others and the autonomy afforded by self-trust. Considering "why it is important to get things right with self-trust and self-distrust," she proposed: "The answer lies in the connection between trusting oneself well and being an autonomous agent." She continued, "People who have autonomy reflect on what they truly believe and value, and they act accordingly. They are also competent and committed to engage in such reflection and to act on the results. Furthermore, they have a positive attitude toward their own competency and commitment" (p. 103).

Remember, however, that self-trust requires social support, and autonomy requires depending on trustworthy others for that support. McLeod took pains to articulate how health care providers are obligated to support autonomy by promoting self-trust along with reasonable self-distrust. We psychotherapists have a significant role in this endeavor, especially with patients whose self-trust has been damaged by abuse, neglect, and oppression. The balance of validation and challenge plays a significant role in this endeavor. Self-trust requires accurate mentalizing of the self—with help from accurate therapeutic mentalizing in a trusting relationship. Zagzebski (2012) put it wisely:

> The self is important enough to be aided in its task by wise, knowledgeable, sensitive, and more experienced others. One's current point of view is not a dependable way to accomplish that task. Rather than to conclude that autonomy is not valuable, we should conclude that *autonomy requires dependence on others*. (p. 250, emphasis added)

Cultivating trust in yourself is a lifelong task. This task is made far more difficult by a history of traumatic attachments that have undermined self-trust as well as trust in others, especially insofar as trust in others is crucial for the cultivation of self-trust. Blind self-trust makes no more sense than blind trust in others. Both put you in a precarious position. Conscientious self-trust, as Zagzebski contended, includes trusting in others. Cultivating trustworthiness of yourself and others not only is a lifelong project; it is a collaborative one.

Hoping in Trust

Although I am considering diverse senses of trust in this book, in the context of psychotherapy I have a challenging prototype in mind: a patient with a history of traumatic relationships who comes to a psychotherapist with a justifiably distrusting attitude but who in desperation—must depend on a therapist for help and feels vulnerable in doing so. Hope and trust occupy the common ground of uncertainty. The act of seeking help implies some hope in the therapist's trustworthiness, even if the hope is not felt or acknowledged. As I explicate in this section, hope plays a vital role in developing trust to the extent that fear and doubt about trustworthiness prevail; hence my concern about hope in trust. I stitch these two concepts together, with the emphasis on hope.

For many years, I conducted educational sessions on the topic of hope for hospitalized patients; each time, for group discussion, I raised the question "What gives you hope?" "Nothing!" was a fair reply in this setting, but most group members described some basis for hope. A young woman gave my all-time favorite answer: "I can be surprised." This attitude would be fitting for a patient who is profoundly doubtful about a therapist's trustworthiness. Hope and trust travel together in this context. "I can be surprised" is a minimally hopeful platform for developing trust, in psychotherapy and in other relationships.

I remember fondly a session on hope I conducted for an outpatient educational group focused on trauma. A woman in the group opened the discussion by stating that she had not wanted to attend because she had no hope and she thought she would just get "a load of bullshit" from me. I was pleased that she spoke up and thanked her for doing so. She was anticipating a cheerleading attitude. I, on the contrary, sought to explain why hope is so difficult to develop and maintain in the context of trauma or any other dire straits. I open discussions of trust with the same attitude, emphasizing how hard-won trust can be. When I recounted in a subsequent group this episode of a patient anticipating B.S., a patient confessed that, when hearing that the session would be on hope, she thought, "Hope? Oh shit!" At the conclusion of that discussion, the patients agreed that this sober view of the problems in creating hope rendered hope *more attainable* by being more realistic. Before this session, they had been encouraged by others simply to have hope as if they could just change their mind if they so chose. They had felt invalidated.

I have come to think of hope and trust as deeply intertwined to the extent that we cannot fully understand trust without incorporating hope into our thinking. As I have done for decades, I am relying on a tradition of which I became a part, using the work of my colleagues and mentors Karl Menninger and Paul Pruyser. In addition, in the course of refining my thinking about hope and trust, I was fortunate to discover Adrienne Martin's (2014) book *How We Hope: A Moral Psychology*. She sees herself working in the domain of "philosophy of psychology" (p. 143); she is a trained philosopher and a natural psychologist, and I am weaving her thinking into mine. Her work is especially fitting for my purposes because she writes from a context in which hope is extremely challenging to create. She took up a 2-year fellowship in a hospital research setting where terminally ill patients were receiving experimental drugs for cancer: "The chances of a participant in a phase I trial receiving medical benefit from the experimental drug are typically less than 1%, and participants are informed of this fact" (p. 1). Although not comparable to the general medical setting in many respects, my psychiatric counterpart of suicidal patients feeling hopeless after years of failed treatments also entails severe challenges to developing hope—which requires, first and foremost, facing reality.

Facing Reality

Martin's (2014) paradigm case exemplifies what she calls "*hoping against hope*," that is, "hoping for an outcome that one highly values but believes is extremely unlikely" (p. 5, emphasis in original). Martin and I are on common ground. She writes, "I focus on hope in the context of a 'trial'—an extreme challenge to one's ability to live well or flourish, a circumstance that makes literal or figurative suicide tempting" (p. 9). When I talked with hospitalized psychiatric patients about hope, I asked, "How many of you would say that your life problems are *dire* at this point?" All hands went up. My colleague and mentor Paul Pruyser (1987b) well understood the plight of the person who needs hope:

> Hoping occurs when one feels trapped, is visited by a calamity, or has come to the end of one's rope in understanding or deed…. *Hoping presupposes a tragic situation*; it is a response to felt tragedy, and is a positive outgrowth of a tragic sense of life. To hope, then, one must have…*an undistorted view of reality*, a degree of modesty vis-à-vis the power and workings of nature or the cosmos. (p. 465, emphasis added)

Accordingly, Pruyser asserted that hoping requires "some capacity to abstain from impulsive, unrealistic wishing" and that "[g]iven the human propensity for uninhibited lavish wishing and the strong cultural reinforcement of wish fulfillment strivings, the disposition and capacity for true hoping may be rather scarce" (pp. 465–466). Lavish wishing is presumptuous; there is another alternative to hope: despair.

Between Presumption and Despair

Karl Menninger (1987) asserted that doctors should be careful to inspire the "right amount" of hope:

> It is a responsibility of the teacher to the student, just as it is of the young doctor to his patient, to inspire the right amount of hope—some, but not too much. Excess of hope is *presumption* and leads to disaster. Deficiency of hope is *despair* and leads to decay. Our delicate and precious duty as teachers is to properly tend this flame. (p. 449, emphasis added)

Menninger's reference to presumption and despair originated in the work of Saint Thomas Aquinas, writing in the thirteenth century (Kinghorn 2013). As I understand it, *hope moves in the uncertain space between the diametrically opposed certainties of presumption and despair.* The patients who protested my session on hope anticipated presumption on my part. Presumption implies certainty, and patients rightly take umbrage at presumptuous clinicians who convey breezily, "Don't worry, everything will be fine." Such presumption flies in the face of patients' dire circumstances. Less obviously, despair and hopelessness also imply certainty: the patient *knows* that nothing will change and nothing will help. Hope requires tolerating ambiguity: not knowing the future—a capacity for surprise.

Tolerating uncertainty comes with a price: *hope is haunted by fear and doubt.* I put it to patients this way: If you did not have fear and doubt, you would not need hope. You would just be going about your life. I advocate acceptance of fear and doubt rather than trying to expunge them with hope. Fear and doubt come into play because the hopeful person is facing reality—dire circumstances and the uncertainty that comes with them. But hope itself brings fear into play: Many patients who have felt hopeful in the past have repeatedly experienced setbacks, recurrences of illness, and defeats only to become profoundly disillusioned. They readily acknowledge *fear of hope.* Hopeless despair offers its own painful respite from this fear. I talked to patients in a trauma-education group about fear of hope, which they readily understood. When we switched to the topic of trust, a young man remarked, "I'm not afraid of hope. But trust scares me to death." Analogous to the refuge of hopelessness, distrust affords safety from vulnerability—at the high price of forgoing help.

Martin (2014) helpfully characterizes the continuum of uncertainty inherent in hope, starting with the orthodox definition of hope in philosophy: "*a combination of the desire for an outcome and the belief that the outcome is possible but not certain*" (p. 4, emphasis added). She highlights *desire* as the attraction to the outcome and specifies the uncertainty as the "probability assigned to the hoped-for outcome" (p. 37). This probability ranges from 0 (no chance) to 1 (certainty), the range from despair to presumption; hope navigates in the middle ground. Toward the upper end, the need for hope fades; hope falls by the wayside when you are *expecting* a particular outcome, that is, fully confident of it. Of course, in the face of the unexpected, the need for hope could resurface; toward the lower end, hopelessness beckons, as diagrammed in Figure 3–1.

Invariably, *fluctuating uncertainty* renders hope especially challenging to maintain; hope does not lie still on the continuum. As Pruyser observed, patients

> do not make up their minds once for all for or against illusions, rebelliousness, anxiousness, or hope, in various sequences. The process of illness itself may force a patient to sort out wishing and hoping, to choose between despairing and hoping, and to search for a reasoned and *reasonable hope* that is resistant to disillusionment. We see in many patients oscillations between one state and another, and in some a stepwise progression toward a peaceful acceptance of their condition. (Pruyser 1987b, p. 469, emphasis added)

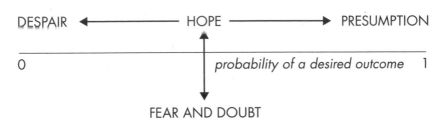

FIGURE 3–1.   Hope moves in the uncertain space between despair and presumption.

Note.   Hope is accompanied by fear and doubt. As hope moves further in the positive direction, it is gradually replaced by confidence in the desired outcome; as hope moves further in the negative direction, it is gradually replaced by hopelessness.

Dating from the thirteenth century, this model of hope fits perfectly the challenges facing the distrusting patient who seeks help from a therapist. The patient hopes for the trustworthiness of the therapist and the treatment. This hope is liable to be haunted by fear and doubt, prominently including *fear of trusting*. Little wonder that highly distrusting patients keep their distance. I remember patients from decades ago, when we were conducting long-term inpatient treatment, who remained on the margins of the therapeutic community for *months* before slowly becoming engaged. Michelle, the patient whom I identified in Chapter 2, "Developing Trust and Trustworthiness," as needing a secure base, continued expressing periodic distrust after 5 years of reasonably trustworthy therapy.

Cultivating Hope in Trust

I find Martin's (2014, 2020) thinking helpful in articulating the psychological and interpersonal process of creating and sustaining hope—and trust alongside it. This process is outlined in Table 3–2. I have set the stage by construing the development of hope as created in the context of a potentially dire *plight*. I am particularly concerned with plights that stem from betrayals of trust and in which trustworthiness and the help that would stem from it constitute the (dimly) hoped-for outcome.

I have worked with many suicidal patients seeking intensive inpatient treatment in desperation after enduring long periods of hopelessness; they have remained mired in a plight, seeing no prospect of moving forward. When they do begin moving forward, they are liable to experience the fluctuating uncertainty that Pruyser (1987b) eloquently described. In treatment, we aspire to help the patient move toward more stable, reasonable hope (and trust). The word *reasonable* allows for the fact that we never achieve the certainty of presumption—the reason we need the concepts of hope and trust. But we can help patients move forward

---

TABLE 3–2. **Moving from hopelessness to hope**

A plight: facing the reality of a challenging or perhaps dire situation in which the stakes are high for a desired outcome and the likelihood of the outcome is low

Licensing hope: allowing yourself to hope; shifting perspective from focusing on low probability to sheer possibility of a good outcome

Incorporating hope into agency: future-oriented feeling (feeling hopeful, anticipating the desired outcome), thinking (imagining a hoped-for future), planning, and action; culminates in taking action that increases the probability of the hoped-for outcome.

---

on the continuum in two steps that Martin (2014) construes as *licensing* hope and then *incorporating* hope into planning and action. Using this broad distinction, we must allow for degrees and fuzzy boundaries: licenses can be revoked, and whatever is incorporated can later be disavowed.

Martin's metaphor, *licensing hope*, points to the critical juncture in the psychological process of creating hope. We can think of hope and hopelessness as live—and rational—options in the face of a desired outcome and slim odds. Here we are in the territory of perspective-taking. Martin (2014) contrasted two patients in experimental drug trials for cancer: "One looks at the situation and says, 'I grant you it is *possible*, but the chance is only one in a thousand!' The other says, 'I grant you the chance is only one in a thousand, but it is *possible!*'" As Martin put it, the "differences are indications of the underlying stances they take toward the probability. There are many ways one can describe or frame a probability" (p. 45, emphasis in original). Both stances are realistic and rational; homing in on *possibility* is grounds for hope, whereas focusing attention on *low probability* can be grounds for despair. Licensing hope is a good way to think about this process: you must give yourself a permit—permission to hope, endorsing and embracing hope, going with the *possibility*, whatever the *probability* might be. Menninger rightly counseled against false hope (wishing or presumption), but Martin argued against ruling out hope in the context of slim chances:

> in a medical setting, where hoped-for outcomes are largely beyond the hopeful person's control, people worry about how to avoid "false" hope without losing all hope.... It is common to think that meeting this challenge means following a blanket rule that directs us to hope and encourage others to hope only for somewhat probable outcomes. Call this *the rule against improbable hope*.... One important result of my proposed analysis of hope is that restricting hopes to somewhat probable outcomes is neither necessary nor sufficient for practical rationality. (Martin 2014, p. 141, emphasis in original)

Hope is influenced by the odds, but, barring the rule against improbable hope, *hope is not fully constrained by the odds*. We must consider perspective-taking and subjectivity. As did Martin, Pruyser (1987b, p. 468) contrasted two hypothetical general medical patients who were gravely ill with a grim prognosis. One patient "may squarely face his fate and ostensibly give up all hope...preparing himself for the demise that is surely and soon to come." The other, while not denying reality, continues to hope and to gratefully receive help, potentially prolonging his life. Reasonableness encompasses latitude. As Pruyser wrote, "reality is not a simple consensually validated world, but an overwhelmingly complex composite of forces that is differently edited and interpreted by different persons." He asked, "Which of the two reactions is more realistic?" He mused, is the second case "an irrational 'hoping against hope,' a flouting of reality, and thus a serious maladaptation?" We should heed his conclusion: "Who can tell, or rather, who is presumptuous enough to answer?" We would best join our patients in tolerating uncertainty, accepting that "hoping is an intimate and private prerogative of each person." So it is with trusting.

As contrasted with the passivity of wishing and the inaction associated with hopeless despair, hoping carries a distinct advantage: as an active and effortful process, hoping increases the probability of the desired outcome. The same goes for trusting, licensed with hope. Hope entails taking in whatever hope-creating experiences emerge and, as Martin put it, *incorporating* these elements into your *agency*, that is, your active engagement in moving forward. Licensing hope, putting possibility in your sights, is the major move from the objective circumstances—the undeniably dire plight—to the subjective transition into hope. In Martin's schema, issuing yourself the license warrants a shift from *allowing* to actively *embracing* hope in future-oriented feeling, thinking, planning, and action. Hope is a *project*, and hope-inspired action is hope's most practical benefit. Hope in trustworthiness enables trust that is essential to the *work* of psychotherapy: open exploration, confiding, seriously considering the therapist's point of view, and collaborating—creating an expandable "we."

I routinely remind patients that by seeking treatment, they have undertaken action that requires effort and sacrifice. I admire patients who have worked hard in psychotherapy for years to overcome lifelong traumatic experiences. Many of them have endured periods of giving up, and many had attempted suicide. If they are alive, and especially if they are engaged in treatment—no matter how reluctantly—I can hold on to hope, and I do. My role is becoming trustworthy as a prerequisite for cultivating trust. Recall a developmental principle from Chapter 2: mentalizing begets mentalizing. We can add that hope begets hope, and trusting begets trust.

Interpersonal Hope

Taking a broad view, Martin (2020) distinguished three forms of hope: *interpersonal* hope (hope in the other person), *intrapersonal* hope (hope in oneself), and *impersonal* hope (e.g., hope for fortunate events in the external world that influence the outcome). Hoping well entails interweaving these three facets of hope. As I see it, interpersonal hope begets trusting in others, intrapersonal hope begets trusting in oneself, and trusting in oneself depends profoundly on help begotten by trusting in trustworthy others. We should never underestimate the importance of life outside the office for the outcome of psychotherapy. As my appreciation for the elasticity in the intentional stance implies (see Chapter 2), I am not averse to thinking about impersonal hope as trusting in the world, which I also think has roots in relationships with trustworthy persons.

I do not remember where I came across the idea of *borrowed hope*—probably from a patient in one of my educational groups. When we lack hope, we can borrow it from others who can feel hopeful for us and see reasons for hope in us that we cannot see in ourselves. Profound depression, a common context for hopelessness, robs its sufferers of emotion and imagination. They cannot remember feeling better. They cannot envision a better future. But they can take heart from others who can remember what they cannot remember and see what they cannot see. When they are unable to feel any self-worth, others continue to see them as worthy, valuable, and lovable. They can borrow hope from others—*provided that they trust* in the other's perspective. The same applies to borrowing trust from a professional or friend in accepting a referral to a therapist.

As I have said of trust, interpersonal hope requires shared goals—creation of a "we" in which each individual plays a different role. In the context of what I think of as *borrowed* hope, Martin (2020) introduces a helpful metaphor: She construes interpersonal hope as the hope that one person *invests* in another. We therapists take on significant roles as investors of hope. To be credible and trustworthy, however, we must accept and endorse the uncertainty inherent in hope, as well as the uncertainty inherent in trusting and trustworthiness. As it is for our patients, our history—and our history of relationships in particular, prominently including our patients—will influence our capacity to feel and invest hope. As Pruyser (1987b) expressed it: "anyone's grounds for hoping do not lie in the facts of reality, but in the ways in which reality has thus far disclosed itself to the person and in the meanings which that person has found in these disclosures" (pp. 468–469). We psychotherapists are in existential territory here, and Pruyser (1974, 1987c) felt at home in it.

Martin (2020) thinks of investing hope as involving *socially extended agency*, a form of interpersonal influence. If I hope for your betterment and hold some vision of it that we share, your experience of my hope might enable you to feel hopeful and, embracing hope, to take action on your own behalf. In this way, a therapist's hope can become therapeutic. Yet this benefit hinges on the patient's trust in the therapist's judgment and authenticity.

As I see it in the context of psychotherapy, socially extended agency goes both ways: My patient invests hope in me; at the least, she does so without extending her agency to me, as in thinking, "I hope he knows what he's doing." Ideally, she might reciprocate fully, hoping to influence my hopeful agency, encouraging me to do my utmost to help her. For example, she might work to engage my attention and interest. Furthermore, she will also help me to understand her fully (by confiding openly) as well as inspiring me to appreciate her efforts and strengths. On the other hand, to the extent that she is in thrall to hopelessness and strives to engender it in me, she might marshal evidence for the intractability of her plight, her inability to cope with it, and my inability to help her.

At best, each of us comes to invest hope in ourselves in conjunction with inspiring hope in each other. As a therapist, my hopes for myself cannot be divorced from my hopes for my patient. I become imaginatively invested in my patient's future and my contribution to it; my imagined future depends on my influencing my patient's agency. Thus, I invest hope in my patient and myself, just as my patient's hope invested in me is commingled with her hope in herself.

Psychotherapy is a skein of hopes, intricately interwoven, and this skein includes trust. To amplify this point, we must reconsider the plight that sets the stage for hope and its context in trust. To the extent that we therapists invest hope in our patients (and in ourselves), we enter into their plight—albeit in attenuated form. We share in our patients' fate. As a therapist (and parent, partner, or friend who is depended on for help), think about sitting with a patient who is in emotional agony, terrified in reliving trauma, paralyzed with depression, or on the brink of suicide. Your plight: You want to have helpful influence, and it is extremely difficult to do so. You need hope. You need to trust in yourself. And your hope will depend on engaging your patient in hope and, in turn, being trustworthy and experienced as such.

I have had ample experience with this plight, which comes with painful feelings of inadequacy, helplessness, and hopelessness. But I know the difference between *feeling* inadequate, helpless, and hopeless and *being* inadequate, helpless, and hopeless. Our patients, potentially incapacitated in the more emotionally excruciating part of this shared plight, will not be able to make this distinction—and hope lies in making it. Often enough, unable to *do* anything, I can be most helpful by tolerating my painful feelings, *being* with the patient, and conveying hope implicitly by not succumbing to despair.

Burdening With Hope

When you are immersed in a plight with patients such as I have just described, you will be incapable of presumption as long as you remain anchored in reality. Yet we should remain cognizant of the potential burden that interpersonal hope can place on the other person—a risk that Martin (2020) delineates. Hope can be experienced as expectation; in turn, expectation can be experienced as demand. The plight of those who invest hope and trust in others—including us therapists—includes the vulnerability to feeling disappointed, let down, or betrayed. To take the extreme, think of investing hope and trust in a person who dies by suicide. As I can attest from my own experience and that of many colleagues, along with sadness come guilt, resentment, and anger.

As Martin (2020) articulates, interpersonal hope requires discernment—rendering her metaphor of *investment* especially apt. Pruyser (1987b) used the term *reasonable hope*, which is consistent with reasonable expectations. Given the context of uncertainty, I find developing reasonable expectations to be one of the most challenging aspects of psychiatric treatment. Hope comes with fear and doubt, more intense as the plight is more dire. As Menninger (1987) implied, we walk a tightrope: When our expectations are unreasonably high, we run the risk of presumption and placing undue burden on patients that will undermine hope. When our expectations are unreasonably low, we run the risk of abetting discouragement or despair. Our personal influence can be profound—even lifesaving—and it can be profoundly limited. And there is much in the fate of a life over which neither we nor our patients have any influence whatsoever.

Neither we therapists nor our patients can navigate the space of hope without accepting the possibility of failure. Hope can go awry, as can trust. I sometimes make the provocative point with patients that giving up is an underrated strategy: When faced with the impossible, give up. Usually, I make this point in the context of problematic and downright traumatic relationships. Here we come back to reasonable hope and reasonable expectations: How do we know when we are faced with the impossible? We rely on judgment, with its own inherent uncertainty.

As I discussed in Chapter 1, some patients do not improve in psychotherapy, and some deteriorate. Moreover, therapists tend to overestimate their effectiveness and to be unaware of deterioration. As all of us sometimes are prone to doing, therapists whose interventions are not working are liable to do more of the same with increasing vigor and doggedness. Persistence is invaluable, but it has its limits. As it is in general medicine, discontinuing the treatment and seeking more effective alternatives is the reasonable strategy. This strategy can be especially difficult in therapy insofar as it entails giving up hope in a valued attachment relationship. In this context, however, giving up the relationship is the pathway to reasonable hope and trust established in other relationships.

From Hope to Faith

I have doubtlessly said a number of stupid things in my career, sadly being oblivious to most. One I remember: In an educational session on hope, a patient asked: "What do you think about blind faith?" At the time, I was talking about psychologist Rick Snyder's (1999) useful idea that hope requires a combination of agency and pathways. In the same vein, Menninger (1987) asserted that "there is no such thing as 'idle hope,'" pointing to the need for a "motive force" and "plan of action" (p. 151). With this authority in mind, I held my ground: blind faith will not work. I remain unenthusiastic about blindness, but I was wrongly dismissive of this patient's plea for faith. I was blind to faith. Working with individual and cultural diversity requires open eyes.

I believe that we must make room for faith in our clinical work, not least because faith is central in the life of many of our patients. When I routinely asked the question "What gives you hope?" in groups, many patients referred to faith. Often, their faith was rooted in religion, which is a predominant source of faith. But religious faith is far from universal, and I wanted to include secular ways of thinking about faith as well. I could not lead these discussions on hope without considering faith, given their kinship. And my broad secular view of faith leaves ample room for religious faith.

Addressing faith authentically in psychotherapy and in educational groups requires not only some conceptual grasp but also having some emotional grasp—feeling it. I find faith elusive but not entirely beyond my conceptual and emotional grasp. Of course, being able to grasp does not prevent losing one's grip. I claim no authority in this spiritual territory, but I have some authority to rely on. Pruyser (1987a, 1987b) made significant contributions to the psychology of religion; Martin (2014) insightfully addressed the relation of hope and faith; and I have long been an admirer of Paul Tillich's work, largely for his breadth of vision that encompasses theology and philosophy as well as his appreciation for existential and psychoanalytic thought (Pauck and Pauck 2015). Pertinent to our present concern, Tillich (1957) wrote a broadminded book, *The Dynamics of Faith*, that became a classic. Marshaling authorities I trust in my somewhat discursive account, I start with Martin, bring in Tillich, return to Pruyser, and conclude with my own secular version of faith in psychotherapy. I am in no position to settle anything here; I merely offer food for thought, and any such thought is inescapably personal.

I am campaigning for therapists to think about faith and to think with their patients about faith when appropriate to patients' concerns. And some therapists might feel a need to go beyond hope to faith, as their patients also might do. Providing some orientation to prevent you from getting utterly lost in the fog in this vaporous territory, I am heading toward the following and admittedly blurry distinction between hope and faith: Hope requires some vision of the desired outcome, coupled with some means of attaining it. Faith affords confidence that you will come through your plight in ways you cannot envision and by means you cannot imagine. "Blind" might not be the best term for faith, but it is not entirely inapt. Faith, whatever its source, provides confidence without any concrete grounds.

Martin (2014), while considering religious forms, also aimed for a secular version of faith, one that would be available to atheists. Hope and faith share the space of not-knowing, but this ambiguity takes different forms. In hope, the uncertainty and not-knowing relate to which one of a number of envisioned possibilities will come to pass (in short, whether the treatment will work or not). Faith encompasses a far more radical form of not-knowing: the outcome is *unimaginable*; that is, unimaginable hope refers to "hope for an outcome that outstrips the hopeful person's concepts in such a way that he cannot imagine or conceive of it" (p. 100). Thinking about the unimaginable is not easy; bear with me.

Martin (2014) offers a simple formula: "faith is hope plus confidence" (p. 105). The confidence of faith is *essentially* sustaining: "it is immune to empirical disappointment. Nothing in the hopeful person's experience need count as a reason to stop desiring the unimaginable outcome" (p. 101). That is, faith entails a robust form of confidence that sustains an attitude of commitment and acceptance that holds fast, regardless of events and adversities. Martin identifies the "mark of faith" as "the confidence that nothing she encounters can give her rea-son to stop hoping" (p. 106). Martin contrasts the contingent sustaining power of hope with the essential sustaining power of faith:

> There are many ways of committing suicide, some literal, some figurative. The temptation our greatest trials present is the idea that suicide of one form or an-other might be the best way to evade being crushed: physically, emotionally, spiritually, evaluatively. I have argued that there are many kinds of hope that counter this idea, that can occupy the conceptual space existential despair re-quires to exist. I have also argued that there is a *more rarified form of hope* that is not only a conceptual counter to existential despair but also a way of lifting oneself out of the world of experience and pinning one's sights on an outcome that one is always justified in hoping for. This unimaginable hope is a plausible candidate for the attitude we call "faith," and under certain conditions it is a ra-tional form of confidence in the possibility of a good outcome to a trial. (p. 117, emphasis added)

We can hardly talk about the *unimaginable* in concrete terms. Yet with the ulti-mate value of a good life in mind, Martin proposes conviction in the *goodness of the world* as one manifestation of faith. Taking a different tack, Tillich (1957) defined faith in relation to one's *ultimate concern*: "the centered movement of the whole personality toward something of ultimate meaning and significance" (p. 123). Whereas Tillich was writing in a broadly religious context, I interpret an ulti-mate concern as referring to what is of ultimate value or significance to you, un-conditional in the sense that you could not give it up without doing profound violence to your integrity and your life. As one of Tillich's commentators sum-marized,

> What distinguishes humans from other animals is that each of us has the capacity to be concerned about something of ultimate importance, something whose loss would divest our lives of meaning and rob us of the courage to be. Whether our ultimate concern is truly ultimate, and not a mere idol instead, can be determined only by observing how adequately it functions to give us courage in the face of fate, death, guilt, and the threat of meaninglessness. (Haught 2009, p. 225)

Contra Martin, and closer to our thinking about hope, Tillich (1957) viewed doubt and uncertainty as intrinsic to faith: "If doubt appears, it should not be considered as the negation of faith, but as an element which was always and will always be present in faith"; moreover, "serious doubt is confirmation of faith. It indicates the seriousness of the concern" (p. 25). The struggles that require courage in sustaining faith in the face of doubt and uncertainty comprise the dynamics of faith, akin to the dynamics of hope that oscillates between pre-sumption and despair. Edging toward Martin's view, Tillich makes room for "a serenity of life in faith beyond the disturbing struggles between faith and doubt," and he recognizes that attaining such a state "is a natural and justified desire of every human being." Nonetheless, "the element of doubt, though conquered, is not lacking." And he cautions that unshakable faith, as evident in fanaticism, is a symptom of repressed doubt; in robust faith, "[d]oubt is overcome not by repression but by courage" (p. 117).

I am drawn to the heady visions articulated here, but I know that we cannot live on abstractions. How do we think about the unimaginable? The ultimate? I have already alluded to what Tillich (1957) asserted: to reach beyond what we are able to grasp to what we cannot grasp, we rely on *symbols*, which "point beyond themselves to something else" (p. 47). In educating patients about hope, I rely on an appealing abstraction that has concrete associations, Pruyser's (1987b) formulation of grounds for hope: "a belief that there is *some benevolent disposition toward oneself somewhere in the universe, conveyed by a caring person*" (p. 467, emphasis in original). I now see Pruyser's conception as an expression of faith that bridges secular and religious thought. I find it apt because of its implication of attachment and love ("some benevolent disposition" and "a caring person") as a basis for faith. Moreover, benevolence and caring comprise cornerstones of basic trust. Even if it is not explicitly grounded in religion, I think faith moves in the territory of spirituality and transcendence, as Pruyser's formulation does. Located "somewhere in the universe," the benevolent disposition could refer to a personalized God or higher power but might instead be felt in a kinship with beauty and nature. Moreover, passion for science—from physics to biology and psychology—might inspire such kinship.

To sum up, I have construed the context for trusting as depending on trustworthiness when one's well-being is at stake. In a broad sense, I see trust as embedded in faith. Martin construed faith as hope plus confidence. Trust implies confidence, as distrust implies lack of confidence. Martin (2014) referred to *transcendent goodness* in the world. Pruyser (1987b) referred to a *benevolent disposition* in the universe, elaborating on the work of existentially oriented psychiatrist Karl Jaspers: "Jaspers once called the world as a whole 'the encompassing'…which I find a nice term. I would be inclined to be slightly more metaphorical and warm about it, by calling it 'the embracing'" (Pruyser 1974, p. 224). I read faith in Simone Weil's inspiring conviction that

> At the bottom of the heart of every human being, *from earliest infancy* until the tomb, there is something that goes on *indomitably expecting*, in the teeth of all experience of crimes committed, suffered, and witnessed, that *good* and not evil will be done to him. It is this above all that is sacred in every human being. (Miles 1986, p. 51, emphasis added)

Weil's conviction is consistent with the primordial sense of basic trust that I endorsed earlier in this chapter, and I agree with her sentiment about the sacredness of goodness. Sadly, I do not agree that the primordial expectation of goodness is indomitable; on the contrary, the seeming extinction of this expectation in the context of unthinkable trauma is the bane of psychotherapy and all other potentially therapeutic relationships: hope, trust, and faith in goodness are most needed when they are most wanting.

For those of us fortunate enough to have access to it, we might view *faith as generalized trust*, which in my view is potentially generalized from concrete experience of benevolence and goodness in early caregiving to the broader world, perhaps represented by nature or a godlike figure or process. Going back to basic trust, such faith could be instantiated in a feeling of being "at home" in the world or the universe, potentially including the sense of serenity that Haybron (2008) gave a prominent role in his concept of *attunement*—the highest form of happiness as it contributes to well-being and a good life (see Chapter 1).

Coming back down to earth, I am inclined to see a faith-like version of trust in the form of distributed caregiving that characterizes small-scale societies (see Chapter 2). Consider what it would feel like for a mother to be free of concern when she has no idea where her toddler is in the community—and what it is like for the toddler. They are at home in the community. Now consider what it is like to feel unsafe at home or in the community or utterly alienated from the world, without hope, trust, or faith. That is a context for suicide. In that context, faith would be an unimaginable luxury. We therapists focus more practically on cultivating hope, with at least some inchoate vision of a better future and some way to bring it about. Our patients need to develop hope in our trustworthiness and in their own. But, coming down from the clouds, I see a relatively prosaic role for therapists' faith in psychotherapy, at least as I have come to develop it.

Faith in Psychotherapy

My experience in psychotherapy that called for hope and faith was all too concrete—viscerally palpable. I never felt comfortable working with patients who felt profoundly hopeless and suicidal, despite how experienced I became in doing so. All too often, I was apprehensive or downright fearful. But I became accustomed to the work and the feelings. When patients were referred to me, I received a thorough psychiatric evaluation, which typically included a cluster of serious psychiatric disorders. More daunting than these disorders, however, were the tragic life circumstances in relation to which the disorders developed—plight after plight. Commonly, the history of traumatic stress and loss was staggering. I could not imagine a pathway forward when I reviewed such a history. However, impersonal clinical narratives can be inadvertently damning, and meeting the patient in person often was reassuring. The presence of a living soul calls for hope. Yet such patients' helplessness and hopelessness can be contagious. In most such instances, however, over the course of therapy, a pathway opened up; the patient and I developed hope, including hope in each other. Almost invariably, the pathway went from conflict and alienation to reconnection in relationships. I learned from this recurrent experience that my inability to imagine what a good-enough outcome would be or how it could come about did not warrant hopelessness on my part. Never presumptuous, never cheerleading, I could be reasonably hopeful. I could invest some hope—gently and cautiously.

Similarly, for more than a decade I served as a co-leader of what we called a peer supervision group in the hospital. We could have called it a support group. This was a self-selected group of nurses, social workers, psychologists, and psychiatrists who came together weekly to discuss patients with whom they were struggling mightily. This group greatly extended my personal experience, as many colleagues (and I) described frustrating, alarming, and seemingly hopeless stalemates and situations. We provided each other with a great deal of consolation, sympathy, empathy, and support, along with occasional good advice or suggestions. Often, we were in emotional distress, but we were not alone in it, practicing what we preached. We created a forum for reflection and understanding. But I learned from this group time and again how a previously unimaginable way forward typically emerged in the treatment. For us all, this experience helped us hold on to hope in the face of the seemingly hopeless. Nonetheless, to prevent the group from being demoralized in the face of our relentless trials, we decided at one point to begin each session with an inspiring instance of progress or a good treatment outcome. We never failed to come up with one, and these examples were often unexpected.

From my own experience and that of my colleagues, I learned that I could be surprised; paradoxically, I came to *count on being surprised*. Perhaps there is a bit of faith in this confidence—counting on the unimaginable. I am no Pollyanna. I learned, along with my colleagues, that I also could be blindsided by suicide and that treatment sometimes failed in other ways. But suicide was, thankfully, extremely rare, and treatment failure was by far the exception rather than the norm. Science played a role: we gathered systematic treatment outcome data that buttressed our extensive encouraging clinical experience (Allen et al. 2017; Oh et al. 2020).

On a daily basis, all of us clinicians face what feels like a low probability but some possibility of a good but unimaginable outcome. Success is never guaranteed or inevitable. We all experience varying degrees of failure and disappointment. None of us is immune to the prospect of suicide, and many of us—myself included—have had to contend with it. We all have influence but no control. Life outside the hospital, most prominently, events in the family, are a powerful force, for better or for worse—not only for patients but also for therapists. But the better prevailed by far over the worse in my fortunate four-decade career in the hospital. Wisdom supports investing hope in possibility and acting on behalf of hope not only *for* my patients but also *in* my patients.

Looking back, I believe that I also developed hope in myself; I could be of help in ways I could not foresee at the outset. Taking a cue from Martin, faith might be a more fitting concept than hope. With Tillich, I would like to think that, for most of us, psychotherapy is embedded in our ultimate values—what matters most—commitment to which calls for faith and courage. All of us need hope, and some of us might be lucky enough to find faith in ourselves along with faith in our work and our patients. We and our patients assume different roles, but we remain immersed in uncertain life together. Hope—and sometimes faith—sustains us all. And we will accomplish nothing without trusting and trustworthiness.

Summary of Key Points

- In the psychotherapy context, the patient is suffering in a plight that requires depending on the therapist. The patient is *counting on* the therapist, and the trustworthy therapist is motivated by responsiveness to *being counted on.*

- Depending and counting on a person renders one vulnerable to being let down, but counting on trustworthy persons decreases vulnerability by providing needed help and support. With trustworthiness, depending on others is a solution, not a problem.

- We can trust in a person's actions (he or she will do as promised), and we can trust in the person as such. Trust in the person develops over the course of his or her trustworthy actions.

- Trusting in psychotherapy requires that the therapist be caring (for the patient's well-being) and competent (knowledgeable and skillful). Caring requires its own competence (interpersonal skill).

- We must learn to trust well (in proportion to trustworthiness) and to distrust well (in proportion to untrustworthiness). Distrust comes in degrees, ranging from vigilance to suspicion to outright distrust.

- A working assumption for therapists: distrusting patients have learned to distrust well in the past but might be overgeneralizing by missing opportunities to trust those who are trustworthy in the present.

- Gottman identified a problematic trajectory in couple relationships: from *trustworthiness* (looking out for your partner's interests) to *untrustworthiness* (no longer looking out for your partner's interests but instead focusing solely on your own interests) to *betrayal* (looking out for your own interests at the expense of your partner's interests). In this trajectory, the couple's relationship becomes devalued, and alternative relationships become more valued.

- Trusting and distrusting yourself parallel trusting and distrusting others: Both should be matched to your trustworthiness to yourself. Self-trust flourishes or is undermined in relationships with others; because we must depend on others, self-trust requires trusting others who are trustworthy.

- Hope and trust are intertwined insofar as both arise in the context of a plight in which the desired outcome is uncertain, such that hope and trust are fraught with fear and doubt. Trust entails hope in a therapist's trustworthiness (care and competence), which is essential in the hoped-for treatment outcome.

Recommendations for Clinical Practice

- When we talk with our patients about their distrust, we can begin by validating the risk they take when they trust, acknowledging their feelings of vulnerability to being let down or betrayed. Then we can point out that they need to trust because they require help and that they will be less vulnerable when they can avail themselves of help—the potential benefit of what they are doing in seeking therapy. But I quickly point out that vulnerability hinges on trustworthiness and that judging others' trustworthiness can be difficult, especially when you have a history of misjudging people who have proven to be untrustworthy.

- Talking with patients about their distrust in you can be difficult—especially but not only for the patient. You might best enter into this potentially fraught territory by inviting patients to talk about what they are counting on you for. In raising this concern, you are implicitly conveying your trustworthiness: you intend to be responsive to being counted on. Moreover, you are first easing into the less personal domain of three-place trust—trusting in your actions or knowledge—as contrasted with two-place trust, which entails trusting you as a person. Patients are likely to find it easier to talk about doubting your helpfulness than their doubt about you. By discussing being counted on, you are providing an implicit frame for more difficult conversations about trust. Moreover, this context provides an opportunity to clarify boundaries and the limits of the extent to which you are willing to be available and helpful—

also an indication of your trustworthiness. And you might also talk about what you are counting on your patient for, implicitly entering the territory of his or her trustworthiness to you. Focusing initially on being counted on will open the door to patients to talk about their trust and distrust in you, as a person.

- When you follow my suggestion of refocusing from the patient's trust to your own trustworthiness, you put yourself in the territory of self-trust. Telling a patient, "You can trust me," would be appealing to presumption. Taking your trustworthiness as a therapist for granted is presumptuous. Instead, think about the extent to which you can be counted on and for what. You could think of yourself as committing to providing a treatment. I think you also are committing to establishing a trusting relationship, and—unlike the treatment method—you are doing so without knowing what you are getting into. I speak from much experience.

- I recommend that you enrich your thinking about trust by taking hope into consideration. Trusting implies hope: tolerating uncertainty, fear, and doubt in trustworthiness while avoiding the polarized alternatives of presumption or despair. If your patient felt confident in counting on you, trust would not be a concern. In the context of a plight—the occasion for seeking treatment—you need to share in your patient's uncertainty regarding hope and trust without succumbing to presumption or despair. You need to invest hope in your patient, and in trusting your patient you are confronted with the uncertainty of hope. Just think about working with suicidal patients. To stay the course when you cannot imagine how the patient (and you) will get out of the plight, you might need faith. If you come across a manual for this unfathomably complex and inherently relational process of creating hope and faith in psychotherapy, don't trust it.

4

Becoming Trustworthy

Peter Fonagy and colleagues observed that "clinicians have historically linked non-responsiveness to therapeutic intervention to *characteristics of their patient* rather than *features of their own relationship to the patient*" (Fonagy et al. 2017, p. 5, emphasis in original). As described in Chapter 1, "From Trusting Therapies to Trusting Therapists," the psychotherapy research literature indicates that we have put far too much emphasis on theories, brands, and techniques, given that the therapeutic relationship carries the lion's share of the influence. Moreover, individual differences among therapists carry more weight than the type of therapy they practice (Wampold and Imel 2015).

As discussed in Chapter 1, I am advocating shifting the balance from developing therapies to the development of therapists. Given the central importance of trusting in psychotherapy, I am thinking about therapists' development from the perspective of trustworthiness. I use *becoming* trustworthy in two developmental senses: first, becoming trustworthy over the course of a particular relationship, with the focus on patient-therapist relationships; second, becoming personally and professionally trustworthy over the course of individual development, including a professional career.

I am not disparaging therapists' character here. On the contrary, I would consider the vast majority of therapists I have known to be trustworthy in the ordinary sense of the word. But I aim to go beyond our ordinary way of thinking to consider trustworthiness as a developmental process, in both the short term and the long term. As is evident throughout this book, becoming trustworthy in psychotherapy is especially challenging in requiring us to integrate our personal and professional knowledge in our potentially fraught relationships with patients who come into the process with a history of well-earned distrust and whom we endeavor to help become more trusting.

Philosopher Nancy Nyquist Potter is a rare exception in the literature on trust, having devoted an entire book to trustworthiness, *How Can I Be Trusted?* In addition to her academic work, she served as a crisis counselor for a large metropolitan agency. She "refocuses the subject of trust by *making central our responsibility to be trustworthy.*" She regarded her work as "a project of ethics" and took a critical stance: "That discussions of trust have so frequently neglected the question of how we can *become trustworthy* seems to me an indictment of much moral inquiry" (Potter 2002, p. xi, emphasis added). Accordingly, in what could be a charge for psychotherapists, she argued that "our moral responsibility to cultivate trust leads to the need for us to cultivate a *trustworthy character*" (p. xv, emphasis added). I agree but would add that, to the extent that we develop a trustworthy character, we do it relationship by relationship, inside and outside therapy, beginning early in life and continuing throughout thereafter. I am mainly interested in the developmental process and am attentive to the relationship-specific aspect of trustworthiness.

We therapists should think of trusting and trustworthiness not only as relationship-specific but also as variable within a therapy relationship, as it can be with other relationships. We should give patients who have suffered a history of trauma in attachment relationships credit for being reasonable when they distrust us, and we should side with their need for evidence of our trustworthiness. They will put us to the test, repeatedly. To varying degrees, we will fail—inevitably. Taking our trustworthiness for granted is a big mistake; when we fail to be trustworthy, putting the onus on the patient's problem with trust is a bigger mistake.

Following Fonagy and colleagues (2019a), I emphasize the importance of trusting not only for the *process* of therapy but also as an optimal *outcome* of therapy. In this chapter, I urge readers to keep in mind that cultivating *patients' trustworthiness* also should be considered crucial not only for the process but also to the outcome. In short, I believe that we have given insufficient attention to trust, neglected therapists' trustworthiness even more, and almost entirely neglected patients' trustworthiness. If trustworthiness is the proper basis for trusting, and trusting is foundational to good relationships, cultivating trustworthiness in patients is a proper goal of any psychotherapy that focuses on problems in relationships. Trustworthiness plays a role in patients' caregiving relationships—parenting not least—and in all their other close relationships. Finally, cultivating trust in psychotherapy requires some degree of trusting and trustworthiness in therapists and patients from the start. We cannot make something out of nothing.

In this chapter, I set the stage with a philosophical perspective on trustworthiness, using Immanuel Kant's argument for balancing love and respect along with Peter Strawson's seminal work on moral reactive attitudes and Christine Swanton's nuanced articulation of what it means to be nonjudgmental. All these ethical perspectives provide a framework for thinking about therapeutic neutrality, a controversial topic that I believe gets to the heart of trustworthiness. I capitalize on psychoanalyst Jessica Benjamin's theoretical and clinical writing to illustrate the enormous challenges of becoming trustworthy in intensive treatment with patients whose distrust is well founded in traumatic relationships. A central theme of these first two sections is the need for therapists to be open and honest with their patients, just as they aspire to enable their patients to be with them. I use my work on written formulations to illustrate one form of such transparency. Our patients' trust entails uncertainty, but it need not be blind.

The Ethical-Moral Basis of Trustworthiness

As described in Chapter 1, professional organizations and state licensing boards that provide oversight of clinical practice strive to promote practitioners' trustworthiness by promulgating ethical principles and codes. Although I agree that knowledge of professional ethics is essential to trustworthiness, I continue with the different tack I have taken in this book, valuing ethical thought exemplified in philosophy as foundational to the conduct of psychotherapy. Nowhere is this foundational role more evident than in the context of trust and trustworthiness.

Love and Respect

As an anchor for my thinking about the moral basis of relationships, I have adopted an ostensibly simple contrast articulated by eighteenth-century German philosopher Immanuel Kant (1797/1966). He proposed that *love* and *respect* are two great moral forces. *Love entails coming close and respect requires keeping distance.* Kant emphasized that love and respect are in tension, and Christine Swanton (2003) proposed that highlighting this tension was Kant's most important contribution. Swanton construed the tension as an equilibrium point and asserted that the "real problem" of balancing love and respect is "the substantive problem of delineating the equilibrium point" (p. 106). I add that the equilibrium point will vary continually in accordionlike fashion within any given relationship, including psychotherapy relationships; at some times, we need to move closer, and at others, we need to keep our distance. Moreover, the balance and expression of closeness and distance varies across cultures.

Kant's (1785/2012) most famous ethical principle is the categorical imperative: "*act according to the maxim that can make itself at the same time a universal law*" (p. 48, emphasis in original), which I understand (crassly) as this: what if everybody did it? More pertinent to our concerns and Kant's overall ethical philosophy is the *formula of humanity* as an end in itself: "*So act that you use humanity, in your own person as well as in the person of any other, always at the same time as an end, never merely as a means*" (p. 41, emphasis in original). The key word in this formula is "merely." Of course, we must use (rely on) others for our own purposes, we are profoundly social. As discussed in Chapter 3, "Trusting," we trust others for instrumental reasons. But we also consider trusting relationships to have intrinsic value. To Kant, every person has profound intrinsic value: "unconditional, incomparable worth" (p. 47). We each have our own ends, evident in our autonomy, which must be respected. In reading Kant's formula of humanity, I think of Appiah's (2008) construal of the central ethical task described in Chapter 1: Each of us is striving to make a good life, and each of us must respect others doing so. In a moral world, when we serve others' needs or desires (instrumentally), we do so freely.

As Swanton asserted, Kant's (1797/1966) main contribution to our thinking about love and respect is the *relationship* between these two great moral forces:

> we consider ourselves in a moral (intelligible) world where, by analogy with the physical world, *attraction* and *repulsion* bind together rational beings (on earth). The principle of mutual love admonishes them constantly to *come closer* to one another; that of the respect they owe one another, to keep themselves *at a distance* from one another. (p. 198, emphasis in original)

We need love, and we need space.

Kant (1797/1966) used the word *love* in its broad sense to refer to benevolence and beneficence: "Benevolence is satisfaction in the happiness (well-being) of others; but beneficence is the maxim of making others' happiness one's end" (p. 201). With an eye toward equality in the worth of every person, Kant included self-love: "making benevolence a duty will include myself, as an object of benevolence" (p. 200). Alerted by Swanton's (2003) understanding of self-love as "*bonding* with oneself" (p. 134, emphasis in original), I think of self-love in the context of a secure attachment relationship with oneself (Allen 2005). Self-love provides a foundation for basic trust in yourself.

Kant (1797/1966) asserted, "The *respect* that I have for others or that another can require from me…is therefore recognition of a *dignity*…in other human beings, that is, of a worth that has no price, no equivalent." He continued, "Every human being has a legitimate claim to respect from his fellow human beings and is *in turn* bound to respect every other" (p. 209, emphases in original). In Kant's way of thinking, respect undergirds the formula of humanity according to which every individual must be regarded as an end and not merely a means. The opposite of respect is contempt, which entails "[j]udging something to be worthless" and thus without dignity. Kant would not be surprised that Gottman (2011) found contempt to be the death knell of love relationships (see Chapter 3). In the context of attachment trauma, neglect is a failure of love (coming close), and abuse is a failure of respect (keeping distance).

Distinguishing love and respect as well as their counterparts, neglect and abuse, should not obscure their entanglement. When they are in balance, love and respect are intertwined; with loving connection comes interest in promoting the other's

TABLE 4–1.   Polarities in the vital balance between love and respect

Love	Respect
Closeness	Distance
Togetherness	Separateness
Relatedness	Autonomy
Safe haven	Secure base
Engagement	Detachment
Absence evident in neglect	Absence evident in abuse

well-being, including separateness and autonomy, safeguarded by respect. In this sense, respect is loving—implicit in nonpossessive love. Failures in respect, by undermining well-being, compromise love. Similarly, neglect and abuse overlap insofar as caring and emotional engagement promote respect and are thus incompatible with abuse. To make another link that underscores commonality and contrast: love and respect require mentalizing, whereas neglect and abuse are among the worst concomitants of nonmentalizing and the height of untrustworthiness.

I propose that the vital balance between love and respect stakes out the basic ethical territory of trustworthy relationships. This polarity is consistent with relatedness and autonomy constituting two fundamental developmental lines (Blatt 2008) and the safe haven and secure base comprising the essential constituents of secure attachment (Bowlby 1988). Several polarities in this vital balance are listed in Table 4–1. Balancing love and respect goes to the heart of a fundamental principle of *therapeutic neutrality*, a challenging and hotly debated topic most thoroughly developed in the psychoanalytic literature that I discuss at a later point.

Moral Reactive Attitudes

In bringing ethics—and the more loaded word morals—into my thinking about how I conduct psychotherapy, I had to contend with a nagging science-minded conscience that made me question my way of thinking. Yet my nagging conscience failed to stem my increasing conviction that I was on the right track. In the course of my philosophical explorations, I found substantial validation in Peter Strawson's (1982) classic paper "Freedom and Resentment." Strawson was concerned with our natural human emotional reactions to each other. In the (psychoanalytic) psychotherapy literature, these reactions come under the banner of countertransference, which (in its narrow sense) refers to emotional responses to the patient's (ill-fitting) transferences. In broader senses, countertransference can refer to the therapist's problematic emotional responses based on personal problems or even emotional responses more generally. Of course, patients, therapists, and everyone else engage in emotionally evocative behavior that has myriad sources: transferences, personal problems, and reasonable reactions among them.

Strawson (1982) identified a source of natural emotional reactivity that grabbed my attention: "*moral* reactive attitudes" (p. 73, emphasis added). He focused on the "very great importance that we attach to the attitudes and intentions toward us of other human beings and the great extent to which our personal feelings and reactions depend upon, or involve, our beliefs about these attitudes and intentions" (p. 62). Now for the moral part: Strawson highlighted "how much we actually mind, how much it matters to us, whether the actions of other people—and particularly *some* other people—reflect attitudes towards us of goodwill, affection, or esteem on the one hand or contempt, indifference, or malevolence on the other" (p. 63, emphasis in original). Of course, others' goodwill or ill will can be influenced by transferences, psychiatric disorders, and myriad other factors. Our moral reactive attitudes are not necessarily disentangling these influences when we feel the emotions. Moreover, we respond vicariously with reactive attitudes toward the way people treat other people and the way they treat themselves (e.g., punitively, destructively).

Crucially, Strawson (1985) contrasted these reactive attitudes with the objective and detached attitude that we also can adopt, for example, for the purpose of scientific inquiry. He asserted that we *can suspend* the moral reactive attitudes, but we *cannot eliminate* them or be reasoned out of them; they are "*a condition of our humanity*" and "as deeply rooted in our natures as our existence as social beings" (p. 33, emphasis added). So much for the idea that, in our role as therapists, we should not feel irritated, frustrated, disgusted, shocked, anxious, threatened, helpless, or sexually enticed as well as admiring, affectionate, compassionate, and loving. In the context of psychoanalytic treatment, Strawson (1982) made the key point that we must *straddle* the moral-reactive and objective-detached stances, employing both perspectives. I think we can *alternate* these stances to some degree, but we also can *integrate* them to varying degrees (reflecting while reacting). What I took from Strawson is the attitude that these moral-reactive responses are not only proper and unavoidable; they are intrinsic to our social humanity. And, as psychoanalysis has emphasized throughout its history, these emotions-laden responses are *informative* to the treatment. Of course, all of us know the experience of overwhelming emotions clouding our thinking, but this experience is generally the exception; "we humans do some of our best thinking while having feelings of varying quality and intensity" (Renik 1996, p. 511).

Being Nonjudgmental

Christine Swanton (2003) clarified a related point for me. I imagine that virtually every psychotherapist has heard that we should be *nonjudgmental*. Keep in mind that being nonjudgmental is challenging in the face of our moral-reactive attitudes. I find Swanton's nuanced perspective vital and packed with wisdom, so I quote her at length:

> "Not being judgmental" is a vague idea, but it involves several things. First, it involves not being too ready to evaluate, particularly negatively. We shouldn't think that the most salient requirement of "coming into the presence of a person" is to evaluate them, as opposed to being receptive to them, for example. Furthermore, not only must one not be too ready to *find fault*, one should not treat a person as a "phenomenon," a person with "interesting" features, the understanding of which is motivated chiefly by *curiosity*. Finally, insofar as one is engaged in evaluation, one is animated in large measure by a desire to *find some good*. (pp. 126–127, emphasis added)

I highlight three points in this passage. First, the best synonym for judgmental would be fault-finding. The main point I emphasize is that being nonjudgmental does not mean refraining from making judgments, including moral judgments. Analogous to Strawson's reasoning, I believe that making judgments is unavoidable, natural, and useful. Second, there is more in this passage, namely, a concern about "curiosity," which drew my attention because curiosity has been a core concept in the inquisitive stance long advocated in the mentalizing approach (Bateman and Fonagy 2016). Curiosity in isolation is potentially problematic. It is not uncommon for patients to protest that they feel like lab rats or specimens under a microscope. Here we have too much detachment and too little emotional engagement—too much distance, too little closeness. As Kant saw, we need balance, and these attitudes are often in tension. Finally, we must be mindful of overdoing our needed clinical focus on psychopathology and give our full attention to the good. Getting this balance right is crucial to therapeutic relationships for us all, inside or outside psychotherapy.

We all feel more open to critical judgment in the broader climate of respectful and compassionate acceptance. And our own lack of self-acceptance can lead us to perceive others' reasonable judgments as judgmental. I recall vividly my first psychotherapy session as a patient decades ago when all my concern was focused on the fee and my therapist observed, "You are anxious" (i.e., about getting into the relationship). I believe that she said this with compassionate acceptance, but I heard it as a criticism. Looking back later, I appreciated her compassionate acceptance, and my memory of this event became a model for my own more compassionate acceptance of my anxiety. It is entirely reasonable to be anxious during your first therapy session (not to mention many thereafter).

Adopting the way of thinking that I have taken from Kant, Strawson, and Swanton leaves us psychotherapists in a state of tension: balancing love and respect, straddling emotional engagement and detachment, making judgments without being judgmental—and applying all these tensions to our relationship with ourselves as well as others. How we manage these tensions will be a mark of our trustworthiness, toward ourselves and others, including our patients. I think that psychoanalysis, over the course of its history, deserves much credit for articulating these inherent tensions in the fraught context of intensive treatments in a way that is relevant to all but the most prescriptive and technical therapeutic procedures. The tension in the professional debates about neutrality mirrors the tensions inherent in finding the ethical-moral balance in relationships that Kant elucidated. In my view, we cannot escape the messiness of psychotherapy once we engage with patients' problems in living and become their partners in experiencing and working with these problems.

Therapeutic Neutrality

I am unqualified to offer any expert opinion on psychoanalytic theory or practice; as just stated, I present this literature because I believe the struggles with neutrality are fundamental to trustworthiness in psychotherapy more generally. This controversy has an extremely long history and a huge literature, and my discussion is necessarily selective. I am biased in favor of the relatively recent relational psychoanalytic perspective, especially as represented by Owen Renik (1995, 1996, 1999, 2006) as well as Irwin Hoffman (1996), Stephen Mitchell (2000), and Hans Loewald (1960), who have criticized what has become a stereotype of psychoanalytic distance. I also rely on William Meissner (1998, 2002) for a thoughtful and expert critique of the critics. Albeit from somewhat differing perspectives, all advocate what they believe to be a trustworthy balance between closeness and distance.

Leaning Toward Distance

Psychoanalysis has long been attacked as unscientific. Ironically, from the perspective of hindsight, its advocacy of neutrality was associated with scientism: adhering narrowly to scientific ("analytic") objectivity as an ideal. As Loewald (1960) characterized it, "The ideal image of the analyst is that of a detached scientist," which was consistent with Freud's view of "the most advanced form of human development," to be attained by the analyst as well as the patient: "the maturity of scientific man who understands himself and external reality not in animistic or religious terms but in terms of objective science." Accordingly, the analysis becomes a "scientific project." Loewald protests, "It is not self-explanatory why a research project should have a therapeutic effect on the subject of study" (p. 19).

As Renik (1995, p. 509) pointed out, we generally think of neutrality as impartiality regarding two sides of a political or military conflict, but Freud's application of the German word *Indifferenz*, which was translated as neutrality, connotes being emotionally detached or uninvolved—at worst, a stiff formality. In practice, such neutrality is exemplified by excessive silence, reluctance to make judgments, and refusals to affirm a patient's point of view. Neutrality also has come to encompass anonymity and minimal self-disclosure. Analogies include surgery (in an antiseptic atmosphere) and engineering as well as hewing religiously to a scientific method, connoting (in my mind) an impersonal approach. As should be obvious from this description, psychoanalytic neutrality lends itself to caricature, and none of several psychoanalysts who taught and supervised me decades ago exemplified emotional indifference in their work; they were devoted to caring.

Of course, some therapists can practice in a manner that corresponds to the caricature. Consider the clinical experience reported by Italian psychoanalyst Antonio Ferro (Ferro and Nicoli 2017) that he said was "one of the few cases in which I…dismissed a candidate during the final exam of training." The analytic candidate reported an event with a pregnant patient who, on entering his office, stumbled and fell on the floor. In his account of the session, the candidate wrote, "Of course I stood motionless and did not touch the patient." Ferro commented that this behavior was not analytic neutrality; it was "nonsense" (p. 35). I think "nonsense" is charitable. Ferro went on to point out that the analyst "should have neither a phobia of emotional contact nor a phobia of physical contact," adding, "If a patient at the end of analysis gives you a kiss on the cheek, you just take it and smile" (p. 37). I had a patient (who was Italian) do just that suddenly when we said goodbye at the end of our last session. I was a bit startled; I hope I smiled. When I said goodbye to my therapist (who was from Greece) when she was leaving the clinic, she kissed me on the cheek. I smiled.

The psychoanalytic emphasis on neutrality developed purposefully in the context of the theory and technique of treatment, namely, establishing the anonymity of the analyst as a "blank screen" for projections to promote transferences that could be interpreted and resolved. Having never practiced psychoanalysis, I am concerned with generalist psychotherapy, in which I believe neutrality to be equally important. More specifically, I think there is a solid ethical justification for therapeutic neutrality: *respect for the patient's autonomy*. A number of words appear repeatedly in this literature in reference to the failures of neutrality, and they begin with the letter "i": intruding, impinging, infringing, interfering, and imposing. Highly relevant to neutrality is the word *boundaries*, which is ubiquitous in the professional literature; boundary violations are serious breaches of neutrality. We remain in the territory of ethics in its broadest sense; as Hoffman (1996) asserted, "There can be no intimacy, of course, without boundaries in *any* relationship" (p. 115, emphasis in original). Respect implies distance, metaphorically and physically. Exploitation is another serious breach of neutrality. Decades ago, I interviewed a graduate school applicant who told me he wanted to become a clinical psychologist so he could learn how to "control" people. We did not accept him.

I spent a number of years conducting educational groups for patients in which we discussed different types of relationships (Stein et al. 2003). In addition to covering relationships with acquaintances, friends, romantic partners, and family members, we discussed relationships with therapists, one of our favorite topics that was highly engaging for patients. This session provided a rare opportunity (on relatively neutral ground) for patients to talk with us therapists about their relationships with their therapists, past and present. Some patients complained about their experience with therapists who were too pushy or opinionated, for example, imposing their views or values on them. But these patients were a distinct minority. By far the most pervasive complaint was that therapists were too passive, too quiet, and too reluctant to say what was on their mind.

I am partial to the i-word *influence*. With neutrality in mind, therapists rightly worry about *undue* influence. Should we also worry about *too little* influence? In our reluctance, we might be confusing influencing with the other i-words I used: intruding, impinging, interfering, infringing, and imposing. We are dealing with shades of gray here, and they are important.

Leaning Toward Closeness

Over the course of my career, I gravitated to a conviction that psychotherapy is a highly individualized process in which—for better or for worse—my personal characteristics play a significant role. Ultimately, I accepted the idea that when I was effective, I was having a *personal influence* on my patients. I was aware that this view went against the grain of my scientific-professional upbringing that was also tinctured by my early psychoanalytic milieu. On reflection, I concluded that my earlier attitude made no sense. We must intend to influence our patients. Why else would we take on this arduous professional (and highly personal) vocation? Granting an intention to influence, would we endeavor to have an *impersonal* influence? Are we merely vehicles for technique? Therapy apps on our smartphones are now available for impersonal influence.

Admiring Renik's open-minded attitude, I found his position on therapeutic influence to be profoundly validating. In his article "The Perils of Neutrality," he asserted, "Psychoanalysts have studied the problem of influence more explicitly than have other caregivers, but we have not been more successful in dealing with it" (Renik 1996, p. 495). He argued that we must take into account that "*personal influence* by the analyst is at the heart of technique" (p. 496, emphasis added). Putting it forcefully, he acknowledged "the highly personal nature of each individual analyst's work" and asserted, "What acceptance of our non-neutrality underlines is that the analyst's *affectively driven intention toward personal influence* is inextricable from our clinical method," going on to characterize clinical psychoanalysis as a "dialectic between two non-neutral participants" (p. 515, emphasis in original). Consider the alternative, for example, how you feel working with profoundly depressed or suicidal patients when you have *no personal influence*. I feel frustrated, helpless, inadequate, guilty, anxious, and incompetent. I much prefer influence, without shading into the other i-words.

Renik (1995, 1996) argued that neutrality (as classically advocated) is an impossible ideal that has become counterproductive; the term *neutrality* is misleading, and the aspiration to be neutral should be abandoned. (For a thoughtful contrary view, see Meissner 1998, 2002.) Renik identified a range of potential problems with neutrality. The ideal of an authoritatively objective analyst is liable to promote idealization. Neutrality implies that if patients were exposed to the analyst's thinking, they would be unable to think for themselves. Anonymity is tantamount to a sphinxlike posture that is distracting to patients, who will become preoccupied with clues that will enable them to guess or decipher what is going on in the analyst's mind. At worst, such opacity could abet distrust in the form of heightened vigilance if not outright suspiciousness.

I find Renik's (2006) argument for openness to be compelling in its respect for patients: "The best safeguard against infringing on a patient's autonomy is for an analyst to acknowledge the highly personal nature of his or her participation in the treatment, so that the patient feels free to evaluate the analyst's contributions for what they are" (p. 80). Hoffman (1996) made a similar point in arguing against the possibility that the patient is "simply putty in the analyst's hands," countering that it is "precisely respect for the patient's agency that opens the door to overcoming our *phobic* attitude toward our own personal influence on our patients' lives" (p. 123, emphasis in original). He added that getting beyond the phobia leaves plenty of room for anxiety about the responsibility entailed in influencing our patients' lives. Similarly, Renik (1996) asserted that the high level of emotional involvement puts a premium on "the analyst's *integrity*, for which a myth of neutrality cannot substitute" (p. 507, emphasis added). In this view, our problems are more ethical than technical. Of course, the power differential also puts a premium on the ethical dimension of influence, and Renik's implication that the patient can objectively evaluate the analyst's contributions should not minimize the impact of the power differential. The patient's greater objectivity might be an ideal outcome of the analysis.

What is the alternative to strict neutrality? Renik (2006) advocated "playing your cards face up" (p. 53), ensuring that the patient understands the analyst's activity "*as fully as possible*" by presenting the patient with "a clear and explicit picture of the analyst's conscious view of his or her purposes and methods," aiming for "comprehensibility, not inscrutability" (Renik 1995, p. 482, emphasis in original). He questioned the prohibition of "rendering personal judgments concerning the way a patient manages his or her crucial life struggles" (Renik 1996, p. 508). Hoffman (1996) was forthright on this point: "we are intimately involved in our patients' struggles to make better lives for themselves, and we cannot ignore our own vision of the better life in our participating in those struggles" (p. 131). I couldn't agree more, as exemplified by my argument for thinking reflectively about ethics with an eye toward explicating the nature of a good life.

Renik (1995) advocated explicitly taking sides sometimes and refraining from taking sides at other times. For example, he told a patient that he thought her guilt toward her sister was unwarranted, that she was less critical of her parents than was warranted, and that she had a right to be more sexually active. He was aware of the influence of his personal history and feelings in taking these sides. On the other hand, when he commented to a patient that his girlfriend was being very disdainful, the patient thought Renik was suggesting that he break up with her, and he asked Renik for his opinion about their relationship. Renik demurred, stating that his personal opinion was not relevant to the work regarding the patient's denial of his girlfriend's disdain. Sensibly, Renik remarked (to the reader), "since she is not my girlfriend, it is not my opinion of her that counts" (p. 480).

Julian Rotter, one of my influential teachers in college, lamented that clinical psychology became allied with medicine rather than education. I do not regret spending most of my career in hospitals, but I agree with Hoffman (1996): "whether we like it or not, we are inevitably involved in some measure as *mentors* to our patients" (p. 108, emphasis in original). I am not averse to giving advice when I (rarely) have it, but I am keenly aware that I do not have to live with the consequences of the decision the patient must make. Patients ask, "What do you think I should do?" or "What would you do in my situation?" A reasonable response would be, "I'm not sure what I would do, and what I might do would not necessarily be the best thing for you to do." Furthermore, as I assume is characteristic of virtually all therapists, I take sides in the patient's conflict about completing suicide, although I also make every effort to engage with both sides of the conflict, understanding and empathizing with the patient's compelling reasons for taking this drastic action while exploring more viable ways of living (Allen 2011).

Self-Disclosure

Debate about therapists' self-disclosure looms large in the literature about neutrality. All therapists are likely to struggle with how much to disclose about themselves to their patients. Meissner (2002) made a crucial distinction between self-*disclosure* and self-*revelation*. Self-revelations are pervasive and unavoidable: "Everything about us and how we comport ourselves is self-revelatory. How we dress, how we talk, where we have our offices, how we decorate them, our mannerisms, our body language, our sex, and even our race—all are self-revelatory" (p. 833). Any public information, including chance meetings in public spaces, is self-revelatory. Our patients know a great deal about us as persons that is largely beyond our control—even if our voluntary, verbal disclosure of information about ourselves is minimal.

Renik (1995) advocated an "ethic of candor" (p. 95). I am inclined to reveal a great deal of what I think and much of what I feel about the patient and the treatment, particularly for the purpose of comparing my perspectives with those of the patient. We therapists are not *imposing* our perspectives; rather, we are offering them for our patients' consideration. In the process, our perspectives might *influence* the patient, just as the patient's perspective influences us therapists. The therapist's perspective is not more *valid*; it is *different* and, hopefully, worth considering: Our "job is not to be *right*; it is to be *useful*" (Renik 1996, p. 516, emphasis in original). We should keep in mind, however, that the inherent power differential in the relationship is liable to render our influence more forceful than we intend.

All self-disclosure pertaining to the therapeutic interaction requires discretion, as does disclosure of personal information that pertains to matters outside the treatment context. Implicitly mentoring their patients, some therapists disclose personal experiences that they believe will be instructive for the patient. There is plenty of room for disagreement in all variations of self-disclosure; bright lines are hard to discern. Beyond the therapeutic values of self-disclosure, Renik (1996) sees an advantage for a more openly engaged approach in psychoanalysis: "we can more comfortably acknowledge our commonality with other [nonpsychoanalytic] therapists" (p. 516). Theoretical approaches aside, we therapists can all agree that burdening patients with our personal problems is counterproductive—disrespectful, in fact.

In decades of practice, I found that most patients were sensitive to boundaries and rarely expressed interest in my personal life. I do have a memorable exception. I worked with Ella, a young woman whose thinking was extremely disorganized and who was continually complaining about the hospital treatment and the therapy with me, all of which was distinctly unhelpful to her. She frequently contradicted my observations and was put off by my questions. Yet she was transparently anguished and distraught, which she typically denied. Although she complained that the therapy was useless, Ella always attended her sessions and showed no inclination to quit. She did acknowledge that she found it somewhat helpful to "vent" her feelings. As I routinely do, I aspired to find a focus to structure our work, to no avail. We were getting nowhere in the first several sessions.

One day, in the middle of a session, apparently frustrated by my questioning, Ella proposed, "How about if I interview you?" I agreed to this role reversal, with the dubious rationale that nothing else was working. Ella asked me where I went to school, and I told her. She asked a few questions about my graduate training, which I answered. Then she asked a more pointed question: "What was most difficult for you in graduate school?" I thought seriously about the question and then answered (truthfully) something to the effect that learning to do psychotherapy was most difficult because there was no clear procedure to follow. Ella happily exclaimed, "Now I see why you like structure!" We both laughed, and, for a significant portion of the session, Ella was more comfortable revealing some painful past experiences. Alas, this interchange did not alter the generally ineffective course of therapy, although we did arrive at some understanding of her fears about the therapy with me before she left the hospital abruptly.

Aiming for Balance

I hope that this brief review of the challenges of neutrality attests to its messiness. I agree with Renik that the term *neutrality* is liable to be more harmful than helpful. He observed that "the technique of beginning analysts tends to suffer more from stiffness than from an excess of spontaneity" (Renik 1999, p. 416). I think this influence extends beyond psychoanalysis. Even in recent years, after the caricature of neutrality had been long abandoned, I found in supervising postdoctoral fellows and psychiatric residents that many of them seemed unduly inhibited and constrained, as if they felt they have to adopt some special "therapeutic" demeanor when they walk into the office with a patient. I found my major task to be helping them to be more natural and responsive to their patients. When I spoke with Len Horwitz about this persistently pernicious influence of the stereotypical psychoanalytic stance (personal communication, July 2020), he countered, "That's not neutrality. They're afraid of making mistakes, so they keep their mouth shut." Point taken.

In his teaching of the mentalizing approach, Anthony Bateman put it succinctly: be ordinary. When I am with a patient, I do not feel any sense of personal difference in my general demeanor, except that I am concentrating on an emotionally and cognitively demanding form of work. Occasionally, patients have remarked that they felt put off by my "staring" at them, although I try to avoid doing so. When this happens, I apologize and tell the patient that I've learned that I tend to stare when I'm thinking hard—which I am highly prone to doing.

"Be ordinary" is good advice. But I am keenly aware that therapy relationships are unique in being profoundly shaped by the treatment context, no matter how ostensibly ordinary the demeanor of the therapist might be. In the context of patients idealizing their analysts, Renik (1995) put it bluntly: the treatment context "permits analysts to treat their patients better in some ways than analysts treat other people in their lives" (p. 479). For example, patients are likely to appreciate our (relatively) consistent attentiveness, empathy, caring, and consideration. Hoffman (1996) elaborated this point instructively: "Regard for the analyst is fostered by the fact that the patient knows so much *less* about him or her than the analyst knows about the patient" (p. 119, emphasis in original). Accordingly, the treatment situation is "likely to promote the most tolerant, understanding, and generous aspects of his or her personality." Concomitantly, "the analyst's regard for the patient is fostered by the fact that he or she knows so much about the patient, including the origins of the patient's difficulties and his or her struggles to deal with them." Here, the boundaries exert a dramatic influence: "neither party has to live with the other...so that each is afforded quite a bit of protection from the other's more difficult qualities" (p. 119). It is little wonder that we therapists are idealized, and such idealization should not go to our heads.

From the literature on neutrality I have reviewed, I see a broad consensus that we must establish a middle ground between closeness and distance, although different individuals—patients and therapists alike—occupy different locations in that wide middle ground. There is a great emphasis on mutuality and a sense of equality and partnership in the relational approach, but everyone recognizes the vital function of a fundamental asymmetry of roles and responsibilities, without which treatment would be impossible. All agree on the cardinal importance of promoting patients' autonomy while differing on the optimal way of doing it. All agree on acknowledging and discussing mistakes. All agree that, whatever stance the therapist takes on neutrality, all interventions, from silence to self-disclosure, are intended to promote the treatment goals with the patient's welfare first and foremost in mind. We could not disclose everything even if we so desire; we must be selective and guided by what is relevant to the treatment. Mitchell (1991) put this point forcefully: "what keeps the analytic situation analytic, what distinguishes the analytic relationship from all other relations, is precisely that one of the participants, the analyst, is responsible for *keeping* it analytic, always, at all moments" (p. 131, emphasis in original). All agree that therapists' personal styles and preferences do and should influence how they navigate this complex interpersonal space. No one advocates "wild analysis" or a free-for-all. In Mitchell's experience, "relational clinicians tend to be a quite thoughtful, careful lot, who operate with a great deal of restraint." He acknowledged a "blurt-it-out school" in which practitioners feel bound by authenticity to "say whatever is on their minds." However, "for the vast majority, in our actual practice, clinical work is quite disciplined, saturated with considerations of caution" (p. 127).

The term *neutrality* is problematic in its connotations. But we therapists must have some way of referring to the necessary balance between closeness and distance, whether we use the word neutrality or not. Loewald (1960), in the context of his therapeutic endeavor to cultivate a relationship with the patient's emerging core self (i.e., relatively free of distortions), characterized the "essence" of neutrality as "*love and respect* for the individual and for individual development" (p. 20, emphasis added). Kant would concur.

Relational Trustworthiness

Jessica Benjamin (2018) describes her clinical work in detail, masterfully illustrating the challenges of becoming trustworthy in treatment relationships with patients who have become highly distrusting in the context of attachment trauma. Benjamin explicates a clinical theory that guides her therapeutic approach, and her theory goes hand in hand with Tomasello's (2019) account of shared intentionality, in which I have anchored my understanding of trust. In addition, like Tomasello, Benjamin integrates her understanding of interpersonal relationships and their broader social context with an explicit ethical-moral framework in her aspiration to foster "a psychoanalytically informed ethics" (p 245).

To elaborate my understanding of trust in this psychotherapeutic context, I introduce a technical term, *the Third*, a term employed in the relational psychoanalytic literature, that plays a prominent role in Benjamin's thinking. Bear with me here; the Third will take a bit of explaining, but you are well prepared in understanding shared intentionality and the experience of interacting as a "we." After we have made the effort to grasp it, I think our uniquely human capacity to interact in the Third, which comes and goes, enables us to trust. In the following subsections, I highlight Benjamin's thinking about *recognition* to clarify the Third and to enrich our understanding of trust. Continuing to develop the theme of ethical thought being integral to psychotherapeutic practice, I conclude this brief foray into Benjamin's theoretical contribution by introducing her concept of the *moral Third*. Finally, I use two of Benjamin's case examples to illustrate how she employs these concepts in practice and their relation to becoming trustworthy in psychotherapy—in fits and starts.

In and Out of the Third

If you can accept the metaphor of *mental space*, you can understand the Third and how we go in and out of it when interacting with each other. Take a moment to pay attention to the mental space you are in right now. Then imagine being with someone else, each of you in a different mental space. We have gone from one mental space to two mental spaces. Now imagine starting a conversation with the other person, deciding what you will do together. Each remaining in your own mental space, you have created a Third, shared mental space. As Benjamin put it, "sharing must be in the Third position, [in which] both partners [are] able to be both receptive and active" (personal communication, February 2021). I find this psychoanalytic language, "the Third," odd, but the experience is entirely ordinary—when we are cooperating. Picture the triangle with you and I at the base and "we" at the apex: separateness conjoined with togetherness. We can use different words, but we cannot comprehend trust without this basic concept: trusting in psychotherapy requires that the patient and therapist create a shared mental space in which they become trusting of each other and trustworthy to each other, committed to cooperating in ameliorating the patient's suffering and enhancing the patient's well-being.

I hasten to make a crucial point here: In my mind, the Third is not merely an alternative term that adds nothing substantive to the concepts we already have reviewed. As I understand it, *the living experience of being in the Third catalyzes the development of trust* as well as maintaining it and restoring it when it is lost. Shared goals are crucial to trust, but the sharing must be experienced in the Third.

To cement the concept of the Third, it helps to concretize it a bit more. To do so, let's go back to conversation. More specifically, think of a stimulating conversation in which you are creating new ways of thinking and understanding with another person. The ongoing joint creation shapes each individual's thinking and feeling, potentially creating new ways of thinking and feeling that each can share. Think of psychotherapy, when it is going well. In trusting relationships, the meeting of minds changes the minds. I needed another kind of concrete experience to fully experience what I think the relational psychoanalysts are getting at here, and the Third captures this concept.

It is no accident that Benjamin uses musical analogies throughout her writing, alluding to rhythm, harmony, and dance as well as improvisation and—more broadly—play. As I wrestled to understand the Third, an intuitive grasp came to me from my experience playing piano for several years in a jazz trio with my friends Barton Jones (bass) and Chris Grimes (drums), both of whom are also psychotherapists. Playing jazz gives us a tangible experience: We hear the music and we can record it. But the creation is fluid and dynamic, and the music lies in the evolving pattern; it cannot be reduced to the playing of any individual, much less any of the measures, chords, or notes. Most important, the *lived experience of the conjoint creation,* enduring over time, guides the creative contribution of each individual at every moment. At our best, each of us becomes fully immersed in the ongoing creation as we make our individual contributions to it. You might think of it this way: the creation creates the creators. Our responsiveness to the creation exemplifies mutual recognition, as I elaborate next. Of course, we also lose the Third in moments of noncooperation, for example, when one of the jazz trio (usually me) falls out of the rhythm or tries to impose a shift in tempo, rhythm, or key that the others resist. Getting out of sync is a rupture that calls for repair. The greatest joy is our spontaneously shifting the pattern together; this connection feels magical.

Think back to the stimulating conversation: The ever-shifting topic and perspectives on the topic shape the thinking of the conversation partners. Like music, conversations have their own tempos and rhythms. This dynamic flow contributes to the intimate feeling of being with another person, together and separate in relation to the shared creation—including in psychotherapy. It is no accident that Daniel Stern (2004) identified *moments of meeting* as pivotal events in psychotherapy.

Commonplace as it might be, think of creating the Third as an achievement. As we get into Benjamin's clinical examples, you will appreciate how hard won this achievement can be. Or think of resolving an argument or impasse in one of your close relationships, for example, when you are feeling stonewalled. I think Benjamin deserves credit for a brilliant book title: *Beyond Doer and Done To.* She enumerates various noncooperative ways of relating in different roles wherein the Third is lacking: dominance-submission, dominance-resistance, perpetrator-victim, hurtful-helpless, demanding-complying, right-wrong, blaming-shamed, tit-for-tat, and the like. Noncooperative interactions also can be symmetrical, as in mutual blaming or fighting.

In discussing Tomasello's account of shared intentionality, I made the point that he has given us an understanding of the *capacity* that we humans have evolved, a capacity that is fundamental to trust. It was Fonagy's work on mentalizing that initially drew me into this fascinating psychological and interpersonal territory. Making this point about our uniquely human capacity starkly, Tomasello contrasts us humans with our primate cousins, chimpanzees, whom he describes as using each other as social tools. However, I emphasize our residual human proclivity for treating each other as objects rather than equal subjects. Benjamin makes this same contrast succinctly in her book title. She has provided us with a mantra for treating attachment trauma, which Benjamin terms "early childhood relational trauma" (personal communication, February 2021). We must find a way to help our patients get beyond doer and done to in psychotherapy and in their other relationships. We do so, regardless of which terminology we use, by the means of creating the Third, relating as "we" without losing the sense of you and I. In psychotherapy, we aim to create this experience of being together recurrently, time after time, to cultivate trust. We do the same in our other relationships; psychotherapy is not exceptional, but it can be exceptionally difficult. And creating this shared space can be especially difficult to do with patients for whom the doer and done to way of relating predominated in their early attachment relationships and for those who have faced pervasive social injustice and oppression.

We can now turn our attention to the linchpin of the Third—and of trust—with Benjamin's return to ordinary language with extraordinary insight.

Recognition

Benjamin (2018) defined recognition as follows:

> Acts of recognition confirm that I am seen, known, my intentions have been understood, I have had an impact on you, and this must also mean that I matter to you; and reciprocally, that I see and know you, I understand your intentions, your actions affect me and you matter to me. Further, we share feelings, reflect each other's knowing, so we also have shared awareness. This is recognition. (p. 4)

We typically think of recognition as unidirectional: one individual recognizes another; the recognized individual is the subject of recognition and the object of the recognizing individual. Benjamin's definition starts there; the recognized individual is seen, known, understood—and matters. Notice the subtle complication that takes us to the essence of recognition. The significance of Benjamin's definition lies in reciprocity and mutuality: the process of recognition is bidirectional inasmuch as *the person recognized also recognizes the recognizer as recognizing.* Recognition constitutes the Third required for trust. Unrecognized recognition has no value; without mutuality of recognition, there is no Third to form the basis of trusting and trustworthiness. In acts of recognition, we have two subjects, each with subjective experience—their own subjectivity—and we have two recognized objects, who are recognized as separate subjects with their own subjectivity. We have closeness with distance, love with respect—the balance of separateness and togetherness in the Third. We could think of Tomasello's 9-month revolution as the dawning of recognition, when an infant becomes dimly aware that he can be the object of joint attention shared with his mother, whom he recognizes as attending to him. This is the developmental nexus of shared intentionality and trust.

The feeling of connection in the act of recognition is of great intrinsic value, something we seek for its own sake. Benjamin captures beautifully the desire to be known: "The need to feel one exists 'inside' the other's mind" (p. 10). The separateness and difference of the other, including difference of perspective and understanding, is paramount to this process: what we cannot recognize or know in ourselves can be recognized and known by others. To reiterate, we must recognize the recognizer's recognition, and we might find something we have not recognized in ourselves in it. As Benjamin puts it poetically, one "can go out into the other's mind and return enriched" (p. 12). Here she has in mind the act of recognizing as well as the experience of being recognized; both are essential, and both are enriching. Recognition can be, in itself, therapeutic.

I put mutual recognition on the front line of trusting and trustworthiness. If we are to count on anyone for anything, we must *count on recognition* for starters. To be deprived of the reciprocal experience of recognition is to feel alone and alienated, and it can be profoundly traumatic, limiting and damaging to the sense of self and relatedness and blocking the flourishing of social connection and learning. I do not think it is an exaggeration to think that recognition is the fundamental precondition for making a good life for oneself and others, especially when we don't need to obsess about it as psychotherapy might require us to do.

A final point that is crucial to our work as psychotherapists and our relatedness more generally: if the Third is elusive, it is because it comes and goes in the form of lived experience that can be hard to put into words. As I stated, playing jazz concretized it for me; I feel it when we go out of sync and back in and love it when we simultaneously go from one form of being in sync to another. More generally, in all kinds of interactions, we are aligned, misaligned, and realigned in a continual flux. We tune in to each other and tune out. We can start a conversation and then get into an argument, each trying to dominate the other. As described earlier, we therapists can strive to *influence* (in the Third) without resorting to *control* (in noncooperative doer–done to interactions). To amplify my earlier point: *without the experience of recognition, the shared goals needed for trust would not come to life.*

The Moral Third

Recall from the discussion in Chapter 2, "Developing Trust and Trustworthiness," that shared intentionality includes joint and collective intentionality; joint intentionality develops in the first 3 years of life, and collective intentionality develops thereafter. Joint intentionality develops in dyads, the "we" of you and I; collective intentionality develops in groups and societies, the "we" as a shared way of living according to accepted norms. As Benjamin (2018) puts it, the moral Third, which entails recognition, is "the principle whereby we create relationships in accord with ethical values" (p. 28). Here basic trust expands into social trust. As I have emphasized repeatedly, psychological understanding and clinical work cannot be divorced from the ethos of the broader cultural-social-political context. In Benjamin's words, "I do not believe it is possible even theoretically to sunder the psychology of reciprocal recognition at the level of individual attachment from reciprocal recognition at the level of social rights and obligations" (p. 239).

Lawfulness is fundamental here, but neither in the juridical sense of being governed by decrees nor in the scientific sense of strict predictability: we must create "a sense of moral order that derives from harmonious or predictable connections at early developmental levels," which entails "upholding the expectation of a *lawful caring world*" (Benjamin 2018, pp. 51–52, emphasis added). The moral Third is an "orientation to a larger principle of lawfulness, necessity, rightness or goodness" (p. 37). In the morally lawful world, "when the unexpected or painful wrongness occurs," the "need to put things right" emerges; moreover, "what cannot be put right is acknowledged" (p. 6).

I have highlighted the experience of feeling alone and invisible in pain in the genesis of trauma. From this perspective, the foundation of psychotherapeutic treatment of trauma is *creating visibility in pain through recognition*: a sense that "This other person is reaching toward me, receiving my message, making it right with me—even *holding my pain in her heart*" (p. 12, emphasis added). Consistent with the trauma literature, Benjamin (2018) adopts the term *witnessing* for this vital healing process. Witnessing requires courage because it entails facing not only the reality of horrific suffering but also the reality of our individual and collective capacity for inflicting suffering. Concomitantly, we must face our capacity for denying, disowning, and dissociating the worst in ourselves: "a kind of madness is created when people feel that the truth of what is being done to them is being blacked out by the world" (p. 235).

As the foregoing attests, we therapists should not take our capacity to witness pain and suffering for granted. When I was involved in educating parents of hospitalized patients about the value of mentalizing—which entails recognition and witnessing—I came across the following passages from Simone Weil's writing (quoted by Miles 1986), and I included them in my presentation:

> Affliction is by its nature inarticulate. The afflicted silently beseech to be given the words to express themselves. There are times when they are given none; but there are also times when they are given words, but ill-chosen ones, because those who choose them know nothing of the affliction they would interpret.
>
> A stag advancing voluntarily step by step to offer itself to the teeth of a pack of hounds is about as probable as an act of attention directed towards a real affliction, which is close at hand, on the part of a mind which is free to avoid it. (p. 65)

Accordingly, witnessing can be emotionally challenging and requires courage, as does the other primary way of establishing moral lawfulness, *acknowledgment*, which entails recognizing our contributions to our patients' suffering and striving to repair the damage. As Benjamin construes it, acknowledgment simultaneously entails "an admission of the other's worthiness as well as an admission of the subject's unworthy action" (p. 19). Such acknowledgment is the moral framework for apology. As Weil recognized, one way in which we are likely to fail is in witnessing. Acknowledging such failures is crucial in the context of the experience of invisibility associated with trauma. Benjamin (2018) proposes that

it becomes all the more critical to find a way to acknowledge the failure in witnessing, that is, the analyst not having fully taken in the depth of pain and terror,
and in this way to gradually distinguish between failing to be fully present and
actually denying or perpetuating abuse. The analyst needs to show the voice or
face of the witness who is moved rather than that of the unmoved bystander
upon whom the patient's suffering has no impact. (p. 61)

The role of the failed witness is not easy to manage; moving through it entails "neither denying it nor getting stuck there," sometimes requiring that "we
must sometimes muddle ungracefully through such moments of breakdown"
(p. 61). When we fail in witnessing or in other ways, we restore the moral Third
by acknowledging our hurtful actions, seeking to understand their basis—
sometimes in active collaboration with the patient—apologizing, and hoping at
least for forbearance if not forgiveness. We cannot be counted on to entirely
avoid hurting our patients emotionally, but we should be counted on to acknowledge our errors of omission and commission and to make reparation. We
should not take our trustworthiness for granted; rather, we should aspire to
trustworthiness in our best efforts to restore the moral Third. In short, trustworthiness does not entail avoiding conflict but rather entails reliable efforts to
face and resolve it. As I stated in Chapter 3, I think what we should value first
and foremost is *commitment to the trusting relationship*.

Renik provides an instructive example of acknowledgment in a vignette
about sexual tension in the therapy relationship. His patient had been describing her sex life in great detail, in a way that suggested she was trying to have
an impact on him. Then, lying on the couch, she raised a leg to adjust her
stocking to her garter belt in such a way that her skirt fell completely away. Renik asked her what she was doing, to which she replied that her stocking was
slipping. Both of them knew that she was lonely, was attracted to him, and was
trying to turn him on. The patient also knew that Renik was unavailable. All
this was in the context of mutual respect and appreciation. Finding a way to
address the situation, he said to her, "I must be torturing you, because you're
sure trying to torture me." She queried, "Am I succeeding?" To which he responded, "Yes, but I can stand it." She went on to talk about how she wanted
to find a nice young doctor to go out with. Grateful for his helpful forthright-
ness and integrity, as she left the office, she said, "Thank you," with tears in her
eyes (Renik 2006, p. 164).

Benjamin points out that acknowledgment and its failures, most conspicuously in the context of trauma, take on vital significance in psychotherapy owing to the asymmetry of roles and the special responsibility that the power
differential entails: "Although it is true that human infants start out very asym-
metrically dependent on the powerful caretaker, and that many of our patients
have not found a viable way out of that asymmetry, it is a limited way of life and
they enter analysis to overcome it" (Benjamin 2018, p. 73). Although a trauma
history renders patients especially vigilant and sensitive to failures of trustworthiness, the power differential in psychotherapy provides a relative advantage:

by virtue of psychotherapy's potential to provide an experience of trusting in relationships with an inherent imbalance of power, patients have an opportunity to experience trustworthy asymmetry in relationships with persons in positions of authority who hold more power. Accordingly, with keen awareness of the analyst's responsibility for much of what goes on in the relationship, Benjamin advocates that when ruptures occur and acknowledgment is required, *the analyst goes first*, taking the lead in restoring the lawful moral Third.

Clinical Examples

I am using Benjamin's (2018) work to illuminate the challenges of trustworthiness in psychotherapy in part because I find her theoretical framework appealing in its resonance with my plea for explicit attention to ethical thought alongside its remarkable compatibility with developmental understanding of trust and its expansion of my understanding. Benjamin's theoretical contribution is thoroughly illuminated in her transparent writing about the clinical challenges of working with patients for whom distrust is paramount in their history and in the treatment process. Her book presents this clinical material in considerable detail; I merely present here abstracts of her work with two patients along with excerpts from her writing to give a glimpse of how the core concepts summarized earlier are evident in her clinical practice: mutual recognition in the Third, the collapse of the Third into noncooperative interactions along with efforts by both patient and analyst to restore it, and the significance of the moral Third in conjunction with witnessing and acknowledgment. Above all, Benjamin's efforts to create a sense of alignment in the Third with her patients and to restore it after collapse exemplify the challenges of *becoming* trustworthy in these intensive treatment processes. Thanks to Benjamin's transparency with her readers, these clinical examples exemplify the highly personal nature of the work and the integrity with which it must be performed. In presenting these summaries, I intersperse my own thoughts about her examples to explicate links to some of the main themes of this book.

At this juncture, however, I want to remind you of the critique of attachment theory from a cross-cultural perspective presented in Chapter 2. The examples I present from Benjamin's work highlight patients' problematic relationships with their mother, which brings to my mind our cultural ideology of intensive mothering (Hays 1996). We must bear in mind the likely plight of the mothers, who themselves might have been entangled in the intergenerational transmission of trauma. Moreover, compared with small-scale societies in which attachment evolved as well as contemporary societies with a more communal orientation, our individualistic ideology shifts the responsibility of the community onto mothers, who are liable to be overburdened by little access to the support of alloparents. These points are consistent with Benjamin's ethical orientation to the moral Third, in which she urges us to not neglect the broader social context in which we conduct the work of psychotherapy.

Jeannette

Benjamin's (2018) work with a patient named Jeannette is instructive for its challenges to Benjamin's becoming trustworthy in the relationship and to her capacity to trust herself in navigating a rupture in which Jeannette threatened to buy a gun to kill her. Benjamin worked with Jeannette early in her career, at a time when expertise in trauma and dissociation was scarce. Moreover, she needed to work with Jeannette in a way that departed from her more traditional training as a psychoanalyst. Here Benjamin gives us a glimpse of her own professional development, expanding her ways of thinking and working in an integrative direction, consistent with the increasingly broad minded view of neutrality that evolved in the relational psychoanalytic approach. As is evident from her retrospective understanding, Benjamin was working from an implicit moral Third before she had come to formulate it explicitly.

Early on, Benjamin saw that Jeannette's overtly submissive and deflated demeanor barely concealed exceptional intelligence and a determined, strong-willed character. Jeannette was working in a professional mental health system serving an underprivileged clientele. For 2 years, Jeannette had been in a sado-masochistic relationship with a boyfriend in which she served as his slave. She sought treatment with Benjamin after reading a book Benjamin had written that described erotic domination. Perhaps Benjamin already had started to become trustworthy to Jeannette through her writing, which might have promoted Jeannette's hope of being understood. As a child, Jeannette engaged in obsessive religious practices, for example, staying up all night on her knees, cutting herself and waiting for death. In light of the religious hypocrisy with which she said she grew up, Jeannette entered therapy with a profound mistrust of faith, including faith in therapy. Thankfully, having known Benjamin through her writing, Jeannette had enough hope to walk through the door to her office.

Here we have the significance of social context: Jeannette's parents lived in a community of large, impoverished, and violent families in a northeastern mill town. Her father was described as ignorant, bigoted, and violent; he kept a gun under his pillow and threatened his children with it. Jeannette also was subjected to her mother's murderous attacks in the context of her mother's obsession with Jeannette's sexuality. Jeannette succeeded in extricating herself from the household at age 18 and identified three dissociated selves: one was engaged with the real world in an outwardly normal way, competent and compliant; a second, rageful self was evil and all-powerful, the self who engaged in the tortured-torturer bonding; a third self, a protective fairy godmother, kept Jeannette alive and provided a model for Benjamin's role.

Consistent with a need for a self-constructed integrative approach, as Benjamin described it, "Being present with Jeannette was not consonant with being an analyst, in any way I had yet known" (Benjamin 2018, p. 202). In the face of Jeannette's continual testing, "my job was to survive, to hang in there and to learn what I could while making constant mistakes" (p. 202). Jeannette put the pressure on, expressing contempt for Benjamin's professional mask and striving to uncover

Benjamin's "real self," in which Jeannette could never believe. Benjamin stated that she needed to respond directly and "not conceal my ignorance" (p. 202). Putting Benjamin in a bind, Jeannette could not tolerate the real Other that she demanded; she could not be in the presence of another mind. Disavowing her dependency, Jeannette declared, in effect, that the analysis would be tolerable if it did not involve another person. Jeannette was as far as could be from creating a Third, and Benjamin's trustworthiness entailed somehow making it safe for Jeannette to be with her in the Third. Benjamin set the stage for creating the Third in a paradoxical fashion: Seeing the treatment as characterized by negation, Benjamin creatively provided recognition by accepting Jeannette's continual negating by finding "a way to play with 'No' together" (p. 203). Benjamin sided with Jeannette's assertion that she could keep Benjamin out. The Third could be held by encompassing its own negation. We can see how a therapist might easily fall into an untrustworthy, noncooperative way of relating in this situation, fighting the negation rather than recognizing, accepting, and joining with it.

The therapy was profoundly threatening to Jeannette in two ways: she was threatened not only by the presence of another person but also by the potential eroding of the protection provided by the dissociation of selves that could not live together in peace, particularly in light of her dangerous rage. Jeannette knew that she had erected a wall against rage to protect herself from its dangerous expression, and she knew more generally that she could not destroy any of her compartmentalized selves without destroying all of them. In my view, Jeannette showed an extraordinarily helpful level of insight about her dissociative experience and the barriers to overcoming it.

Benjamin understood that Jeannette could overcome the terror of annihilation only through a Third that would require "a different kind of experience with an other. This someone should be knowing of the dangerous world of death yet also connected to the world of life and loving" (Benjamin 2018, p. 204). Benjamin sensed that traditional analysis would not be sufficient and that the relationship would need to be created in action: Jeannette "would have to show and tell what she knew, and so actually know it to be true herself" (p. 205). Moreover, "Jeannette would intuitively construct for me the role of healer" (p. 206). As it played out, the enactment was dangerous, triggered by Jeannette's showing Benjamin a journal entry that included an early childhood memory of her mother coming home, finding her in bed wearing no pajama bottoms, and throwing her against the wall, accusing her of being a whore.

Benjamin thought Jeannette was handing her the journal pages to keep, and Jeannette did not protest when she held on to them, mistakenly implying to Benjamin that they were interacting in the Third, being in agreement that she was *giving* the pages to Benjamin rather than *showing* them to her. But Jeannette belatedly revealed that she was in the noncooperative mode when, in the next session, she expressed the feeling that Benjamin had set a trap in obtaining her writing and was merely regarding her as case material for her own use—far from the Third.

In this session, when Jeannette gave Benjamin her writing, she identified it as a copy for her. Correspondingly opening up a space for the Third, Benjamin acknowledged her mistake in keeping the first journal entry, which she saw as an inadvertent boundary violation, and she viewed Jeannette's marking of the second set of writings as a repair of that rupture: "She was interested in sharing her thoughts but not relinquishing them" (Benjamin 2018, p. 208). This quotation aptly encapsulates the experience of the Third as preserving separateness in togetherness, balancing closeness with distance. Helpfully, in what I think of as a mentalizing mode, Jeannette was able to open up space in her own mind for the development of the Third. Specifically, Jeannette reflectively associated her outburst with her rageful self and provided Benjamin with a list of defiant deeds in her childhood that included stealing from her mother, beating her siblings with the belt her mother used to beat her, cutting herself with razor blades, and turning on the gas with the intention of blowing up the house. As a young adult, she endangered others with her car and fantasized about dangerous crimes. She identified her rageful self with her mother and herself.

Jeannette moved toward overcoming the dissociation that kept the warring selves separate, envisioning herself as multifaceted and accepting the need for other relationships. To use my language, Jeannette was appreciating that minds need other minds. But the threat of closeness was powerful, and the Third was precarious. Jeanette's growing trust in Benjamin heightened her internal sense of vulnerability: she continued to be wary of being lured into a trap. Nevertheless, she could identify the origins of her suspicion in her relationship with her mother. In addition, she was able to directly acknowledge her fear. Jeannette was not alone in her fear. Benjamin also felt a sense of dread—and rightly so. In a subsequent session, Jeannette revealed a dream in which she had been hunted down by men with rifles who intended to kill her, and at the end of the hour, she told Benjamin in a worryingly detached manner that she was considering buying a gun to shoot Benjamin and that she had called gun stores toward this end. As I understand it, fearful of the developing closeness, Jeannette was seeking to push separateness to the extreme by annihilating Benjamin.

Benjamin was alarmed but did not respond immediately. She had anticipated that Jeannette would need to express her plight through action, although perhaps not to this extreme. In consultation with a colleague, Benjamin decided that she needed to take the revelation extremely seriously—not as a real threat but rather as a drama in which she had a delicate part to play. In my view, this is a context in which the stakes of mutual trusting and mutual trustworthiness were as high as can be. Jeannette had created the extreme of the "doer–done to" mode, to use Benjamin's book title; the only way back to trust was through restoring the Third, which the two of them managed to do. Benjamin called Jeannette that night and let her know that she wanted to keep working with her but that to do so, Jeannette must agree to not buy a gun, not harm anyone else or herself with her car, and call her in the future if she had any similar ideas so that Benjamin could keep the therapy safe for herself and Jeannette. The risk of being truthful was alarming to Benjamin, and it brought forth her need to trust herself: "I wondered if I was equal to this life and death struggle. This was the moment to honestly ask myself if I could be a healer who in some way did know about life and death, knew such terrible things could happen. I was not sure." She went on, "Yet to be a witness, not to fail…I was obliged to try my best" (Benjamin 2018, p. 211).

After this limit setting, Jeannette felt humiliated and ashamed, but she left Benjamin a phone message stating that she needed to be confronted with limits and needed Benjamin to act from her "own instincts, authentically" and not just from "therapeutic rules." In my language, Jeannette was expressing her need to trust *Benjamin*, not the therapy. As I think of it, Jeannette was frightened of accepting Benjamin's personal influence, which was precisely what she would need to do to heal. This dilemma was just where they had started, and, as Benjamin had anticipated, she was put to the test of trustworthiness, albeit in an extreme way. Again, opening space for the Third, Jeannette was able to mentalize, reflecting on her pleasure in her progress, recognizing that dissociating her rage had backfired in becoming intensified as she had projected it onto Benjamin. Jeannette subsequently expressed a profound shift in relatedness to Benjamin, indicating that she was feeling warmly connected along with a newfound sense of space. Bearing directly on her experience of this relationship as trustworthy, Jeannette spoke of her appreciation for Benjamin's acknowledgment of her mistakes, her determination to overcome obstacles in their relationship, and her authenticity. Jeannette ultimately was able to distinguish the real relationship from her idealizations and frightening projections

In this context, Benjamin articulated the moral Third as follows: "I learned about the meaning of *witnessing*: that at times the most meaningful thing we can do is to express some version of the moral power that *acknowledges* and affirms what is *lawful*, what is wrong, what should never happen to a child, to a human being" (Benjamin 2018, p. 213, emphasis added). Benjamin went on to observe that "dealing with real damage and harm, there is bound to be ambiguity and sometimes *dire uncertainty*" (p. 214, emphasis added). Here I thought of the need for hope in the context of a plight and the ambiguity of the space between despair and presumption. I also thought of faith—and Jeannette's initial mistrust of all faith—when Benjamin commented on her "sense that the script we enacted was somehow being revealed to us as well as created by us" (p. 213).

Wendy

In her work with a patient named Wendy, Benjamin presents a clear example of the need for mutual trusting and trustworthiness in effective therapy and illustrates the way in which Benjamin's relationship with her own mother played a role in understanding the problems with trust and working through them with Wendy.

Wendy was extremely distressed and virtually impossible to comfort or soothe in therapy, continually conveying that Benjamin was failing in her efforts. Wendy's mother had been anxious, emotionally dysregulated, apparently frightened about taking care of Wendy when she was a baby, and alternately dismissing of Wendy's distress and demanding attention for herself. Wendy's father was the "angry, agitated, chaotic giant of her family" (Benjamin 2018, p. 106). In striving to recognize Wendy's distress, Benjamin was in a bind: validating Wendy's feelings only confirmed that Wendy was irreparably damaged. Benjamin construed the dilemma in attachment terms: As if in response to her alternately avoidant and ambivalent mother, Wendy criticized Benjamin's efforts, which was "the equivalent of the baby leaning as far away as possible from mother crying and pushing away" (p. 91). Wendy found Benjamin's soothing responsiveness to be unsettling and to amplify her distress.

As she had striven to do with her mother, Wendy coached Benjamin by demonstrating the persona of a Tough Mama. To an extent, Benjamin's efforts to adopt this more tough persona were successful in creating the Third by accepting the fear that something is terribly wrong without becoming swamped by it. They were able to understand Wendy as identifying with a mean girl, critical of herself and everyone else, fearing that Benjamin would either come unglued or angrily retaliate, leaving Wendy "feeling destructive and alone" (p. 92). Yet the Third they established was precarious, as evidenced by a major rupture, repair of which required mutual recognition and trusting.

In a session on a Friday before a weekend in which Wendy was anxious about completing a work assignment on time, Benjamin felt that they had "found a place of shared understanding and warm connection" (Benjamin 2018, p. 105), the Third wherein Wendy had met her hopes for soothing along with increased confidence in getting her work done. They discussed how Wendy's anxiety had been associated with her fear that Benjamin would find her bothersome or needing too much. However, the following Monday, having lost the Third, Wendy came back in a state of agitation; she had been unable to finish the work and was afraid that Benjamin would be unable to help. Also faltering in the Third, Benjamin "could feel how the part of me that is organized around trying to be different from my angry, dismissive mother was activated." At the same time, Benjamin was aware of her inclination to suppress her hostile reaction to Wendy's accusation along with her worry about being unable to contain Wendy's aggression. Nonetheless, in conjunction with these conflicts, Benjamin maintained her intention to get back to the Third, cognizant of her own "need to repair and make things good again" (p. 105).

In the following session, "Wendy marched in determined to deal with our messy encounter and make repair," and Benjamin "felt a similar determination" (Benjamin 2018, p. 105). Both had felt the loss of their connection in the Third that they had established on Friday, and they were aligned in their desire to restore it. But restoration was not easy. Wendy let Benjamin know how emotionally flooded she was feeling along with her belief that Benjamin would feel equally flooded. Benjamin acknowledged the truth of Wendy's observation but also commented on how Wendy had pulled away from her, in contrast with their connection in the session before the weekend. Benjamin wondered aloud, "What do you think happened to the Friday Wendy?" (p. 106). Wendy responded dismissively. They were back in the noncooperative relationship in which Wendy was too destructive, left alone without help, and protesting—"refusing to be satisfied with this miserable excuse for mothering." To Benjamin's invitation to restore the Third of Friday, Wendy countered that Benjamin had been unable to hold on to Friday Wendy and that on Monday, being unable to soothe her, Benjamin would feel badly about doing a poor job as a therapist.

Without hesitation, Benjamin responded to Wendy's challenge: "Touché. You got me there." She then asked Wendy if she wanted to hear how Benjamin saw their interaction, and Wendy agreed to listen, opening the pathway back to the Third. Trusting Wendy, Benjamin "felt safe enough to be vulnerable and admit the part that felt shameful to me." She acknowledged to Wendy that she felt she was "not do-ing a good enough job," and, moreover, "it is a feeling I know quite well." Wendy then came to a significant realization, acknowledging her feeling that Benjamin hated her for being such a mess and that she hated Benjamin in turn, thus accusing her of doing a poor job. This was a major revelation because Wendy had not recog-nized the extent of her own hatred and had not previously had the experience of her hatred being accepted and acceptable. Benjamin described how all this experience became organized in a narrative from the Third, in which Wendy had been

> left alone, unsoothed and ashamed of her neediness as a young child; boiling with her helpless feeling of hate; trying to be good, helpful and show her mother what to do; when this failed, dealing with frustration by becoming in turns bossy and enraged with her mother, hating herself. (p. 107)

Making use of self-disclosure in the service of the Third, Benjamin also de-scribed how her own acknowledgment contributed to Wendy's crucial realization:

> My willingness to be vulnerable in front of her (and only a bit retaliatory) con-vinced her that I was not afraid of her hate, indeed, that her efforts to repair and correct me, make a better mother of me, might not even be seen as hateful by me. Further, I could hold my own vulnerability and keep my mind intact. I could acknowledge my own tendencies to dysregulation and shame, not so dif-ferent from her own, while remaining willing to hear how angry she had been with me. My risking knowing about my badness, my failure, opened her to a similar but different risk of intersubjective vulnerability. This meant that feel-ings good and bad were not "unthinkable." (p. 107)

Following this creation of the Third with mutual trusting and trustworthiness, Wendy came to her sessions without fear of damage to her mental health, and she became less fearful in general. As Benjamin summarized, "Wendy actually came to trust that I would carry out my responsibility for her, play my role without in-struction, value our co-created thirdness and her part in shaping it" (p. 109).

Reflections

As should be evident from my discussion of neutrality and Benjamin's writing, I find the psychoanalytic theoretical and clinical literature invaluable in illuminating the challenges of becoming trustworthy in the process of psychotherapy. The literature on neutrality illustrates the challenge of balancing closeness and distance, reconciling the two great moral forces of love and respect, as Kant (1797/1966) framed the challenge more than two centuries ago. I find Benjamin's thinking about her work especially valuable in her aim to promote a psychoanalytically informed ethics. With Fonagy's and Tomasello's conceptualization in mind, I can see in Benjamin's clinical work the confluence of developmental science, explicit ethical principles, a well-established treatment approach, and acceptance of the profoundly personal nature of the work. We also see the confluence of personal and professional development as they bear on creating mutual trusting and trustworthiness in the relationship. To reiterate a point I made earlier, the mastery of a craft is the work of a lifetime. Kant might also have said the same about our need to find a balance between love and respect.

Writing Personal Formulations

Among the many concepts pertinent to trustworthiness in psychotherapy, I would rank *transparency* high. We routinely encourage transparency in our patients. In teaching undergraduates about psychotherapy in a course on clinical psychology, I used Sheldon Korchin's (1976) text, in which he wrote that the patient's fundamental obligation was to be *open and honest*. Psychoanalysis takes openness and honesty to the limit in its aspiration to achieve spontaneity in free association, but much of the therapeutic work relates to all the obstacles to such openness (e.g., transference, resistance). Perhaps this psychoanalytic ideal—of great value in any form of therapy—would require the rarity that Hawley (2012) identified: absolute trust.

Throughout this book, I have advocated reciprocity: trusting and trustworthiness go both ways. Should we not value therapists' openness and honesty equally? The affirmative response to that question accounts for much of the appeal to me of the mentalizing approach (Bateman and Fonagy 2016) and the flexible thinking about neutrality in the relational psychoanalytic literature summarized earlier in this chapter. In the context of promoting epistemic trust, Fonagy and colleagues (2017, 2019a) have pointed to the importance of the therapist's understanding the patient's experience in a way that the patient feels to be accurate as well as well intended and helpful. Without diminishing the importance of a sense of being understood at an emotional, nonverbal level, I believe that explicating our understanding in a thoroughgoing way also is important. Such explication allows our patients to benefit from our knowledge as well as to evaluate what we think and correct us when we are off course. We therapists can conjure all sorts of ideas and come to believe them without restraint if they remain in our heads. Often, we urge our patients who worry what others think about them to "check it out," that is, ask what they are thinking. Good advice that we therapists also should heed. I take explication one step farther beyond voicing our thoughts relatively freely. I think there is substantial benefit in providing patients with a systematic *written* formulation as a working document.

A Clinical Process

In the latter years of my career, I made a practice of writing detailed formulations after a series of initial sessions, as summarized in Table 4–2. With the benefit of the hospital setting, these formulations were informed by clinical assessments and conversations with colleagues, but I constructed them primarily from my own fairly detailed psychotherapy records. I went through my documents carefully: underlining, making notes, and developing an outline—jogging my memory in the process. Although I did not think of it at the time, this was an example of deliberate practice (see Chapter 1). It is hard work and time consuming—a luxury sadly unavailable to many therapists inundated with heavy caseloads.

I thought of these as *personal* formulations—not clinical formulations—using a minimum of jargon and diagnostic language. They were written akin to a letter or as if I were speaking directly to the patient in a personal way, as I strive to do in the therapy process. Barring something urgent, I gave the formulation to patients at the beginning of the session and asked them to read it so that we could discuss it on the spot. I offered these formulations with the intention of letting patients know how I was thinking about them and their treatment so as to compare my thinking with theirs. Sometimes I wrote a formulation in response to a patient's expressed desire to know more about my thinking. Often, I offered a formulation spontaneously to ensure that the patient and I were in accord. I corrected and amended the formulations as needed and sometimes revised them as the treatment proceeded. One memorable patient kept finding fault with my account of her history, so I made several revisions. She observed that I was "frustrated." I confirmed her observation but pointed out that she was helping me with the work of therapy, which was partly to clarify how her history was affecting her in the present, and we needed to get it right. For all patients, I updated the formulation at the end of therapy by writing a discharge summary in the same personal style. Writing something that patients understand increases the likelihood that other clinicians also will understand it.

I was not stinting with praise. I made a point of recognizing patients' efforts in therapy as well as their lifelong successes, talents, and character strengths. Nonetheless, some patients felt that I had not appreciated their gains or strengths sufficiently, and, after helpful discussion, I revised the formulation accordingly. For example, when one patient with whom I had worked quite well read my discharge summary, he casually tossed what I had written onto the floor rather than placing it on the table by his elbow. He then talked about how his treatment team had not appreciated his strengths. I wondered with him if he

---

TABLE 4–2. Key features of written personal formulations

Introduced after a series of initial sessions

Convey the therapist's understanding of the patient and the treatment

Typically include a developmental perspective

Employ a minimum of technical and diagnostic language

Introduced routinely, or in response to a patient's request, and to repair a rupture in the alliance

Revised on the basis of the patient's feedback and updated as needed

Can be used by patients to inform and educate partners and family members

Provide a framework for a discharge summary that can be given to the patient

---

felt the same about my discharge summary. He said he did and elaborated on his former competence and the substantial gains he made in treatment. I picked up my summary from the floor, tossed it in my desk drawer, and told him I would rewrite it to give the fuller picture he had conveyed to me. I gave him the revised version before he left the hospital.

At times, I wrote a formulation to sort out a muddle or to dig myself out of a hole I had dug. For example, I worked with one patient who was profoundly and chronically addicted to alcohol, with a history of continual relapses. She was objecting to recommendations for structured aftercare treatment. She was disheartened by my unconcealed skepticism about the benefit of the therapy and her prognosis. She was especially troubled because I was reputed to be an expert therapist, and even I might not be able to help her. At one point she declared, "You are not God!" I was not acting like God, and she was not criticizing me. But I was feeling pressured to be omnipotent, and she was helpfully acknowledging my limitations to herself and to me. I wrote a formulation that included explicit delineation of what treatment could offer and what was up to her. As it played out, she did not do her bit after discharge, and she was certainly right about my limitations.

In an example of digging myself out of a hole, I had seen a highly obsessive and perfectionistic professional man for a handful of sessions during which he had conveyed pessimism about getting any help from therapy. I felt inadequate to help him. With his permission, I talked with his outpatient psychiatrist, who conveyed similar feelings of inadequacy. We agreed that I should focus on the patient's way of relating to potential helpers as a problem to address, and I broached the subject with the patient in the next session. He exclaimed that he had never felt so "despairing" in his entire life, and I felt extremely guilty. He heard me saying he could not be helped, and he felt "ganged up on" by me and his psychiatrist. I pleaded with him not to quit the therapy, and he returned for another session. Having recovered my emotional equilibrium to a degree, I wrote an elaborate formulation, summarizing my understanding of his plight while advocating (from an attachment perspective) that he was missing emotional connections and confiding relationships that could help assuage his distress. I pointed out that he was starting to develop some such connections in relationships with his peers in the hospital program devoted to treating professionals. Moreover, I indicated that he had engaged in the therapy in the most productive way by expressing his despair so poignantly in our previous session. He spent quite a while poring over the formulation, using a marker to highlight various passages (which I feared he would be criticizing). When he finished, he said, "That sounds about right. I needed someone who could think about my struggles from a different perspective, and you have." This was not rocket science: he was thinking about cognitive coping strategies and I was thinking about relationships. More simply, I was finding it hard to outthink him (which he knew to be a losing battle) and decided instead that he might have an easier time with his anxious misery if he were not so alone with it. The formulation got us back on track, and he used the therapy and the rest of treatment productively, with a solid outpatient plan going forward.

These formulations contained no revelations; they merely summarized what the patient and I had discussed in a systematic fashion, most often from a developmental perspective. As much appreciation as I have for unconscious processes, I am quite content with getting the patient's conscious experience right. Sometimes the patients found the formulation distressing, for example, when I had made plain the sheer extent and magnitude of trauma over their lifetime. Most patients found that putting the understanding we had achieved into writing was helpful, and some shared the formulations with their partners or family members to help them better understand their problems and treatment. More important than the substance, however, was patients' appreciation of the time and effort that I had put into thinking about them. Yet quite often, notwithstanding that I was reiterating the content of our sessions, patients found the formulations revealing in their seeming perspicacity. Never underestimate the potential value of writing. Explicating what we had discussed discursively in a coherent and succinct manner provided a new perspective as well as a blueprint for the patient going forward. I am reminded of a passage from Karl Menninger's article on hope:

> In a way it seems curious that the psychoanalytic process, which is so obviously diagnostic, has generally come to be called treatment. Diagnosis is the hopeful search for a way out; but the setting forth on the way which one discovers and the unflinching persistence in making the effort—*that* is the treatment; that is the self-directed, self-administered change. (Menninger 1987, p. 460, emphasis in original)

I have no formula for writing formulations; they must be personal, as therapy must be. Manuals notwithstanding, we therapists are not interchangeable. I can offer only an example, not a model. In the following case example, I start with the patient's history and then present the formulation to show how I summarized it for her.

Case Example: Marianne
Clinical History

Marianne, a 34-year-old nurse, told her psychiatrist she had saved a stash of pills; she accepted hospitalization when she was on the brink of suicide. I served as Marianne's psychotherapist during her hospital stay. She opened her first session by declaring, "I hate people. I don't trust anyone." She said this not with hostility but with resignation. She soon added, "The only way I can stand being alive is knowing that I'll kill myself when I get out of this place. I agreed to come here so that my aunt would know she did everything she could and wouldn't blame herself when I do the deed." She added, "I'm sick of fighting, so I'll cooperate with you guys while I'm here, knowing that my escape hatch is in place." That said, she conveyed her history remarkably openly and authentically.

Throughout her school years, Marianne was an anxious, "nerdy" child who was teased and ostracized by peers, especially the "in crowd," although she was liked by a number of teachers who appreciated her quirky interests (e.g., bugs and reptiles) and her diligence. She felt inferior to her older sister, who was "prettier" and "part of the gang." She was withdrawn in her home owing to fighting between her alcoholic parents and between her mother and her sister. She preferred playing alone in the woods and when at home kept to her room—sometimes hiding in the closet during fights. Her only refuge was visiting her paternal aunt, who lived alone, welcomed her company, appreciated her interests, and helped her with her schoolwork. But her aunt avoided talking about Marianne's painful family experience.

Marianne had been eager to go to college to escape the turmoil at home and hoped to enjoy life with more "mature" peers. But she quickly rejected the "party animal social scene," kept emotional distance from her roommates, and "spent hours in the library" by herself, including weekends. Marianne saw her parents and sister only on "obligatory" holidays but continued to visit her aunt on some weekends. In her junior year, she developed a confiding relationship with a classmate, Rafaela, that became the closest relationship of her life. She welcomed Rafaela's warmth and affectionate manner, developing a close attachment. Their affectionate contact gradually evolved into a valued sexual relationship, about which Marianne felt ambivalent and guilty.

In her senior year of college, Marianne decided to pursue a career in nursing. She moved away from Rafaela, with the intention of maintaining the relationship. They continued to see each other on weekends periodically. After several months apart, Rafaela confessed to Marianne that she had a boyfriend and that she didn't think it was fair to Marianne to continue their relationship. Marianne accepted this declaration but was "devastated" and vowed that she would never again open herself up like that to another person. She became a "hermit," except for her continuing visits with her aunt.

Anxious and depressed, Marianne sought psychotherapy, which she said "kept me going," although she remained isolated. She kept her "nose to the grindstone" in nursing school, and she said that after graduation, "I made my work my life." She appreciated the social contact with patients and peers at work: "It kept me from totally spacing out in my own world."

Marianne was "blindsided" when she met Kim, with whom she quickly became "infatuated," and "fell head over heels in love." Kim, however, became possessive, jealous, and "smothering"—all of which was overwhelming to Marianne, who was more comfortable with distance. When Marianne started pushing back against Kim's demands, the relationship became stormy. Marianne had quit therapy in the early weeks of her relationship with Kim, believing that she had become settled in "love and work." She continued to see her psychiatrist periodically and was prescribed medication, but she minimized the problems she was having in her life. Hence, she felt alone and "out on a limb" in managing the turmoil with Kim. The fights that ensued were reminiscent of the battles in her family that she had striven so hard to leave behind when she went to college. Moreover, feeling self-conscious about her romantic relationships with women, she had distanced herself from her aunt.

Marianne said that the "straw that broke the camel's back" and precipitated her suicidal state was her discovery that, throughout much of their relationship, Kim had resumed her romantic relationship with an ex-boyfriend and had gone to great lengths to conceal it. When Marianne confronted Kim, she first denied it and then came clean, blaming Marianne for being "unavailable" so much of the time. Mortified, Marianne grabbed her stash of pills and went to a hotel room, where she grappled with killing herself. Ultimately, she went to the bar, had a few drinks, returned to the room, and "crashed," falling asleep. When she woke up, Marianne felt confused and eyed the stash of pills on the nightstand, but the thought of her aunt gave her pause. She was able to get an emergency appointment with her psychiatrist, and they called her aunt, who arranged for Marianne to come and stay with her immediately. Her aunt investigated treatment options and arranged for Marianne to be hospitalized.

As her rich account in psychotherapy indicated, despite herself, Marianne became engaged with the therapy. Similarly, she was open with her psychiatrist, and she was willing to talk with her social worker and aunt, whom she regarded as her "only family." Helpfully, for the first time, her aunt was able to open up about the painfulness of feeling intimidated by her brother and her guilty feelings not being more emotionally involved in Marianne's family struggles growing up. Marianne said she was starting to "feel heard." She added, "But it's not enough. I'm done. If I let myself trust anyone, I'll just be crushed again."

The hospital treatment put a premium on patients confiding and feeling emotionally connected with their peers. Marianne said she felt it was like being "back in school." She added, "I'm just going to keep my mouth shut. What am I going to say? 'I hate you all?'" Moreover, she believed, "It's all a big show. They all make nice, pretending they care about each other, and they probably just can't wait to get out of here either."

In session with Marianne, I used the metaphor that she had retreated to a cave, that she had been digging herself deeper into the cave over the years, and that she had come close to sealing the entrance. I remarked that she had let Rafaela into the cave and then kept everyone out after feeling betrayed by Kim. I thought it was good that she had devoted herself to work, which allowed her to come out of the cave a little during the day, knowing that she could withdraw at night. Her infatuation with Kim broke her isolation in the cave. For a time—as with Rafaela—Marianne felt "loved." But this second betrayal was more than she could stand.

After the initial series of sessions, I wrote a formulation of my understanding of the therapeutic challenge Marianne and I faced.

Personal Formulation for Marianne

I thought it might be helpful for me to summarize my understanding of you and your treatment so far. We are in a quandary: You have firmly decided, after much thought, to kill yourself, although you "pushed the pause button," as we say. You said you'd "cooperate" while you're here, knowing that you're "out of here—permanently," when we're done. Yet, in my view, you've done more than cooperate. Living up to what your aunt had hoped, you've been sincere in your willingness to undertake treatment, largely motivated by your concern for her feeling that she'd done all she could to help you stay alive. You've unwittingly put yourself in a bit of a bind: you'd made up your mind about suicide, but your willingness to engage with us implies some openness to living. Another sticking point: after a lifetime of pain, your decision to kill yourself provided relief and tempered the pain, making it more bearable; my aim in therapy would be to help you reconsider the prospect of living, which, as you see it, would then open you back up to (seemingly endless) pain. Somehow, in the middle of this tangled web, I think you've used this therapy as productively as anyone could.

From what you've described, here's the picture I've developed of your early life. You've said that you and your sister were "not cut out of the same cloth." Speculating, I'd give temperamental factors a significant role. These factors could make you prone to a high level of anxiety and introversion as well as compliance and conscientiousness. Naturally, feeling isolated from your family, you found the attention and interest of your teachers to be rewarding. But you paid the price of being labeled a "teacher's pet" and a "nerd." Your aunt's home provided a "lifesaving" refuge, but the kindness and interest of adults didn't offset the pain of being so alienated from your peers. Your aunt and high school guidance counselor reasonably assured you that college would provide a fresh start socially, with more acceptance in the offing. Unfortunately, it was not long before you became disillusioned—as you put it, "back in the same old social shit." Your peers' high level of alcohol consumption, in particular, was all too painfully familiar. But your consistent academic work over the many years of your education paid off in a career that was both fulfilling and a source of stability—indeed, "sanity," as you experienced it.

We've talked about trauma, and I have a broad view of it, namely, the lasting effects of having experienced unbearable emotional pain while feeling alone (in the sense of lacking relationships in which you feel understood and cared about). By this definition, the experience we've discussed has been traumatic. You've said that growing up in your family was frequently "hair-raising." Considering that you sometimes feared that your father would seriously injure your mother and, at the very least, drive her away, would be frightening if not terrifying—especially when you were very young. You also saw your sister endanger herself by getting between your father and mother in futile efforts to break up their fights. Although you knew how distressed your mother was by your witnessing the violent episodes, you couldn't help feeling let down by her failure to protect you.

You said that what kept you from feeling completely hopeless was your vision of leaving home and taking charge of your own life. You did well to set the stage for charting your own course by your success in college and in establishing a solid career in nursing, where you felt appreciated for your work. But you continued your long-standing pattern of keeping emotionally distant and fending for yourself. Given your early experience and your apprehension, I think you showed considerable strength and resolve in establishing an intimate relationship with Rafaela, wherein you could feel loved and lovable as well as loving. Sadly, in the long run, you felt that you were "punished" for taking the risk. Naturally, you retreated. Nonetheless, you took care of yourself in seeking the help of psychotherapy and in maintaining your work and the social connection it provided. But you said you kept your distance even in the therapy, in part because you were wary of feeling close to another woman. As you put it, the therapy served mainly to keep you afloat. In the aftermath of your relationship with Rafaela, I don't think I'm exaggerating to describe your relationship with Kim as "tragic." In fact, the way it evolved—and especially the way it ended—could have killed you, and you're not out of those woods yet.

You started this therapy by declaring, "I hate people!" and that you trusted no one. No wonder. And, as we discussed, you sought refuge in a "cave" for much of your life, and you've kept digging your way in deeper. But the cave has become a prison, and it's become frightening, as you've sometimes felt you're losing your mind when you're "so far gone" into your mind that you could "float away and disappear." To say that you became distrustful in the face of your experience of being disappointed, let down, and betrayed is an understatement. I have no doubt that you were ready to give up and quit life and that you haven't gotten off that path.

But I am heartened by another side of you that seems far from hating people—at least all of them. Perhaps this side has kept you going all these years. I see you as being good-hearted. You talked about how caring you felt toward some of your patients and how careful you are in all your work. You've been grateful to your aunt and sensitive to not wanting to let her down or hurt her by your suicide. You were profoundly grateful to Rafaela and treasured the caring that each of you felt for each other. For all the frustration in your relationship with Kim, you saw through her storms how much she depended on you, and you stuck with her until she blew it all up. You have complained about your peers here being "phony" and "just playing the game," but you have not wanted to spoil their treatment and alienate yourself by confessing, "I hate you all and think you're full of it." You've been cordial and respectful, if distant. To use your word, you've been "cooperative" in the groups. But I think you've gone further in your individual relationships—with me, your social worker, and your psychiatrist. Despite your conviction that this treatment would be of no help, you've been all-in, open and engaging. Either you're out of the cave, or you've let me and others in—at least partway.

So here's the bind we're in as I see it. To a large extent (although your roommate here in the hospital might be an exception), your experience with the other patients has only reinforced your long-standing view that social relationships are "a sham." On the other hand, you've felt understood by your psychiatrist, your social worker, and me. Moreover, your social worker has used her understanding to your benefit, enabling you to feel more connected with your aunt. Feeling more connected to your aunt, however, has made you feel even more reluctant to hurt her, interfering with your "escape hatch" of suicide. So, as this treatment has gone on, you're feeling more agitated and trapped, caught between the connections you're making through feeling understood and cared for, on the one hand, and wanting to exit life, on the other. I've done my best to understand your desire to die, and I can sympathize with it. I also recognize that you've "given life a fair shot," as you put it. Nevertheless, to put it starkly, I see so much good in you that it's hard for me to take the side of your decision to die.

But the dilemma we face is this: You've been badly hurt—traumatized—by what you have most needed throughout your life—loving, caring relationships. You took risks in those relationships, and you're taking a risk here by confiding in some of us as well as your aunt. I don't know if you will allow yourself to risk again beyond these relationships. If you do, you'll need to do it cautiously. You'd need to have confidence that you can manage the potential pain if you take the risk. Toward that end, you've been willing to work with medication here, and you've recognized that there might be some value in "coping skills" being taught here, despite your disdain for the "platitudes" you hear in the educational groups. I think you've shown some openness in considering that some of the patients do seem to really care about each other, despite your skepticism. You know what it's like to care and to feel cared about, and you can see it here.

I've been worried about the possibility of your suicide all along, and I remain so. To your credit, you've been straight about it. You rightly pride yourself on your truthfulness, which has been a great help to this therapy. I feel worried, but not hopeless. Ironically, you've given me hope—not just by all you've done in your life but also by your commitment to this treatment and the trust you've shown in confiding in us. Perhaps most significantly, you said at the end of our last meeting that you have a bit of hope that you can develop hope as time goes on. What could be more reasonable at this point?

Hospital Treatment Outcome

As the treatment progressed beyond the point of this formulation, Marianne took advantage of the therapeutic community, beginning to trust some of her peers and to open up in the groups. She came to appreciate the patients' genuineness in caring about each other and in valuing the treatment and the community. Her hope that she would have hope was founded in an enduring capacity for trust that she had not allowed herself to recognize for fear of being hurt yet again. She left the hospital with a plan to live with her aunt for a time while resuming psychotherapy, for which she had developed a greater appreciation.

Summary of Key Points

- Therapists should not take their trustworthiness for granted but rather should think about becoming trustworthy to the patient over the course of the therapy and restoring trustworthiness when it is disrupted.

- Kant distinguished between love as coming close and respect as keeping distance. This distinction corresponds to the two fundamental developmental lines of relatedness and autonomy as well as the synergy of the safe haven and secure base in attachment theory. Maintaining the balance between love and respect lies at the heart of a long-standing debate about therapeutic neutrality, which is essential to the trustworthy conduct of psychotherapy.

- The personal influence of the therapist plays a key role in the change process, and emotional responses guided by ethical-moral judgments are intrinsic to this influence. Being nonjudgmental does not entail refraining from making judgments but rather involves refraining from fault finding and looking for the good.

- Self-revelation (e.g., through body language, sex, race, public information) is inescapable, but self-disclosure (verbally) is voluntary and a matter for careful consideration.

- Individual differences among therapists and patient-therapist dyads influence the balance between closeness and distance, but balance is essential and must be guided by keeping the treatment goals and patient's welfare foremost in mind.

- The concept of the Third refers to the patient and therapist experiencing a shared mental space. This experience is the basis for cooperation and commitment to shared goals, and it catalyzes the development of trust and trustworthiness in the relationship. The experience of the Third is a mutual creation that naturally comes and goes, being lost in noncooperative interactions and restored continually in the cultivation of trust.

- Recognition builds and sustains the Third, and it is a reciprocal process: not only is the recognized individual seen and known, but the recognizing person must be seen and known in the act of recognizing.

- Several overlapping concepts refer to shared mental space: joint intentionality, the "we," recognition, and the Third. Regardless of the terminology, trusting in psychotherapy requires that the patient and therapist create a mental space in which they become trusting of each other and trustworthy to each other, committed to cooperating in ameliorating the patient's suffering and enhancing the patient's well-being.

- Transparency exemplifies trustworthiness, and writing personal formulations to articulate the therapist's understanding of the patient and the therapy is a potential means of promoting trust.

- The conduct and effectiveness of psychotherapy cannot be isolated from its broader social context: without a predictably moral-ethical society, trusting and trustworthiness cultivated in psychotherapy cannot flourish.

Recommendations for Clinical Practice

- Over the course of my career, I increasingly became aware of the inescapably personal nature of conducting psychotherapy. Accepting that you are exerting personal influence entails a kind of responsibility that is different from mastering treatment methods. I felt a need for expertise in this ethical-moral territory and found it in the philosophical literature. I needed some conceptual handholds, and I commend three that I have found most grounding: appreciating our need to continually

balance love and respect, accepting that moral reactive attitudes are intrinsic to our humanity and cannot be sidelined in
our relationships with patients, and recognizing that we can
make judgments without being judgmental. *Neutrality* seems
a rather pale word for navigating this profoundly messy territory, but there is something right in this long-held aspiration.

- I've filled this book with more than 100,000 words, but you
will need to translate it into experience if it is to be of any value. I prefer *mentalizing* to its original usage, *mentalization*, to
emphasize that it is something we must do. *The Third* allows
for no such rendering, but I have said that finding our way into
the Third—the feeling of "we" with our patients—is essential to
establishing trust. We establish the Third and then lose it in
the noncooperative, "doer–done to" mode. We mentalize and
then lose mentalizing. These concepts are useful in directing
your attention to the flux in relating. A trusting relationship
does not require continuous experience of mentalizing, the
Third, or a sense of being together in the "we." Establishing
trust entails a joint commitment to finding your way back
when you become lost—no longer together. As a therapist, you
are a guide, and you sometimes must rely on your patient's
guidance.

- I recommend that you write personal formulations for your
patients, but I do so hesitantly, knowing the time it takes and
the burden of heavy clinical practice. Occasionally, I have giv-
en a patient a list of bullet points (e.g., highlighting problems
in our interactions) or a paragraph (e.g., highlighting the way
a traumatic relationship in the past is influencing a problematic pattern of relating in the present). Less formally, I keep a
pad handy and jot down a few ideas (akin to the key points
herein), make a list (e.g., of cumulative stressors), or draw a
diagram of a recurring cascade (e.g., feeling alone, you engage
in stress-relieving but risky alcohol abuse that draws your
partner's concern but also engenders her resentment; she
gradually distances herself more, which escalates your anxiety about a breakup along with increasing feelings of isolation, leading to increasingly dangerous binges, and so on). As
should be obvious, I put a lot of stock in writing; it can help us
think—and remember.

Parting Thoughts

You might have noticed throughout this book that I have not offered any methods for cultivating trust or becoming trustworthy as a therapist. As I wrote at the end of Chapter 3, if you come across a manual, don't trust it. Instead, I intended to help you think about trusting in psychotherapy in a more refined way than is characteristic in the literature. I have used a lot of science, but more in the service of understanding than in action. Science informs our practice but cannot rule it. At the outset, I praised Huston Smith's (1992) assertion that in our effort to know reality, we should start with science but not end with it. But we do not start with science; we integrate it with whatever personal knowledge we have acquired from childhood onward. And we certainly cannot end by replacing our personal knowledge with science. As much as we might wish for it when everything goes haywire, there is no manual for life—our patients' or our own.

We therapists have no alternative to charting our own developmental course as we work on mastering the craft of psychotherapy. As it is for the patient, much of the therapist's developmental course is shaped by happenstance; much of the developmental influence is unconscious; and deliberation along the way plays a contributing role to varying degrees. To generalize, as research does: the patient's characteristics and social context play a larger role in the treatment outcome than does the therapist's influence. I hope to have persuaded you that the method you employ plays a mere supporting role in comparison with the relationship you and your patient create together. But you must have a method, and you and your patient must find it credible—trusting in it. As I interpret decades of psychotherapy research, the profession is in no position to prescribe the methods you choose.

You need confidence, but it is best to hold it lightly. As I reported in Chapter 1, some research hints that therapists' self-doubt is associated with better outcomes. I am put off by therapists brimming with enthusiasm and confidence when they lecture about their methods. Have they never felt bewildered, helpless, and inadequate in their work? Have they not yet lost a patient to suicide? I find audiences more responsive to empathizing with the sheer difficulty of conducting psychotherapy and articulating the reasons for the difficulty. We therapists and our patients need trust, along with hope and faith, because we practice in the potentially perilous realm of uncertainty. Presumption is no better than despair.

On the whole, psychotherapy and psychotherapists are effective in providing help. We relieve suffering, and we can help our patients improve their life. If our patients are to be believed, we sometimes save lives. We cannot do it without building and restoring trust, and that is worth thinking about—carefully.

References

Ainsworth MDS, Blehar MC, Waters E, et al: Patterns of Attachment: A Psychological Study of the Strange Situation. Hillsdale, NJ, Erlbaum, 1978

Allen JG: The spectrum of accuracy in memories of childhood trauma. Harvard Rev Psychiatry 3:84–95, 1995

Allen JG: Traumatic Relationships and Serious Mental Disorders. Chichester, UK, Wiley, 2001

Allen JG: Coping With Trauma: Hope Through Understanding, 2nd Edition. Washington, DC, American Psychiatric Publishing, 2005

Allen JG: Coping With Depression: From Catch-22 to Hope. Washington, DC, American Psychiatric Publishing, 2006

Allen JG: Evil, Mindblindness, and trauma: challenges to hope. Smith Coll Stud Social Work 77:9–31, 2007

Allen JG: Psychotherapy: the artful use of science. Smith Coll Stud Social Work 78:159–187, 2008

Allen JG: Mentalizing suicidal states, in Building a Therapeutic Alliance With the Suicidal Patient, Edited by Michel K, Jobes DA. Washington, DC, American Psychological Association, 2011, pp 81–92

Allen JG: Hope in human attachment and spiritual connection. Bull Menninger Clin 77:302–331, 2013a

Allen JG: Mentalizing in the Development and Treatment of Attachment Trauma. London, Karnac, 2013b

Allen JG: Restoring Mentalizing in Attachment Relationships: Treating Trauma With Plain Old Therapy. Arlington, VA, American Psychiatric Publishing, 2013c

Allen JG: Should the century-old practice of psychotherapy defer to science and ignore its foundations in two millenia of ethical thought? Bull Menninger Clin 80:1–29, 2016

Allen JG, Fonagy P: Mentalizing in psychotherapy, in The American Psychiatric Association Publishing Textbook of Psychiatry, 7th Edition. Washington, DC, American Psychiatric Association Publishing, 2019, pp 1019–1040

Allen JG, Coyne L, Colson DB, et al: Pattern of therapist interventions associated with patient collaboration. Psychotherapy 33:254–261, 1996

Allen JG, Fonagy P, Bateman A: Mentalizing in Clinical Practice. Washington, DC, American Psychiatric Publishing, 2008

Allen JG, O'Malley F, Freeman C, et al: Promoting mentalizing in brief treatment, in Handbook of Mentalizing in Mental Health Practice. Edited by Fonagy P, Bateman AW. Washington, DC, American Psychiatric Publishing, 2012, pp 159–196

Allen JG, Fowler JC, Madan A, et al: Discovering the impact of psychotherapeutic hospital treatment for adults with serious mental illness. Bull Menninger Clin 81:1–38, 2017

American Psychological Association: Ethical Principles of Psychologists and Code of Conduct. Washington, DC, American Psychological Association, 2017

APA Presidential Task Force on Evidence-Based Practice: Evidence-based practice in psychology. Am Psychol 614:271–285, 2006

Appiah KA: Experiments in Ethics. Cambridge, MA, Harvard University Press, 2008

Armony JL, LeDoux JE: How the brain processes emotional information, in Psychobiology of Posttraumatic Stress Disorder (Vol 821). Edited by Yehuda R, MacFarlane AC. New York, New York Academy of Sciences, 1997, pp 259–270

Arnott B, Meins E: Links between antenatal attachment representations, postnatal mind-mindedness, and infant attachment security: a preliminary study of mothers and fathers. Bull Menninger Clin 71:132–149, 2007

Baier A: Trust and antitrust. Ethics 96:231–260, 1986

Barkham M, Lutz W, Lambert MJ, et al: Therapist effects, effective therapists, and the law of variability, in How and Why Are Some Therapists Better Than Others? Understanding Therapist Effects. Edited by Castonguay LG, Hill CE. Washington, DC, American Psychological Association, 2017, pp 13–36

Bartlett RC, Collins SD: Aristotle's Nicomachean Ethics. Chicago, IL, University of Chicago Press, 2011

Bateman A, Fonagy P: Effectiveness of partial hospitalization in the treatment of borderline personality disorder: a randomized controlled trial. Am J Psychiatry 156:1563–1569, 1999

Bateman A, Fonagy P: Treatment of borderline personality disorder with psychoanalytically oriented partial hospitalization: an 18-month follow-up. Am J Psychiatry 158:36–42, 2001

Bateman A, Fonagy P: Mentalization-Based Treatment for Borderline Personality Disorder: A Practical Guide. New York, Oxford University Press, 2006

Bateman A, Fonagy P: Randomized controlled trial of outpatient mentalization-based treatment versus structured clinical management for borderline personality disorder. Am J Psychiatry 166:1355–1364, 2009

Bateman A, Fonagy P: Mentalization-Based Treatment for Personality Disorders: A Practical Guide. New York, Oxford University Press, 2016

Bateman A, Fonagy P (eds): Handbook of Mentalizing in Mental Health Practice, 2nd Edition. Washington, DC, American Psychiatric Association Publishing, 2019

Beebe B, Jaffe J, Markese S, et al: The origins of 12-month attachment: a microanalysis of 4-month mother-infant interaction. Attach Hum Dev 12:3–142, 2010

Bellah R, Madsen R, Sullivan WM, et al: The Good Society. New York, Random House, 1991

Bellah R, Madsen R, Sullivan WM, et al: Habits of the Heart: Individualism and Commitment in American Life. Berkeley, University of California Press, 2008

Benjamin J: Beyond Doer and Done To: Recognition Theory, Intersubjectivity and the Third. New York, Routledge, 2018

Beutler LE, Edwards CJ, Kimpara S, et al: Coping style, in Psychotherapy Relationships That Work. Volume 2: Evidence-Based Therapist Responsiveness, 3rd Edition. Edited by Norcross JC, Wampold BE. New York, Oxford University Press, 2019, pp 56–85

Bishop MA: The Good Life: Unifying the Philosophy and Psychology of Well-Being. New York, Oxford University Press, 2015

Blatt SJ: Polarities of Experience. Washington, DC, American Psychological Association, 2008

Bleiberg E, Safier E: Couples therapy, in Handbook of Mentalizing in Mental Health Practice, 2nd Edition. Edited by Bateman A, Fonagy P. Washington, DC, American Psychiatric Association Publishing, 2019, pp 151–180

Bloom P: Just Babies: The Origins of Good and Evil. New York, Broadway Books, 2013

Bogin B, Bragg J, Kuzawa C: Childhood, biocultural reproduction, and human lifetime reproductive effort, in Childhood: Origins, Evolution, and Implications. Edited by Meehan CL, Crittenden AN. Albuquerque, University of New Mexico Press, 2016, pp 45–74

Bohart AC, Tallman K: Clients: the neglected common factor, in The Heart and Soul of Change: Delivering What Works in Psychotherapy, 2nd Edition. Edited by Duncan BL, Miller SD, Wampold BE, et al. Washington, DC, American Psychological Association, 2010, pp 83–112

Boswell JF, Kraus DR, Constantino MJ, et al: The implications of therapist effects for routine practice, policy, and training, in How and Why Are Some Therapists Better Than Others? Understanding Therapist Effects. Edited by Castonguay LG, Hill CE. Washington, DC, American Psychological Association, 2017, pp 325–341

Boswell JF, Newman MG, McGinn LK: Outcome research on psychotherapy integration, in Handbook of Psychotherapy Integration, 3rd Edition. Edited by Norcross JC, Goldfried MR. New York, Oxford University Press, 2019, pp 405–431

Bowlby J: Attachment and Loss, Volume 2: Separation. New York, Basic Books, 1973

Bowlby J: Attachment and Loss, Volume 3: Loss: Sadness and Depression. New York, Basic Books, 1980

Bowlby J: Attachment and Loss, 2nd Edition, Vol 1: Attachment. New York, Basic Books, 1982

Bowlby J: A Secure Base: Parent-Child Attachment and Healthy Human Development. New York, Basic Books, 1988

Brassard A, Johnson SM: Couple and family therapy: an attachment perspective, in Handbook of Attachment: Theory, Research, and Clinical Applications. Edited by Cassidy J, Shaver PR. New York, Guilford, 2016, pp 805–823

Budge SL, Moradi B: Gender identity, in Psychotherapy Relationships That Work, in Psychotherapy Relationships That Work. Volume 2: Evidence-Based Therapist Responsiveness, 3rd Edition. Edited by Norcross JC, Wampold BE. New York, Oxford University Press, 2019, pp 133–156

Burston D, Frie R: Psychotherapy as a Human Science. Pittsburgh, PA, Duquesne University Press, 2006

Carlson EA: A prospective longitudinal study of attachment disorganization/disorientation. Child Dev 69:1107–1128, 1998

Caspar F: Professional expertise in psychotherapy, in How and Why Are Some Therapists Better Than Others? Understanding Therapist Effects. Edited by Castonguay LG, Hill CE. Washington, DC, American Psychological Association, 2017, pp 193–214

Cassidy J, Shaver PR (eds): Handbook of Attachment: Theory, Research, and Clinical Applications, 3rd Edition. New York, Guilford, 2016

Castonguay LG, Hill CE (eds): How and Why Are Some Therapists Better Than Others? Washington, DC, American Psychological Association, 2017a

Castonguay LG, Hill CE: Preface, in How and Why Are Some Therapists Better Than Others? Understanding Therapist Effects. Edited by Castonguay LG, Hill CE. Washington, DC, American Psychological Association, 2017b, pp xiii–xv

Castonguay LG, Constantino MJ, Xaio H: Integrating research and practice, in Handbook of Psychotherapy Integration. Edited by Norcross JC, Goldfried MR. New York, Oxford University Press, 2019, pp 432–447

Chapman NA, Black SW, Drinane JM, et al: Quantitative performance systems: feedback informed treatment, in The Cycle of Excellence: Using Deliberate Practice to Improve Supervision and Training. Edited by Rousmaniere T, Goodyear RK, Miller SD, et al. Chichester, UK, Wiley, 2017, pp 123–144

Coan JA: Toward a neuroscience of attachment, in Handbook of Attachment: Theory, Research, and Clinical Applications, 3rd Edition. Edited by Cassidy J, Shaver PR. New York, Guilford, 2016, pp 242–269

Constantino MJ, Boswell JF, Coyne AE, et al: Who works for whom and why? Integrating therapist effects analysis into psychotherapy outcome and process research, in How and Why Are Some Therapists Better Than Others? Understanding Therapist Effects. Edited by Castonguay LG, Hill CE. Washington, DC, American Psychological Association, 2017, pp 55–68

Cooper M, Norcross JC: A brief multidimensional measure of clients' therapy preferences: The Cooper-Norcross Inventory of Preferences (C-NIP). Int J Clin Health Psychol 16:87–98, 2016

Cowen EL: Help is where you find it: four informal helping groups. Am Psychol 37:385–395, 1982

Crittenden AN: Children's foraging and play among the Hazda: the evolutionary significance of "work play," in Childhood: Origins, Evolution, and Implications. Edited by Meehan CL, Crittenden AN. Albuquerque, University of New Mexico Press, 2016, pp 155–172

Csikszentmihalyi M: Flow: The Psychology of Optimal Experience. New York, HarperCollins, 1990

Cuijpers P, Reijnders M, Huibers MJH: The role of common factors in psychotherapy outcomes. Annu Rev Clin Psychol 15:207–231, 2019

Cushman P: Constructing the Self, Constructing America: A Cultural History of Psychotherapy. New York, Perseus, 1995

Darwall S: Trust as a second-personal attitude (of the heart), in The Philosophy of Trust. Edited by Faulkner P, Simpson T. New York, Oxford University Press, 2017, pp 35–50

de Waal F: Mama's Last Hug: Animal Emotions and What They Tell Us About Ourselves. New York, Norton, 2019

Dennett DC: The Intentional Stance. Cambridge, MA, MIT Press, 1987

Dennett DC: From Bacteria to Bach and Back: The Evolution of Minds. New York, Norton, 2017

Domenicucci J, Holton R: Trust as a two-place relation, in The Philosophy of Trust. Edited by Faulkner P, Simpson T. New York, Oxford University Press, 2017, pp 149–160

Doyle TP: Roman Catholic clericalism, religious duress, and clergy sexual abuse. Pastoral Psychol 51:189–231, 2003

Dunbar R: Grooming, Gossip, and the Evolution of Language. Cambridge, MA, Harvard University Press, 1996

Duncan BL: Prologue: Saul Rosenzweig: the founder of common factors, in The Heart and Soul of Change: Delivering What Works in Psychotherapy, 2nd Edition. Edited by Duncan BL, Miller SD, Wampold BE, et al. Washington, DC, American Psychological Association, 2010, pp 3–22

Dutton D, Painter SL: Traumatic bonding: the development of emotional attachments in battered women and other relationships of intermittent abuse. Victimology 6:139–155, 1981

Edwards CJ, Beutler LE, Someah K: Reactance level, in Psychotherapy Relationships That Work. Volume 2: Evidence-Based Therapist Responsiveness, 3rd Edition. Edited by Norcross JC, Wampold BE. New York, Oxford University Press, 2019, pp 188–211

Edwards-Stewart A, Norcross JC: Integrating self-help and psychotherapy, Handbook of Psychotherapy Integration. Edited by Norcross JC, Goldfried MR. New York, Oxford University Press, 2019, pp 357–384

Elliott R, Bohart AC, Watson JC, et al: Empathy, in Psychotherapy Relationships That Work. Volume 1: Evidence-Based Therapist Contributions, 3rd Edition. Edited by Norcross JC, Wampold BE. New York, Oxford University Press, 2019, pp 245–287

Ellis TE, Green KL, Allen JG, et al: Collaborative assessment and management of suicidality in an inpatient setting: a pilot study. Psychotherapy 49:72–80, 2012

Erikson EH: Childhood and Society. New York, Norton, 1963

Eubanks CF, Goldfried MR, Norcross JC: Future directions in psychotherapy integration, in Handbook of Psychotherapy Integration, 3rd Edition. Edited by Norcross JC, Goldfried MR. New York, Oxford University Press, 2019a, pp 474–485

Eubanks CF, Muran JC, Safran JD: Repairing alliance ruptures, in Psychotherapy Relationships That Work, Volume 1: Evidence-Based Therapist Contributions, 3rd Edition. Edited by Norcross JC, Wampold BE. New York, Oxford University Press, 2019b, pp 549–579

Exline JJ: Religious and spiritual struggles, in APA Handbook of Psychology, Religion, and Spirituality. Volume 1: Context, Theory, and Research. Edited by Pargament KI, Exline JJ, Jones EP. Washington, DC, American Psychological Association, 2013, pp 459–475

Farber BA: Gaining therapeutic wisdom and skills from creative others (writers, actors, musicians, and dancers), in How and Why Are Some Therapists Better Than Others? Understanding Therapist Effects. Edited by Castonguay LG, Hill CE. Washington, DC, American Psychological Association, 2017, pp 215–232

Farber BA, Suzuki JY, Lynch DA: Positive regard and affirmation, in Psychotherapy Relationships That Work. Volume 1: Evidence-Based Therapist Contributions, 3rd Edition. Edited by Norcross JC, Wampold BE. New York, Oxford University Press, 2019, pp 288–322

Faulkner P: Knowledge on Trust. New York, Oxford University Press, 2011

Faulkner P: The problem of trust, The Philosophy of Trust. Edited by Faulkner P, Simpson T. New York, Oxford University Press, 2017, pp 109–128

Fernyhough C: The Voices Within: The History and Science of How We Talk to Ourselves. New York, Basic Books, 2016

Ferro A, Nicoli L: The New Analyst's Guide to the Galaxy: Questions About Contemporary Psychoanalysis. London, Karnac, 2017

Flanagan O: The Geography of Morals. New York, Oxford Universtiy Press, 2017

Flückiger C, Del Re AC, Wampold BE, et al: Alliance in adult psychotherapy, in Psychotherapy Relationships That Work. Volume 1: Evidence-Based Therapist Contributions, 3rd Edition. Edited by Norcross JC, Wampold BE. New York, Oxford University Press, 2019, pp 24–78

Foa EB, Rothbaum BO: Treating the Trauma of Rape: Cognitive-Behavioral Therapy for PTSD. New York, Guilford, 1998

Fonagy P: A child's understanding of others. Bulletin of the Anna Freud Centre 12:91–115, 1989

Fonagy P: Peter Fonagy on a revolution in mental health care. Interviewer: J. Al-Khalili. BBC Life Scientific, January 28, 2020

Fonagy P, Bateman A: Introduction, in Handbook of Mentalizing in Mental Health Practice, 2nd Edition. Edited by Bateman A, Fonagy P. Washington, DC, American Psychiatric Association Publishing, 2019, pp 3–20

Fonagy P, Steele H, Steele M: Maternal representations of attachment during pregnancy predict the organization of infant-mother attachment at one year of age. Child Dev 62:891–905, 1991

Fonagy P, Luyten P, Allison E, et al: What we have changed our minds about: Part 2. Borderline personality disorder, epistemic trust and the developmental significance of social communication. Borderline Personal Disord Emot Dysregul 4:9, 2017

Fonagy P, Allison E, Campbell C: Mentalizing, resilience, and epistemic trust, in Handbook of Mentalizing in Mental Health Practice, 2nd Edition. Edited by Bateman A, Fonagy P. Washington, DC, American Psychiatric Association Publishing, 2019a, pp 63–78

Fonagy P, Campbell C, Allison E: Therapeutic models, in Handbook of Mentalizing in Mental Health Practice, 2nd Edition. Edited by Bateman A, Fonagy P. Washington, DC, American Psychiatric Association Publishing, 2019b, pp 169–180

Frank JD: Persuasion and Healing. New York, Shocken Books, 1961

Frank JD, Frank JB: Persuasion and Healing: A Comparative Study of Psychotherapy, 3rd Edition. Baltimore, MD, Johns Hopkins University Press, 1991

Gaskins S, Beeghly M, Bard KA, et al: Implications for policy and practice, in The Cultural Nature of Attachment: Contextualizing Relationships and Development. Edited by Keller H, Bard KA. Cambridge, MA, MIT Press, 2017, pp 321–334

George C, Solomon J: The caregiving system: a behavioral systems approach to parenting, in Handbook of Attachment: Theory, Research, and Clinical Applications, 2nd Edition. Edited by Cassidy J, Shaver PR. New York, Guilford, 2008, pp 833–856

George C, Solomon J: Caregiving helplessness: the development of a screening measure for disorganized maternal caregiving, in Disorganized Attachment and Caregiving. Edited by Solomon J, George C. New York, Guilford, 2011, pp 133–166

Gergely G: The social construction of the subjective self: the role of affect-mirroring, markedness, and ostensive communication in self development, in Developmental Science and Psychoanalysis. Edited by Mayes L, Fonagy P, Target M. London, Karnac, 2007, pp 45–82

Gergely G, Csibra G: The social construction of the cultural mind: imitative learning as a mechanism of human pedagogy. Interaction Studies 6:463–481, 2005

Gergely G, Watson JS: The social biofeedback theory of parental affect-mirroring: the development of emotional self-awareness and self-control in infancy. Int J Psychoanal 77:1181–1212, 1996

Gergely G, Egyed K, Király I: On pedagogy. Dev Sci 10:139–146, 2007

Gleiser M: The Island of Knowledge: The Limits of Science and the Search for Meaning. New York, Basic Books, 2014

Goldberg SB, Rousmaniere T, Miller SD, et al: Do psychotherapists improve with time and experience? A longitudinal analysis of outcomes in a clinical setting. J Couns Psychol 63:1–11, 2016

Goldberg SB, Babins-Wagner R, Miller SD, et al: Nurturing expertise at mental health agencies, in The Cycle of Excellence: Using Deliberate Practice to Improve Supervision and Training. Edited by Rousmaniere T, Goodyear RK, Miller SD, et al. Chichester, UK, Wiley, 2017, pp 199–218

Goldfried MR, Pachankis JE, Goodwin BJ: A history of psychotherapy integration, in Handbook of Psychotherapy Integration, 3rd Edition. Edited by Norcross JC, Goldfried MR. New York, Oxford University Press, 2019, pp 28–63

Goodyear RK, Rousmaniere T: Helping therapists to each day become a little better than they were the day before: the expertise-development model of supervision and consultation, in The Cycle of Excellence: Using Deliberate Practice to Improve Supervision and Training. Edited by Rousmaniere T, Goodyear RK, Miller SD, et al. Chichester, UK, Wiley, 2017, pp 67–95

Gottman JM: What Predicts Divorce? Hillsdale, NJ, Lawrence Erlbaum, 1994

Gottman JM: The Science of Trust: Emotional Attunement for Couples. New York, Norton, 2011

Grandqvist P, Kirkpatrick LA: Religion, spirituality, and attachment, in APA Handbook of Psychology, Religion, and Spirituality. Volume 1: Context, Theory, and Research. Edited by Pargament KI, Exline JJ, Jones EP. Washington, DC, American Psychological Association, 2013, pp 139–156

Greene B: Until the End of Time: Mind, Matter, and Our Search for Meaning in an Evolving Universe. New York, Knopf, 2020

Groat M, Allen JG: Promoting mentalizing in experiential psychoeducational groups. Bull Menninger Clin 75:315–343, 2011

Haught JF: Tillich in dialogue with natural science, in The Cambridge Companion to Paul Tillich. Edited by Re Manning R. New York, Cambridge University Press, 2009, pp 223–237

Hawley K: Trust: A Very Short Introduction. New York, Oxford University Press, 2012

Haybron DM: The Pursuit of Unhappiness: The Elusive Psychology of Well-Being. New York, Oxford University Press, 2008

Haybron DM: Happiness: A Very Short Introduction. New York, Oxford University Press, 2013

Hayes JA, Owen J, Nissen-Lie HA: The contributions of client culture to differential therapist effectiveness, in How and Why Are Some Therapists Better Than Others? Understanding Therapist Effects. Edited by Castonguay LG, Hill CE. Washington, DC, American Psychological Association, 2017, pp 159–174

Hays S: The Cultural Contradictions of Motherhood. New Haven, CT, Yale University Press, 1996

Henrich J: The WEIRDest People in the World: How the West Became Psychologically Peculiar and Particularly Prosperous. New York, Farrar, Straus & Giroux, 2020

Hesse E: The Adult Attachment Interview: protocol, method of analysis, and selected empirical studies, in Handbook of Attachment: Theory, Research, and Clinical Applications, 3rd Edition. Edited by Cassidy J, Shaver PR. New York, Guilford, 2016, pp 553–597

Hilsenroth MJ, Diener MJ: Some effective strategies for the supervision of psychodynamic psychotherapy, in The Cycle of Excellence: Using Deliberate Practice to Improve Supervision and Training. Edited by Rousmaniere T, Goodyear RK, Miller SD, et al. Chichester, UK, Wiley, 2017, pp 163–188

Hoffman I: The intimate and ironic authority of the psychoanalyst's presence. Psychoanal Q 65:102–136, 1996

Holmes J: Defensive and creative uses of narrative in psychotherapy: an attachment perspective, in Healing Stories: Narrative in Psychiatry and Psychotherapy. Edited by Roberts G, Holmes J. London, Oxford University Press, 1999, pp 49–66

Holmes J: The Search for the Secure Base: Attachment Theory and Psychotherapy. New York, Routledge, 2001

Holmes J: Exploring in Security: Towards an Attachment Informed Psychoanalytic Psychotherapy. New York, Routledge, 2010

Hook JN, Captari LE, Hoyt W, et al: Religion and spirituality, in Psychotherapy Relationships That Work. Volume 2: Evidence-Based Therapist Responsiveness, 3rd Edition. Edited by Norcross JC, Wampold BE. New York, Oxford University Press, 2019, pp 212–263

Horwitz L, Gabbard GO, Allen JG, et al: Borderline Personality Disorder: Tailoring the Therapy to the Patient. Washington, DC, American Psychiatric Press, 1996

Hrdy SB: Mothers and Others: The Evolutionary Origins of Mutual Understanding. Cambridge, MA, Harvard University Press, 2009

Hrdy SB: Development plus social selection in the emergence of "emotionally modern" humans, in Childhood: Origins, Evolution, and Implications. Edited by Meehan CL, Crittenden AN. Albuquerque, University of New Mexico Press, 2016, pp 11–44

Hursthouse R: On Virtue Ethics. New York, Oxford University Press, 1999

James W: The Principles of Psychology, Volume 1. 1890. New York, Dover, 1950

Jobes DA: Managing Suicidal Risk: A Collaborative Approach. New York, Guilford, 2006

Jones K: Trust as an affective attitude. Ethics 107:4–25, 1996

Jones K: Trustworthiness. Ethics 123:61–85, 2012

Jones K: "But I was counting on you!" in The Philosophy of Trust. Edited by Faulkner P, Simpson T. New York, Oxford University Press, 2017, pp 90–108

Kahneman D: Thinking, Fast and Slow. New York, Farrar, Straus & Giroux, 2011

Kant I: The Metaphysics of Morals (1797). New York, Cambridge University Press, 1966

Kant I: Groundwork of the Metaphysics of Morals (1785). New York, Cambridge University Press, 2012

Keller H: Introduction: Understanding relationships—what we would need to know to conceputalize attachment as the cultural solution of a universal developmental task, in Different Faces of Attachment: Cultural Variations on a Universal Human Need. Edited by Otto H, Keller H. Cambridge, UK, Cambridge University Press, 2014, pp 1–24

Keller H, Bard KA (eds): The Cultural Nature of Attachment: Contextualizing Relationships and Development. Cambridge, MA, MIT Press, 2017

Keller H, Chaudhary N: Is the mother essential for attachment? Models of care in different cultures, in The Cultural Nature of Attachment: Contextualizing Relationships and Development. Edited by Keller H, Bard KA. Cambridge, MA, MIT Press, 2017, pp 109–138

Keller H, Otto H: Epilogue: The future of attachment, in Different Faces of Attachment: Cultural Variations on a Universal Human Need. Edited by Otto H, Keller H. Cambridge, UK, Cambridge University Press, 2014, pp 307–312

Keyes CLM: Mental health as a complete state: how the salutogenic perspective completes the picture, in Bridging Occupational, Organizational, and Public Health: A Transdisciplinary Approach. Edited by Bauer GF, Hämmig O. New York, Springer, 2014, pp 179–192

Kinghorn W: "Hope that is seen is no hope at all:" theological constructions of hope in psychotherapy. Bull Menninger Clin 77:369–394, 2013

Kittay EF: The relationality and the normativity of an ethic of care, in The Oneness Hypothesis: Beyond the Boundary of Self. Edited by Ivanhoe PJ, Flanagan O, Harrison VS, et al. New York, Columbia University Press, 2018, pp 120–141

Kolden GG, Wang C-C, Austin SB, et al: Congruence/genuineness, in Psychotherapy Relationships That Work. Volume 1: Evidence-Based Therapist Contributions, 3rd Edition. Edited by Norcross JC, Wampold BE. New York, Oxford University Press, 2019, pp 323–250

Korchin S: Modern Clinical Psychology. New York, Basic Books, 1976

Korsgaard CM: Creating the Kingdom of Ends. New York, Cambridge University Press, 1996

Korsgaard CM: Self-Constitution: Agency, Identity, and Integrity. New York, Oxford University Press, 2009

Krebs P, Norcross JC, Nicholson JM, et al: Stages of change, in Psychotherapy Relationships That Work. Volume 2: Evidence-Based Therapist Responsiveness, 3rd Edition. Edited by Norcross JC, Wampold BE. New York, Oxford University Press, 2019, pp 296–328

Lagerspetz O: Trust, Ethics, and Human Reason. London, Bloomsbury, 2015

Lambert MJ, Whipple JL, Kleinstäuber M: Collecting and delivering client feedback, in Psychotherapy Relationships That Work. Volume 1: Evidence-Based Therapist Contributions, 3rd Edition. Edited by Norcross JC, Wampold BE. New York, Oxford University Press, 2019, pp 580–630

Lancy DF: Ethnographic perspectives on culture acquisition, in Childhood: Origins, Evolution, and Implications. Edited by Meehan CL, Crittenden AN. Albuquerque, University of New Mexico Press, 2016, pp 173–199

Lecours S, Bouchard M-A: Dimensions of menalisation: outlining levels of psychic transformation. Int J Psychoanal 78:855–875, 1997

Levine RA: Attachment theory as cultural ideology, in Different Faces of Attachment: Cultural Variations on a Universal Human Need. Edited by Otto H, Keller H. Cambridge, UK, Cambridge University Press, 2014, pp 50–65

Lichtenberg JD: Psychoanalysis and Motivation. Hillsdale, NJ, Analytic Press, 1989

Lineberry T: The therapeutic alliance with hospitalized patients, in Building a Therapeutic Alliance With the Suicidal Patient. Edited by Michel K, Jobes DA. New York, Guilford, 2011, pp 343–352

Linehan MM: Cognitive-Behavioral Treatment of Borderline Personality Disorder. New York, Guilford, 1993

Loewald H: On the therapeutic action of psycho-analysis. Int J Psychoanal 41:16–33, 1960

Løgstrup KE: The Ethical Demand. London, University of Notre Dame Press, 1997

Lyons-Ruth K, Jacobvitz D: Attachment disorganization: genetic factors, parenting contexts, and developmental transformation from infancy to adulthood, in Handbook of Attachment: Theory, Research, and Clinical Applications, 2nd Edition. Edited by Cassidy J, Shaver PR. New York, Guilford, 2008, pp 666–697

Lyons-Ruth K, Bronfman E, Atwood G: A relational diathesis model of hostile-helpless states of mind: expressions in mother-infant interaction, in Attachment Disorganization. Edited by Solomon J, George C. New York, Guilford, 1999, pp 33–70

MacIntyre A: Dependent Rational Animals: Why Human Beings Need the Virtues. Peru, IL, Open Court, 1999

Maeschalck CL, Prescott DS, Miller SD: Feedback informed treatment, in Handbook of Psychotherapy Integration, 3rd Edition. Edited by Norcross JC, Goldfried MR. New York, Oxford University Press, 2019, pp 105–121

Main M: Metacognitive knowledge, metacognitive monitoring, and singular (coherent) vs. multiple (incoherent) model of attachment, in Attachment Across the Life Cycle. Edited by Parkes CM, Stevenson-Hinde J, Marris P. London, Routledge, 1991, pp 127–159

Main M, Hesse E: Parents' unresolved traumatic experiences are related to infant disorganized attachment status: is frightened and/or frightening parental behavior the linking mechanism? in Attachment in the Preschool Years: Theory, Research, and Intervention. Edited by Greenberg MT, Cicchetti D, Cummings EM. Chicago, University of Chicago Press, 1990, pp 161–182

Main M, Solomon J: Procedures for identifying infants as disorganized/disoriented during the Ainsworth Strange Situation, in Attachment in the Preschool Years: Theory, Research, and Intervention. Edited by Greenberg MT, Cicchetti D, Cummings EM. Chicago, University of Chicago Press, 1990, pp 121–160

Main M, Hesse E, Kaplan N: Predictability of attachment behavior and representational processes at 1, 6, and 19 years of age, in Attachment From Infancy to Adulthood: The Major Longitudinal Studies. Edited by Grossman K, Grossman E, Waters E. New York, Guilford, 2005, pp 245–304

Main M, Hesse E, Goldwyn R: Studying differences in language usage in recounting atachment history: an introducion to the AAI, in Clinical Applications of the Adult Attachment Interview. Edited by Steele H, Steele M. New York, Guilford, 2008, pp 31–68

Malcom N: Ludwig Wittgenstein: A Memoir. New York, Oxford University Press, 1958

Marcus DK, O'Connell D, Norris AL, et al: Is the Dodo bird endangered in the 21st century? A meta-analysis of treatment comparison studies. Clin Psychol Rev 34:519–530, 2014

Martin AM: How We Hope: A Moral Psychology. Princeton, NJ, Princeton University Press, 2014

Martin AM: Interpersonal hope, in The Moral Psychology of Hope. Edited by Bloeser C, Stahl T. Minneapolis, MN, Rowman & Littlefield, 2020, pp 229–248

McGilchrist I: The Master and His Emissary: The Divided Brain and the Making of the Western World. New Haven, CT, Yale University Press, 2019

McLeod C: Self-Trust and Reproductive Autonomy. Cambridge, MA, MIT Press, 2002

McLeod J: Qualitative methods for routine outcome measurement, in The Cycle of Excellence: Using Deliberate Practice to Improve Supervision and Training. Edited by Rousmaniere T, Goodyear RK, Miller SD, et al. Chichester, UK, Wiley, 2017, pp 99–122

Meehan CL, Crittenden AN (eds): Childhood: Origins, Evolution, and Implications. Albuquerque, University of New Mexico Press, 2016

Meehan CL, Helfrecht C, Malcom CD: Implications of lengthy development and maternal life history: allomaternal investment, peer relationships, and social networks, in Childhood: Origins, Evolution, and Implications. Edited by Meehan CL, Crittenden AN. Albuquerque, University of New Mexico Press, 2016, pp 199–220

Meins E: Security of Attachment and the Social Development of Cognition. East Sussex, UK, Psychology Press, 1997

Meissner WW: Neutrality, abstinence, and the therapeutic alliance. J Am Psychoanal Assoc 46:1089–1128, 1998

Meissner WW: The problem of self-disclosure in psychoanalysis. J Am Psychoanal Assoc 50:827–867, 2002

Menninger KA: The Vital Balance. New York, Viking Press, 1963

Menninger KA: Hope. Bull Menninger Clin 51:447–462, 1987

Mercier H: Not Born Yesterday: The Science of Who We Trust and What We Believe. Princeton, NJ, Princeton University Press, 2020

Mercier H, Sperber D: The Enigma of Reason. Cambridge, MA, Harvard University Press, 2017

Mesman J, van Ijzendoorn MH: Cross-cultural patterns of attachment: universal and contextual dimensions, in Handbook of Attachment: Theory, Research, and Clinical Applications, 3rd Edition. Edited by Cassidy J, Shaver PR. New York, Guilford, 2016, pp 852–877

Mikulincer M, Shaver PR: Attachment in Adulthood: Structure, Dynamics, and Change, 2nd Edition. New York, Guilford, 2016

Miles S: Simone Weil: An anthology. New York, Grove Press, 1986

Miller SD, Hubble MA, Chow D: Professional development: from oxymoron to reality, in The Cycle of Excellence: Using Deliberate Practice to Improve Supervision and Training. Edited by Rousmaniere T, Goodyear RK, Miller SD, et al. Chichester, UK, Wiley, 2017, pp 23–48

Mitchell SA: Contemporary perspectives on self: Toward an integration. Psychoanal Diaglogues 1:121–147, 1991

Mitchell SA: Relationality: From Attachment to Intersubjectivity. New York, Analytic Press, 2000

Moradi B, Budge SL: Sexual orientation, in Psychotherapy Relationships That Work, 3rd Edition. Vol 2: Evidence-Based Therapist Responsiveness. Edited by Norcross JC, Wampold BE. New York, Oxford University Press, 2019, pp 264–295

Morelli GA, Chaudhary N, Gottlieb A, et al: Taking culture seriously: a pluralistic approach to attachment, in The Cultural Nature of Attachment: Contextualizing Relationships and Development. Edited by Keller H, Bard KA. Cambridge, MA, MIT Press, 2017, pp 139–170

Morris C: The Runes of Evolution: How the Universe Became Self-Aware. West Conshohocken, PA, Templeton, 2015

Morrison JA: The therapeutic relationship in prolonged exposure therapy for posttraumatic stress disorder: the role of cross-theoretical dialogue in dissemination. Behavior Therapist 34:20–26, 2011

Moss E, Bureau J-F, St-Laurent D, et al: Understanding disorganized attachment at preschool and school age: examining divergent pathways of disorganized and controlling children, in Disorganized Attachment and Caregiving. Edited by Solomon J, George C. New York, Guilford, 2011, pp 25–49

Murdoch I: The Sovereignty of Good. London, Routledge, 1971

Nagel T: The View From Nowhere. New York, Oxford University Press, 1986

Nissen-Lie HA, Monsen JT, Rønnestad MH: Therapist predictors of early patient-rated working alliance: a multilevel approach. Psychother Res 20:627–646, 2010

Nissen-Lie HA, Rønnestad MH, Høglend PA, et al: Love yourself as a person, doubt yourself as a therapist? Clin Psychol Psychother 24:48–60, 2015

Norcross JC, Alexander EF: A primer on psychotherapy integration, in Handbook of Psychotherapy Integration, 3rd Edition. Edited by Norcross JC, Goldfried MR. New York, Oxford University Press, 2019, pp 3–27

Norcross JC, Finnerty M: Training and supervision in psychotherapy integration, in Handbook of Psychotherapy Integration, 3rd Edition. Edited by Norcross JC, Goldfried MR.New York, Oxford University Press, 2019, pp. 377–404

Norcross JC, Lambert MJ: Evidence-based psychotherapy relationships: the third task force, in Psychotherapy Relationships That Work, 3rd Edition, Vol 1: Evidence-Based Therapist Contributions. Edited by Norcross JC, Wampold BE. New York, Oxford University Press, 2019a, pp 1–23

Norcross JC, Lambert MJ (eds): Psychotherapy Relationships That Work, 3rd Edition. Vol 1: Evidence-Based Therapist Contributions. New York, Oxford University Press, 2019b

Norcross JC, Wampold BE: Evidence-based psychotherapy responsiveness: the third task force, in Psychotherapy Relationships That Work, 3rd Edition. Vol 2: Evidence-Based Therapist Responsiveness. Edited by Norcross JC, Wampold BE. New York, Oxford University Press, 2019a, pp 1–14

Norcross JC, Wampold BE: Personalizing psychotherapy: results, conclusions, and practices, in Psychotherapy Relationships That Work, Vol 2: Evidence-Based Therapist Responsiveness, 3rd Edition. Edited by Norcross JC, Wampold BE. New York, Oxford University Press, 2019b, pp 329–342

O'Neill O: A Question of Trust. Cambridge, UK, Cambridge University Press, 2002

Oh H, Lee J, Kim S, et al: Time in treatment: examining mental illness trajectories across inpatient psychiatric treatment. J Psychiatr Res 130:22–30, 2020

Orbach I: Taking an inside view: stories of pain, in Building a Therapeutic Alliance With the Suicidal Patient. Edited by Michel K, Jobes DA. Washington, DC, American Psychological Association, 2011, pp 111–128

Otto H: Don't show your emotions! Emotion regulation and attachment in the Cameroonian Nso, in Different Faces of Attachment: Cultural Variations on a Universal Human Need. Edited by Otto H, Keller H. Cambridge, UK, Cambridge University Press, 2014, pp 215–229

Otto H, Keller H (eds): Different Faces of Attachment: Cultural Variations on a Universal Human Need. Cambridge, UK, Cambridge University Press, 2014

Owen J, Hilsenroth MJ: Interaction between alliance and technique in predicting patient outcome during psychodynamic psychotherapy. J Nerv Ment Dis 199(6):384–389, 2011 21629016

Pargament KI: Spiritually Integrated Psychotherapy: Understanding and Addressing the Sacred. New York, Guilford, 2007

Pargament KI, Mahoney A, Exline JJ, et al: Envisioning an integrative paradigm for the psychology of religion and spirituality, in APA Handbook of Psychology, Religion, and Spirituality. Vol 1: Context, Theory, and Research. Edited by Pargament KI, Exline JJ, Jones EP. Washington, DC, American Psychological Association, 2013, pp 3–19

Pauck W, Pauck M: Paul Tillich: His Life and Thought. Eugene, OR, Wipf & Stock, 2015

Peluso PR, Freund RR: Emotional expression, in Psychotherapy Relationships That Work, 3rd Edition. Vol 1: Evidence-Based Therapist Contributions. Edited by Norcross JC, Wampold BE. New York, Oxford University Press, 2019, pp 421–460

Perry RB: The Thought and Character of William James. Nashville, TN, Vanderbilt University Press, 1996

Polanyi M: The Study of Man (1959). Chicago, IL, University of Chicago Press, 2014

Polanyi M: Personal Knowledge: Towards a Post-Critical Philosophy. Chicago, IL, University of Chicago Press, 1962

Polanyi M: The Tacit Dimension. Chicago, IL, University of Chicago Press, 1966

Potter NN: How Can I Be Trusted? A Virtue Theory of Trustworthiness. New York, Rowman & Littlefield, 2002

Prilleltensky I: The Morals and Politics of Psychology: Psychological Discourse and the Status Quo. Albany, State University of New York Press, 1994

Prochaska JO, DiClemente CC: The transtheoretical approach, in Handbook of Psychotherapy Integration, 3rd Edition. Edited by Norcross JC, Goldfried MR. New York, Oxford University Press, 2019, pp 161–183

Pruyser PW: Between Belief and Unbelief. New York, Harper & Row, 1974

Pruyser PW: Changing Views of the Human Condition. Macon, GA, Mercer University Press, 1987a

Pruyser PW: Maintaining hope in adversity. Bull Menninger Clin 51:463–474, 1987b

Pruyser PW: Now what? Bull Menninger Clin 51:475–480, 1987c

Reese RJ, Usher EL, Bowman DC, et al: Using client feedback in psychotherapy training: an analysis of its influence on supervision and counselor self-efficacy. Train Educ Prof Psychol 3:157–168, 2009

Renik O: The ideal of the anonymous analyst and the problem of self-disclosure. Psychoanal Q 64:466–495, 1995

Renik O: The perils of neutrality. Psychoanal Q 65:495–517, 1996

Renik O: Analytic interaction: conceptualizing technique in light of the analyst's irreducible subjectivity, in Relational Psychoanalysis: The Emergence of a Tradition. Edited by Mitchell SA, Aron L. New York, Routledge, 1999, pp 407–424

Renik O: Practical Psychoanalysis for Therapists and Patients. New York, Other Press, 2006

Roberts LW (ed): The American Psychiatric Association Publishing Textbook of Psychiatry, 7th Edition. Washington, DC, American Psychiatric Association Publishing, 2019

Roberts LW, Dunn LB: Ethical considerations in psychiatry, in The American Psychiatric Association Publishing Textbook of Psychiatry, 7th Edition. Edited by Roberts LW. Washington, DC, American Psychiatric Association Publishing, 2019, pp 177–200

Rogers CR: Client-Centered Therapy: Its Current Practice, Implications, and Theory. Boston, MA, Houghton Mifflin, 1951

Rogers CR: The necessary and sufficient conditions of therapeutic personality change. J Consult Clin Psychol 60:827–832, 1992

Röttger-Rössler B: Bonding and belonging beyond WEIRD worlds: rethinking attachment theory on the basis of cross-cultural anthropological data, in Different Faces of Attachment: Cultural Variations on a Universal Human Need. Edited by Otto H, Keller H. Cambridge, UK, Cambridge University Press, 2014, pp 141–168

Rounsaville BJ, Goodyear RK, Miller SD, et al: Nurturing therapeutic mastery in cognitive behavioral therapy and beyond: an interview with Donald Michenbaum, in The Cycle of Excellence: Using Deliberate Practice to Improve Supervision and Training. Edited by Rousmaniere T, Goodyear RK, Miller SD, et al. Chichester, UK, Wiley, 2017, pp 189–198

Sandel MJ: The Tyranny of Merit: What's Become of the Common Good? New York, Farrar, Straus & Giroux, 2020

Sandler J: The background of safety. Int J Psychoanal 41:352–356, 1960

Searle JR: Making the Social World: The Structure of Human Civilization. New York, Oxford University Press, 2010

Seligman MEP: Flourish: A Visionary New Understanding of Happiness and Well-Being. New York, Atria, 2011

Seligman MEP: The Hope Circuit: A Psychologist's Journey From Helplessness to Optimism, Boston, MA, Nicholas Brealey, 2018

Slade A, Grienenberger J, Bernbach E, et al: Maternal reflective functioining, attachment, and the transmission gap: a preliminary study. Attach Hum Dev 7:283–298, 2005

Smith H: Forgotten Truths: The Common Vision of the World's Religions. New York, Harper-Collins, 1992

Snyder CR (ed): Coping: The Psychology of What Works. New York, Oxford University Press, 1999

Solms M: The Hidden Spring: A Journey to the Source of Consciousness. New York, Norton, 2021

Soto A, Smith TB, Griner D, et al: Cultural adaptations and multicultural competence, in Psychotherapy Relationships That Work, 3rd Edition. Vol 2: Evidence-Based Therapist Responsiveness. Edited by Norcross JC, Wampold BE. New York, Oxford University Press, 2019, pp 86–132

Sroufe LA, Waters E: Attachment as an organizational construct. Child Dev 48:1184–1199, 1977

Steele H, Steele M, Fonagy P: Associations among attachment classifications of mothers, fathers, and their infants. Child Dev 67:541–555, 1996

Stein H, Allen JG, Hill J: Roles and relationships: a psychoeducational approach to reviewing strengths and difficulties in adulthood functioning. Bull Menninger Clin 67:281–313, 2003

Stern DN: The Present Moment in Psychotherapy and Everyday Life. New York, Norton, 2004

Sternberg RJ: Race to Samarra: the critical importance of wisdom in the world today, in The Cambridge Handbook of Wisdom. Edited by Sternberg RJ, Glück J. New York, Cambridge University Press, 2019, pp 3–9

Stiles WB, Horvath AO: Appropriate responsiveness as a contribution to therapist effects, in How and Why Are Some Therapists Better Than Others? Understanding Therapist Effects. Edited by Castonguay LG, Hill CE. Washington, DC, American Psychological Association, 2017, pp 71–84

Stone DM, Simon TR, Fowler KA, et al: Vital signs: trends in state suicide rates—United States, 1999–2016 and circumstances contributing to suicide—27 states, 2015. MMWR Morb Mortal Wkly Rep 67:617–624, 2018

Strawson P: Freedom and resentment, in Free Will. Edited by Watson G. New York, Oxford University Press, 1982, pp. 59–80

Strawson P: Skepticism and naturalism: Some varieties. New York, Columbia University Press, 1985

Strupp HH, Hadley SW: Specific vs nonspecific factors in psychotherapy: a controlled study of outcome. Arch Gen Psychiatry 36:1125–1136, 1979

Swanton C: Virtue Ethics: A Pluralistic View. New York, Oxford, 2003

Swift JK, Callahan JL, Cooper M, et al: Preferences, in Psychotherapy Relationships That Work, 3rd Edition. Vol 2: Evidence-Based Therapist Responsiveness. Edited by Norcross JC, Wampold BE. New York, Oxford University Press, 2019, pp 157–187

Taylor JM, Neimeyer GJ: The ongoing evolution of continuing education: past, present, and future, in The Cycle of Excellence: Using Deliberate Practice to Improve Supervision and Training. Edited by Rousmaniere T, Goodyear RK, Miller SD, et al. Chichester, UK, Wiley, 2017, pp 219–248

Tillich P: Dynamics of Faith. New York, HarperCollins, 1957

Tomasello M: The Cultural Origins of Human Cognition. Cambridge, MA, Harvard University Press, 1999

Tomasello M: A Natural History of Human Thinking. Cambridge, MA, Harvard University Press, 2014

Tomasello M: A Natural History of Human Morality. Cambridge, MA, Harvard University Press, 2016

Tomasello M: Becoming Human: A Theory of Ontogeny. Cambridge, MA, Harvard University Press, 2019

Tronick E: The Neurobehavioral and Social-Emotional Development of Infants and Children. New York, Norton, 2007

Vicedo M: The Nature and Nurture of Love: From Imprinting to Attachment in Cold War America. Chicago, IL, University of Chicago Press, 2013

Vicedo M: The Strange Situation of the ethological theory of attachment: a historical perspective, in The Cultural Nature of Attachment: Contextualizing Relationships and Development. Edited by Keller H, Bard KA. Cambridge, MA, MIT Press, 2017, pp 13–52

Vygotsky LS: Mind in Society: The Development of Higher Psychological Processes. Cambridge, MA, Harvard University Press, 1978

Wachtel PL: Relational Theory and the Practice of Psychotherapy. New York, Guilford, 2008

Walsh DM: Organisms, Agency, and Evolution. New York, Cambridge University Press, 2015

Wampold BE: What should we practice? A contextual model for how psychotherapy works, in The Cycle of Excellence: Using Deliberate Practice to Improve Supervision and Training. Edited by Rousmaniere T, Goodyear RK, Miller SD, et al. Chichester, UK, Wiley, 2017, pp 49–66

Wampold BE, Imel ZE: The Great Psychotherapy Debate: The Evidence for What Makes Psychotherapy Work, 2nd Edition. New York, Routledge, 2015

Wampold BE, Ulvenes PG: Integration of common factors and specific ingredients, in Handbook of Psychotherapy Integration, 3rd Edition. Edited by Norcross JC, Goldfried MR. New York, Oxford University Press, 2019, pp 69–87

Wampold BE, Baldwin SA, Holtforth MG, et al: What characterizes effective therapists? in How and Why Are Some Therapists Better Than Others? Understanding Therapist Effects. Edited by Castonguay LG, Hill CE. Washington, DC, American Psychological Association, 2017, pp 37–54

Weinberger J: Common factors aren't so common: the common factor dilemma. Clini Psychol Sci Pract 2:45–69, 1995

Weinberger J, Stoycheva V: The Unconscious: Theory, Research, and Clinical Implications. New York, Guilford, 2020

Weisner TS: The socialization of trust: plural caregiving and diverse pathways in human development across cultures, in Different Faces of Attachment: Cultural Variations on a Universal Human Need. Edited by Otto H, Keller H. Cambridge, UK, Cambridge University Press, 2014, pp 263–277

Williams B: Ethics and the Limits of Philosophy. Cambridge, MA, Harvard University Press, 1985

Williams B: Truth and Truthfulness: An Essay in Geneaology. Princeton, NJ, Princeton University Press, 2002

Zagzebski LT: Epistemic Authority: A Theory of Trust, Authority, and Autonomy in Belief. New York, Oxford University Press, 2012

Index

Page numbers printed in **boldface** type refer to tables or figures